EPIDEMIOLOGY

EPIDEMIOLOGY Fourth Edition

LEON GORDIS, MD, MPH, DrPH

Professor of Epidemiology

Johns Hopkins Bloomberg School of Public Health

Professor of Pediatrics

Johns Hopkins School of Medicine

Baltimore, Maryland

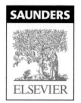

SAUNDERS

ELSEVIER

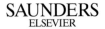

SAUNDERS
ELSEVIER

1600 John F. Kennedy Boulevard
Suite 1800
Philadelphia, PA 19103-2899

EPIDEMIOLOGY   ISBN: 978-1-4160-4002-6

Notice

Neither the Publisher nor the Author assumes any responsibility for any loss or injury and/or damage to persons or property arising out of or related to any use of the material contained in this book. It is the responsibility of the treating practitioner, relying on independent expertise and knowledge of the patient, to determine the best treatment and method of application for the patient.

The Publisher

Previous editions copyrighted 1996, 2000, 2004.

Library of Congress Cataloging-in-Publication Data

Gordis, Leon
    Epidemiology / Leon Gordis.—4th ed.
        p. ; cm.
    Includes bibliographical references and index.
    ISBN 978-1-4160-4002-6
    1. Epidemiology.   I. Title.
    [DNLM: 1. Epidemiology. 2. Epidemiologic Methods. WA 105 G661e 2008]
RA651.G58 2009
614.4—dc22

                                    2007030111

ISBN: 978-1-4160-4002-6

Acquisitions Editor: James Merritt
Developmental Editor: Andy Hall
Publishing Services Manager: Joan Sinclair
Design Direction: Gene Harris

Working together to grow
libraries in developing countries

www.elsevier.com | www.bookaid.org | www.sabre.org

ELSEVIER   BOOK AID
            International   Sabre Foundation

Printed in the United States of America

Last digit is the print number: 9   8   7   6   5   4   3

For Dassy

th by modifying the natural history of disease, the next step is to select an ropriate and effective intervention—a selection that ideally is made using the lts of randomized trials of prevention and treatment (Chapters 7 and 8).

ection II deals with the use of epidemiology to identify the causes of disease. pter 9 discusses the design of cohort studies and Chapter 10 introduces case-trol, nested case-control, case-cohort, case-crossover, and cross-sectional lies. Chapters 11 and 12 discuss how the results of these studies are used to mate risk. We do so by determining whether there is an association of an osure and a disease as reflected by an increase in risk in exposed persons. r a brief review (Chapter 13), Chapter 14 discusses how we move from such lence of an association to answering the important question: Does the asso-ion reflect a causal relationship? In so doing, it is critical to take into account es of bias, confounding, and interaction, which are discussed in Chapter 15. pter 16 describes the use of epidemiology, often in conjunction with molec-biology, to assess the relative contributions of genetic and environmental ors to disease causation.

ection III discusses several important applications of epidemiology to major lth issues. Chapter 17 addresses one of the major uses of epidemiology, which evaluate the effectiveness of health services. Chapter 18 reviews the use of demiology in evaluating screening programs. Chapter 19 considers the place pidemiology in formulating and evaluating public policy. These diverse appli-ons have enhanced the importance of epidemiology, but at the same time e given rise to an array of new problems, both ethical and professional, in the duct of epidemiologic studies and in the use of the results of such studies. A nber of these issues are discussed in the final chapter (Chapter 20).

n each edition of this book, illustrations and graphics have been used exten-ly to help the reader understand the principles and methods of epidemiology to enhance presentation of the examples described in the text.

major change in the fourth edition is publication of the book in color. The of color has made new approaches possible for illustrating important prin-les and methods. I hope that readers will share our excitement about the nsition to color and the positive impact that introduction of color has had on ny aspects of the published book.

Above and beyond the addition of color, the data cited and the examples used e been updated whenever possible, and new examples have been added to ther clarify epidemiologic principles and methods. Some sections have been anded, others added, and numerous revisions and additions have been made oughout the book. Among the new or expanded sections are those discussing son-time, registration of clinical trials, overdiagnosis bias in evaluating screen-programs, and the problem of uncertainty in moving from epidemiologic a to clinical and public health policy. Newer approaches to study design, luding case-cohort and case-crossover studies, have also been introduced. ent issues such as trends in thyroid cancer and the increasing prevalence of sity in the United States and in many other countries have been added. iew questions are included at the end of most chapters or topics.

Preface

In recent years epidemiology has become an increasingly importar
both public health and clinical practice. Epidemiology is the ba
disease prevention and plays major roles in the development and
public policy as well as in social and legal arenas. Together w
research, epidemiology is now used to identify environmental ar
factors for disease and to shed light on the mechanisms involved
genesis of different diseases. The heightened media attention that
has recently received has major implications for health care provic
makers as well as for epidemiologists. As a result of this scrutiny, tl
methodology, and uses of epidemiology have garnered increasing
an ever-broadening group of professionals in different disciplines ;
the public at large.

This book is an introduction to epidemiology and to the
approach to problems of health and disease. The basic principles
of epidemiology are presented together with many of the applicat
miology to public health and clinical practice.

The fourth edition of this book retains the organization and st
previous editions, which consisted of three sections. Section I f
epidemiologic approach to understanding disease and to developir
interventions designed to modify and improve its natural histo
provides a broad context and perspective for the discipline, and (
cusses how disease is transmitted and acquired. Chapters 3 and
measures we use to assess the frequency and importance of diseas:
strate how these measures are used in disease surveillance—one
roles of epidemiology in public health. Chapter 3 discusses measur
ity, and Chapter 4, measures of mortality. Chapter 5 addresses the
of how to distinguish persons who have a disease from those wh
how to assess the quality of the diagnostic and screening tests use

Once persons who have a certain disease have been identifiec
characterize the natural history of their disease in quantitative tern
acterization is essential if we are to identify any changes that take p
in survival and severity, or changes that result from preventive c
interventions (Chapter 6). Because our ultimate objective is to im

The sequence of the three sections of this book is designed to provide the reader with a basic understanding of epidemiologic methods and study design and of the place of epidemiology in preventive and clinical medicine and in disease investigation. After finishing this book, the reader should be able to assess the adequacy of the design and conduct of reported studies and the validity of the conclusions reached in published articles. It is my hope that the fourth edition of this book will continue to convey to its readers the excitement of epidemiology, its basic conceptual and methodologic underpinnings, and an appreciation of its increasingly vital and expanding roles in enhancing health policy for both individuals and communities through effective prevention and treatment.

In closing, a few words about the cover illustration. The photographer and the site of the photograph are not known. The photograph shows a busy intersection with multiple pedestrian crossings. In our everyday lives, we each choose different paths and consequently experience different exposures. But each of us also has different genetic characteristics and different susceptibilities which although not explicitly shown in the picture are perhaps symbolized by the different colors of the umbrellas in the photo. (Of course, only some people develop disease or adverse health effects, also not shown in the picture.) A major role of epidemiology is to elucidate the causal pathways linking exposures and risks of illness so that preventive measures can be developed. Even our everyday decisions such as which pedestrian crossing to use, or choices of different life styles, vary greatly from one person to another. Such choices often seem ordinary, but at times they may influence our futures without our being aware of the significance of our choices. The objective of epidemiology is to enhance human health not only by responding to high visibility situations such as natural disasters and other dramatic threats to the community, but also by preventing and detecting the diseases that arise from many seemingly routine choices that each of us makes in our everyday lives.

Leon Gordis
January 2008

Acknowledgments

This book is based on my experience of teaching two courses in introductory epidemiology—Principles of Epidemiology to students in the Johns Hopkins School of Hygiene and Public Health, now the Bloomberg School of Public Health, and Clinical Epidemiology to students in the Johns Hopkins School of Medicine—for over 30 years. In the words of the Talmudic sage Rabbi Hanina, "I have learned much from my teachers, and even more from my colleagues, but most of all from my students." I am grateful to the over 17,000 students I have been privileged to teach during this time. Through their questions and critical comments they have contributed significantly to the content, style, and configuration of this book. Their invaluable comments regarding the first three editions have been of tremendous help to me in preparing the fourth edition of this book.

I was first stimulated to pursue studies in epidemiology by my late mentor and friend, Dr. Milton Markowitz. For many years he was a guide and inspiration to me. Years ago, when we were initiating a study to evaluate the effectiveness of a comprehensive care clinic for children in Baltimore, he urged me to obtain the training needed to evaluate the program rigorously; even at that time he recognized that epidemiology was an essential approach for evaluating health services. He therefore suggested I speak with Dr. Abraham Lilienfeld, who at the time was chairman of the Department of Chronic Diseases, later the Department of Epidemiology, at the Johns Hopkins School of Hygiene and Public Health. I then came as a student to Abe's department, where he became my doctoral advisor and friend. Over many years, until his death in 1984, Abe had the wonderful talent of being able to communicate to his students and colleagues the excitement he found in epidemiology, and he shared with them the thrill of discovering new knowledge using population-based methods. To both these mentors, Milt Markowitz and Abe Lilienfeld, I owe tremendous debts of gratitude.

In revising this book, I have been fortunate to have had support from many wonderful colleagues and friends. I have had the pleasure of working with the chairman of our Department of Epidemiology, Dr. Jonathan Samet, for the past 14 years. Jon has always been an enthusiastic supporter of this book and of my preparing this fourth edition, and I am very grateful to him. He has always been gracious and generous with his time and effort in reviewing parts of the manuscript and I thank him for invariably being a constructive and caring critic. Having trained in Pediatrics, I am grateful to Dr. George Dover, Chairman of the Department of Pediatrics in the Johns Hopkins School of Medicine, for stimulating discussions we have had and for facilitating my serving as a faculty member in his department.

Over the years many other colleagues and friends have made valuable contributions to the development of this book and to its subsequent revisions. I owe a great debt to the late Dr. George W. Comstock, Professor of Epidemiology at Johns Hopkins, who was my teacher, colleague, and friend until his death in 2007. Although there is always a risk of omission in naming individuals, I want to express my thanks to Drs. Haroutune Armenian, Alfred Buck, Josef Coresh, Manning Feinleib, Kathy Helzlsouer, Michel Ibrahim, Barnett Kramer, Lechaim Naggan, Javier Nieto, Neil Powe, Moyses Szklo, and Paul Whelton, who spent time discussing many conceptual issues with me and in doing so helped me find better ways of presenting them in an introduction to epidemiology. In this edition I have also been able to build upon the many contributions made to the previous editions by my colleague Allyn Arnold. I also appreciate the gracious and expert help of Christine Ruggere, Associate Director and Curator of the Historical Collection of the Johns Hopkins Institute of the History of Medicine. Dr. J. Morel Symons, who assisted me in preparing the previous edition, has enhanced this edition with his fine work in developing the associated website, which includes explanations for the answers to the review questions found at the end of most of the chapters in this book.

Other colleagues, both in our department and elsewhere, have also been very generous with their time and talents in discussing many of the issues that arose first in teaching and then in preparing and revising the manuscript. They have often suggested specific examples that have helped clarify many of the concepts discussed. Their efforts have contributed significantly to improving this volume. I apologize for not naming them individually and am grateful to them. Their many wise suggestions, comments, and perceptive questions have been invaluable.

I have been fortunate to have had the assistance of two outstanding doctoral students in the Johns Hopkins Department of Epidemiology, Keri Althoff and Lindsay Jorgensen. I thank Keri for her tremendous help in many aspects of the preparation of this edition. She has updated many of the examples used in this book and has made many other creative contributions in addition to reviewing the copy-edited manuscript and proofreading the page proofs. She has also helped address many of the new challenges that were involved in the transition to color in this edition. I am also very grateful to Lindsay, who spent many hours carefully reviewing and proofreading the page proofs. In the course of doing this, she has also made many perceptive and valuable suggestions that have significantly improved the quality of this volume. I also appreciate the help of my assistant, Vera Edmonds, throughout the time involved in completing this revision.

Since joining the faculty at Johns Hopkins over 35 years ago, I have been privileged to work under outstanding leaders in both the Johns Hopkins Bloomberg School of Public Health and the Johns Hopkins School of Medicine. Deans John C. Hume, D. A. Henderson, Alfred Sommer, and Michael Klag in the Johns Hopkins Bloomberg School of Public Health and Deans Richard S. Ross, Michael M. E. Johns, and Edward D. Miller in the Johns Hopkins School of Medicine have always enthusiastically supported the teaching of epidemiology in both schools.

I wish to thank my editor at Elsevier, James Merritt. Not only is Jim a talented and expert editor, but he has also been far more than an editor; he has been a caring and supportive friend. Andrew Hall has been invaluable in his role as Senior Developmental Editor for this edition. I thank Andy for all his expertise and support. Denise Roslonski, Electronic Media Specialist at Elsevier, has played a crucial role in moving this book to color through her gracious and caring handling of the format conversions needed for publishing this book and for her concern about issues of legibility and color and her willingness to tolerate graciously multiple requests for modifying the artwork. I also wish to thank Linnea Hermanson, Production Editor, who has coordinated the many critical phases from copy-editing the manuscript, through creation of the pages, proofreading of the page proofs, and final production.

Finally, I have been blessed with a family that has always been a source of love, inspiration, and encouragement to me. My children urged me to write this book and lent enthusiastic support as I prepared each revision. Years ago, my wife, Hadassah, strongly supported my pursuing studies first in medicine and later in epidemiology. Since that time she has been a wise and wonderful friend and advisor, and has constantly encouraged me in all my professional activities, even when they have involved personal sacrifices on her part. She was enthusiastic from the start about my preparing this book. Through her seemingly limitless patience and optimistic outlook, she facilitated my writing it and then my preparing the second, third, and fourth editions. For months on end, she even graciously yielded our dining room table to a virtually endless avalanche of paper involved in the preparation of this revision. With her keen critical mind she has always left me thinking and reconsidering issues that I first thought simple and later came to recognize as being considerably more complex and challenging. She has the wonderful ability to see through to the core issues in any area. She has made my completing and revising this book possible. As we approach our 53rd wedding anniversary, I recognize how truly fortunate I have been over the years in having her love and support, together with her wisdom and understanding. I thank her more than these words can even begin to express.

Leon Gordis
January 2008

SECTION I
The Epidemiologic Approach to Disease and Intervention

SECTION II
Using Epidemiology to Identify the Cause of Disease

Contents

Section *I*
THE EPIDEMIOLOGIC APPROACH TO DISEASE AND INTERVENTION

This section begins with an overview of the objectives of epidemiology, some of the approaches used in epidemiology, and examples of the applications of epidemiology to human health problems (Chapter 1). It then discusses how diseases are transmitted (Chapter 2). Diseases do not arise in a vacuum; they result from an interaction of human beings with their environment. An understanding of the concepts and mechanisms underlying the transmission and acquisition of disease is critical to exploring the epidemiology of human disease and preventing and controlling many infectious diseases.

To discuss the epidemiologic concepts presented in this book, we need to develop a common language, particularly for describing and comparing morbidity and mortality. Chapter 3, therefore, discusses morbidity and how measures of morbidity are used in both clinical medicine and public health, including disease surveillance. Chapter 4 presents the methodology and approaches to using mortality data in investigations relating to public health and clinical practice.

Armed with knowledge of how to describe morbidity and mortality in quantitative terms, we then turn to the question of how to assess the quality of diagnostic and screening tests that are used to determine which people in the population have a certain disease (Chapter 5). After we identify people with the disease, we need ways to describe the natural history of disease in quantitative terms; this is essential for assessing the severity of an illness and for evaluating the possible effects on survival of new therapeutic and preventive interventions (see Chapter 6).

Having identified persons who have a disease, how do we decide which interventions—whether treatments, preventive measures, or both—should be used in trying to modify the natural history of the illness? Chapters 7 and 8 present the randomized trial, an invaluable and critical study design that is generally considered the "gold standard" for evaluating both the efficacy and the potential side effects of new therapeutic or preventive interventions.

Chapter 1

Introduction

I hate definitions.
—Benjamin Disraeli (1804–1881)

WHAT IS EPIDEMIOLOGY?

Epidemiology is the study of how disease is distributed in populations and the factors that influence or determine this distribution. Why does a disease develop in some people and not in others? The premise underlying epidemiology is that disease, illness, and ill health are not randomly distributed in human populations. Rather, each of us has certain characteristics that predispose us to, or protect us against, a variety of different diseases. These characteristics may be primarily genetic in origin or may be the result of exposure to certain environmental hazards. Perhaps most often, we are dealing with an interaction of genetic and environmental factors in the development of disease.

A broader definition of epidemiology than that given above has been widely accepted. It defines epidemiology as "the study of the distribution and determinants of health-related states or events in specified populations and the application of this study to control of health problems."[1] What is noteworthy about this definition is that it includes both a description of the content of the discipline and the purpose or application for which epidemiologic investigations are carried out.

THE OBJECTIVES OF EPIDEMIOLOGY

What are the specific objectives of epidemiology?

First, to identify the *etiology* or *cause* of a disease and the relevant risk factors—that is, factors that increase a person's risk for a disease. We want to know how the disease is transmitted from one person to another or from a nonhuman reservoir to a human population. Our ultimate aim is to intervene to reduce morbidity and mortality from the disease. We want to develop a rational basis for prevention programs. If we can identify the etiologic or causal factors for disease and reduce or eliminate exposure to those factors, we can develop a basis for prevention programs.

Second, to determine the extent of disease found in the community. What is the burden of disease in the community? This question is critical for planning health services and facilities, and for training future health care providers.

Third, to study the natural history and prognosis of disease. Clearly, certain diseases are more severe than others; some may be rapidly lethal while others may have longer durations of survival. Still others are not fatal. We want to define the baseline natural history of a disease in quantitative terms so that as we develop new modes of intervention, either through treatments or through new ways of preventing complications, we can compare the results of using such new modalities with the baseline data in order to determine whether our new approaches have truly been effective.

Fourth, to evaluate both existing and newly developed preventive and therapeutic measures and modes of health care delivery. For example, does screening men for prostate cancer using the prostate-specific antigen (PSA) test improve survival in people found to have prostate cancer? Has the growth of managed care and other new systems of health care delivery and health care insurance had an impact on the health outcomes of their patients and on their quality of life?

Fifth, to provide the foundation for developing public policy relating to environmental problems, genetic issues, and other considerations regarding disease prevention and health promotion. For example, is the electromagnetic radiation that is emitted by electric blankets, heating pads, and other household appliances a hazard to human health? Are high levels of atmospheric ozone or particulate matter a cause of adverse acute or chronic health effects in human populations? Is radon in homes a significant risk to human beings? Which occupations are associated with increased risks of disease in workers, and what types of regulation are required?

CHANGING PATTERNS OF COMMUNITY HEALTH PROBLEMS

A major role of epidemiology is to provide a clue to changes that take place over time in the health problems presenting in the community. Figure 1-1 shows a sign in a cemetery in Dudley, England, in 1839. At that time, cholera was the major cause of death in England; the churchyard was so full that no burials of persons who died of cholera would henceforth be permitted. The sign conveys an idea of the importance of cholera in the public's consciousness and in the spectrum of public health problems in the early 19th century. Clearly, cholera is not a major problem in the United States today; but in many countries of the world it remains a serious threat, with many countries periodically reporting outbreaks of cholera that are characterized by high death rates.

Let us compare the major causes of death in the United States in 1900 and in 2004 (Fig. 1-2). The categories of causes have been color coded as described in the legend for this figure. In 1900, the leading causes of death were pneumonia and influenza, followed by tuberculosis and diarrhea and enteritis. In 2004, the leading causes of death were heart disease, cancer, stroke (or cerebrovascular disease), and chronic lower respiratory diseases. What change has occurred? Over a century there was a dramatic shift in the causes of death in this country.

In 1900, the three leading causes of death were infectious diseases; now we are dealing with chronic diseases that in most situations do not appear to be communicable or infectious in origin. Consequently, the kinds of research, intervention, and services we need today differ from those that were required in the United States in 1900.

The pattern seen in developing countries today is often similar to that seen in the United States in 1900: infectious diseases are the largest problems. But, as countries become industrialized they increasingly manifest the mortality patterns currently seen in developed countries, with chronic disease mortality becoming the major challenge. However, even in industrialized countries, as human immunodeficiency virus (HIV) infection has emerged and the incidence of tuberculosis has increased, infectious diseases are again becoming major public health problems. Table 1-1 shows the 15 leading causes of death in the United States in 2004. The three leading causes—heart disease, cancer, and cerebrovascular disease—account for almost 60% of all deaths, an observation that suggests specific targets for prevention if a significant reduction in mortality is to be achieved.

Another demonstration of changes that have taken place over time is seen in Figure 1-3, which shows the remaining years of expected life in the United States at birth and at age 65 years for the years 1900, 1950, and 2004 by race and sex.

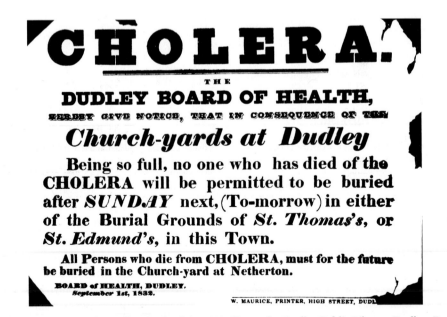

Figure 1-1. Sign in cemetery in Dudley, England, in 1839. (From the Dudley Public Library, Dudley, England.)

Figure 1-2. Ten leading causes of death in the United States, 1900 and 2004. Although the definitions of the diseases in this figure are not exactly comparable in 1900 and 2004, the bars in the graphs are color coded to show chronic diseases (salmon), infectious diseases (purple), injuries (aqua), and diseases of aging (white). (Redrawn from Grove RD, Hetzel AM: Vital Statistics Rates of the United States, 1940–1960. Washington, DC, US Government Printing Office, 1968; and National Center for Health Statistics: National Vital Statistics Report, vol 54, no 19, June 28, 2006.)

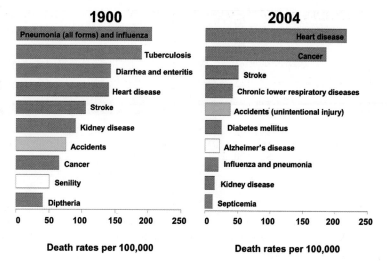

TABLE 1-1. Fifteen Leading Causes of Death, and Their Percents of All Deaths, United States, 2004

Rank	Cause of Death	Number of Deaths	Percent (%) of Total Deaths	Death Rate*
	All Causes	**2,397,615**	**100.0**	**800.8**
1	Heart diseases	652,486	27.2	217.0
2	Cancer	553,888	23.1	185.8
3	Cerebrovascular diseases	150,074	6.3	50.0
4	Chronic lower respiratory diseases	121,987	5.1	41.1
5	Accidents (unintentional injuries)	112,012	4.7	37.7
6	Diabetes mellitus	73,138	3.1	24.5
7	Alzheimer's disease	65,965	2.8	21.8
8	Influenza and pneumonia	59,664	2.5	19.8
9	Nephritis, nephrotic syndrome, and nephrosis	42,480	1.8	14.2
10	Septicemia	33,373	1.4	11.2
11	Intentional self-harm (suicide)	32,439	1.4	10.9
12	Chronic liver disease and cirrhosis	27,013	1.1	9.0
13	Hypertension and hypertensive renal disease	23,076	1.0	7.7
14	Parkinson's disease	17,989	0.8	6.1
15	Assault (homicide)	17,357	0.7	5.9
	All other and ill-defined causes	414,674	17.3	

*Rates are per 100,000 population and age-adjusted for the 2000 US standard population.

Note: Percentages may not total 100 due to rounding. Symptoms, signs, and abnormalities and pneumonitis due to solids and liquids were excluded from the cause-of-death ranking order.

Data from Centers for Disease Control and Prevention: National Vital Statistics Reports, vol 54, no 19, June 28, 2006. Available at: www.cdc.gov/nchs/data/nvsr/nvsr54/nvsr54_19.pdf.

The years of life remaining at birth have dramatically increased in all of these groups, with most of the improvement having occurred from 1900 to 1950, and much less having occurred since 1950. If we look at the remaining years of life at age 65 years, very little improvement is seen from 1900 to 2004.

What primarily accounts for the increase in remaining years of life at birth are the decreases in infant mortality and childhood diseases. In terms of diseases that afflict adults, we have been much less successful in extending the span of life, and this remains a major challenge.

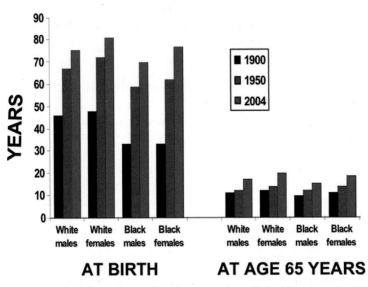

Figure 1-3. Life expectancy at birth and at 65 years of age, by race and sex, United States, 1900, 1950, and 2004. (Redrawn from National Center for Health Statistics: Health, United States, 1987 DHHS publication no 88–1232. Washington, DC, Public Health Service, March 1988; and National Center for Health Statistics: National Vital Statistics Report, vol 54, no 19, June 28, 2006.)

EPIDEMIOLOGY AND PREVENTION

A major use of epidemiologic evidence is to identify subgroups in the population who are at high risk for disease. Why should we identify such high-risk groups? First, if we can identify these high-risk groups, we can direct preventive efforts, such as screening programs for early disease detection, to populations who are most likely to benefit from any interventions that are developed for the disease.

Second, if we can identify such groups, we may be able to identify the specific factors or characteristics that put them at high risk and then try to modify those factors. It is important to keep in mind that such risk factors may be of two types. Characteristics such as age, sex, and race, for example, are not mod-

ifiable, although they may permit us to identify high-risk groups. On the other hand, characteristics such as obesity, diet, and other lifestyle factors may be potentially modifiable and may thus provide an opportunity to develop and introduce new prevention programs aimed at reducing or changing specific exposures or risk factors.

In discussing prevention, it is helpful to distinguish among primary, secondary, and tertiary prevention (Table 1-2). *Primary prevention* denotes an action taken to prevent the development of a disease in a person who is well and does not (yet) have the disease in question. For example, we can immunize a person against certain diseases so that the disease never develops or, if a disease is environmentally induced, we can prevent a person's exposure to the

TABLE 1-2. **Three Types of Prevention**		
Type of Prevention	**Definition**	**Examples**
Primary prevention	Preventing the *initial development* of a disease	Immunization, reducing exposure to a risk factor
Secondary prevention	Early detection of *existing disease* to reduce severity and complications	Screening for cancer
Tertiary prevention	Reducing the *impact of the disease*	Rehabilitation for stroke

environmental factor involved and thereby prevent the development of the disease. Primary prevention is our ultimate goal. For example, we know that most lung cancers are preventable. If we can stop people from smoking, we can eliminate 80% to 90% of lung cancer in human beings. However, although our aim is to prevent diseases from occurring in human populations, for many diseases we do not yet have the biologic, clinical, and epidemiologic data on which to base effective primary prevention programs.

Secondary prevention involves identifying people in whom a disease has already begun but who have not yet developed clinical signs and symptoms of the illness. This period in the natural history of a disease is called the *preclinical phase* of the illness. Once a person develops clinical signs or symptoms, it is generally assumed the person will seek medical care. Our objective with secondary prevention is to detect the disease earlier than it would have been detected with usual care. By detecting the disease at an early stage in its natural history, often through screening, it is hoped that treatment will be easier and/or more effective. For example, most cases of breast cancer in older women can be detected through breast self-examination and mammography. Several recent studies indicate that routine testing of the stool for occult blood can detect treatable colon cancer early in its natural history. The rationale for secondary prevention is that if we can identify disease earlier in its natural history than would ordinarily occur, intervention measures will be more effective. Perhaps we can prevent mortality or complications of the disease and use less invasive or less costly treatment to do so. Evaluating screening for disease and the place of such intervention in the framework of disease prevention is discussed in Chapter 18.

Tertiary prevention denotes preventing complications in those who have already developed signs and symptoms of an illness and have been diagnosed—that is, people who are in the clinical phase of their illness. This is generally achieved through prompt and appropriate treatment of the illness combined with ancillary approaches such as physical therapy that are designed to prevent complications such as joint contractures.

Two possible approaches to prevention are a population-based approach and a high-risk approach.[2] In the population-based approach, a preventive measure is widely applied to an entire population. For example, prudent dietary advice for preventing coronary disease or advice against smoking may be provided to an entire population. An alternate approach is to target a high-risk group with the preventive measure. Thus, screening for cholesterol in children might be restricted to children from high-risk families. Clearly, a measure that will be applied to an entire population must be relatively inexpensive and noninvasive. A measure that is to be applied to a high-risk subgroup of the population may be more expensive and is often more invasive or inconvenient. Population-based approaches can be considered public health approaches, whereas high-risk approaches more often require a clinical action to identify the high-risk group to be targeted. In most situations, a combination of both approaches is ideal.

EPIDEMIOLOGY AND CLINICAL PRACTICE

Epidemiology is critical not only to public health but also to clinical practice. The practice of medicine is dependent on population data. For example, if a physician hears an apical systolic murmur, how does he or she know that it represents mitral regurgitation? Where did this knowledge originate? The diagnosis is based on correlation of the auscultatory findings with the findings of surgical pathology or autopsy and of catheterization or angiography findings in a large group of patients. Thus, the process of diagnosis is population-based (see Chapter 5). The same holds for prognosis. A patient asks his physician, "How long do I have to live, doctor?" and the doctor replies, "Six months to a year." On what basis does the physician prognosticate? He or she does so on the basis of experience with large groups of patients who had the same disease, were observed at the same stage of disease, and received the same treatment. Again, prognostication is based on population data (see Chapter 6). Finally, selection of appropriate therapy is also population based. Randomized clinical trials studying the effects of a treatment in large groups of patients are the ideal means to identify appropriate therapy (see Chapters 7 and 8). Thus, population-based concepts and data underlie the critical processes of clinical practice, including diagnosis, prognostication, and selection of therapy. In effect, the physician applies a population-based probability model to the patient who is lying on the examining table.

Figure 1-4 shows a physician demonstrating that the practice of clinical medicine relies heavily on population concepts. What is portrayed humorously is a true commentary on one aspect of pediatric practice—a pediatrician often makes a diagnosis

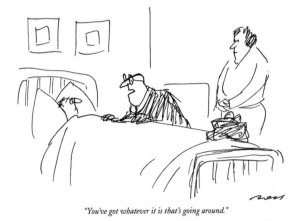

"You've got whatever it is that's going around."

Figure 1-4. "You've got whatever it is that's going around." (© The New Yorker Collection 1975. Al Ross from cartoonbank.com. All rights reserved.)

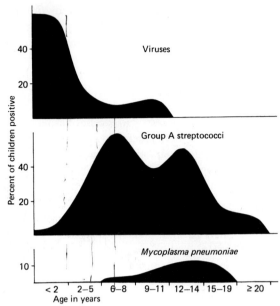

Figure 1-5. Frequency of agents by age of children with pharyngitis, 1964–1965. (From Denny FW: The replete pediatrician and the etiology of lower respiratory tract infections. Pediatr Res 3:464–470, 1969.)

based on what the parent tells him or her over the telephone and which illnesses, such as viral and bacterial infections, the pediatrician knows are "going around" the community. Thus, the data available about illness in the community can be very helpful in suggesting a diagnosis, even if they are not conclusive. Data regarding the etiology of sore throats according to a child's age are particularly relevant (Fig. 1-5). If the infection occurs early in life, it is likely to be viral in origin. If it occurs at ages 4 to 7 years, it is likely to be streptococcal in origin. In an older child *Mycoplasma* becomes more important. Although these data do not make the diagnosis, they do provide the physician or other health care provider with a good clue as to what agent or agents to suspect.

THE EPIDEMIOLOGIC APPROACH

How does the epidemiologist proceed to identify the cause of a disease? Epidemiologic reasoning is a multistep process. The first step is to determine whether an association exists between exposure to a factor (e.g., an environmental agent) or a characteristic of a person (e.g., an increased serum cholesterol level) and the development of the disease in question. We do this by studying the characteristics of groups and the characteristics of individuals.

If we find there is indeed an association between an exposure and a disease, is it necessarily a causal relationship? No, not all associations are causal. The second step, therefore, is to try to derive appropriate inferences about a possible causal relationship from the patterns of the associations that have been found. These steps are discussed in detail in later chapters.

Epidemiology often begins with descriptive data. For example, Figure 1-6 shows rates of gonorrhea in the United States in 2005 by state. Clearly, there are marked regional variations in reported cases of gonorrhea. The first question to ask when we see such differences between two groups or two regions or over time is, "Are these differences real?" In other words, are the data from each area of comparable quality? Before we try to interpret the data, we should be satisfied that the data are valid. If the differences are real, then we ask, "Why have they occurred?" Are there environmental differences between high-risk and low-risk areas, or are there differences in the people who live in those areas? This is where epidemiology begins its investigation.

Many years ago, it was observed that communities in which the natural level of fluoride in the drinking water differed also differed in the frequency of dental caries in the permanent teeth of residents. Communities that had low natural fluoride levels had high levels of caries, and communities that had higher levels of fluoride in their drinking water had low levels of caries (Fig. 1-7). This finding suggested that fluoride might be an effective prevention if it were artificially added to the drinking water supply. A trial was therefore carried out to test the hypothesis. Although, ideally, we would like to randomize a group of people

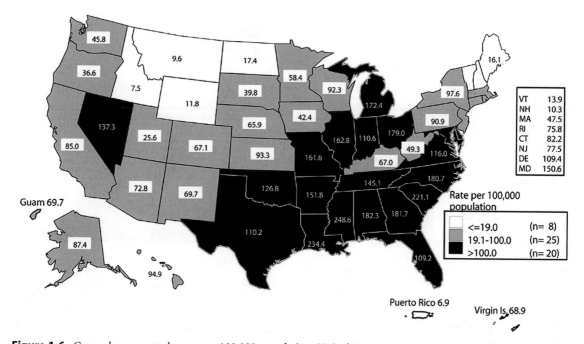

VT	13.9
NH	10.3
MA	47.5
RI	75.8
CT	82.2
NJ	77.5
DE	109.4
MD	150.6

Rate per 100,000 population

☐	<=19.0	(n= 8)
▨	19.1-100.0	(n= 25)
■	>100.0	(n= 20)

Figure 1-6. Gonorrhea: reported cases per 100,000 population, United States and territories, 2005. (Gonorrhea—Rates by State: United States and outlying areas, 2005. www.cdc.gov/std/stats05/figures/fig14.htm)

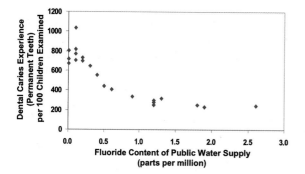

Figure 1-7. Relationship between rate of dental caries in children's permanent teeth and fluoride content of public water supply. (Adapted from Dean HT, Arnold FA, Jr, Elvove E: Domestic water and dental caries: V. Additional studies of the relation of fluoride in domestic waters to dental caries experience in 4,425 white children aged 12 to 14 years of 13 cities in 4 states. Public Health Rep 57: 1155–1179, 1942.)

either to receive fluoride or to receive no fluoride, this was not possible to do with drinking water because each community generally shares a common water supply. Consequently, two similar communities in upstate New York, Kingston and Newburgh, were chosen for the trial. The DMF index, a count of decayed, missing, and filled teeth, was used. Baseline data were collected in both cities, and at the start of

the study, the DMF indices were comparable in each group in the two communities. The water in Newburgh was then fluoridated, and the children were reexamined. Figure 1-8 shows that, in each age group, the DMF index in Newburgh had dropped significantly 10 years or so later, whereas in Kingston, there was no change. This is strongly suggestive evidence that fluoride was preventing caries.

It was possible to go one step further in trying to demonstrate a causal relationship between fluoride ingestion and low rates of caries. The issue of fluoridating water supplies has been extremely controversial, and in certain communities in which water has been fluoridated, there have been referenda to stop the fluoridation. It was therefore possible to look at the DMF index in communities such as Antigo, Wisconsin, in which fluoride had been added to its water supply and then, after a referendum, fluoridation had been stopped. As seen in Figure 1-9, after the fluoride was removed, the DMF index rose. This provided yet a further piece of evidence that fluoride acted to prevent dental caries.

FROM OBSERVATIONS TO PREVENTIVE ACTIONS

In this section, three examples are discussed that demonstrate how epidemiologic observations have

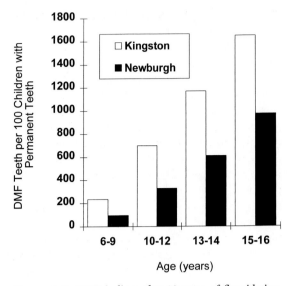

Figure 1-8. DMF indices after 10 years of fluoridation, 1954–1955. DMF, decayed, missing, and filled teeth. (Adapted from Ast DB, Schlesinger ER: The conclusion of a 10-year study of water fluoridation. Am J Public Health 46:265–271, 1956. Copyright 1956 by the American Public Health Association. Adapted with permission.)

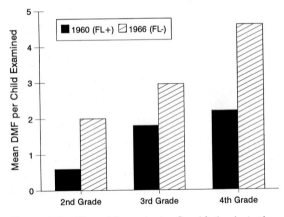

Figure 1-9. Effect of discontinuing fluoridation in Antigo, Wisconsin, November 1960. DMF, decayed, missing, and filled teeth; FL+, during fluoridation; FL−, after fluoridation was discontinued. (Adapted from Lemke CW, Doherty JM, Arra MC: Controlled fluoridation: The dental effects of discontinuation in Antigo, Wisconsin. J Am Dental Assoc 80:782–786, 1970. Reprinted by permission of ADA Publishing Co., Inc.)

led to effective preventive measures in human populations.

Ignáz Semmelweis and Childbed Fever

Ignáz Semmelweis (Fig. 1-10) was born in 1818 and began as a student in law school until he left his studies to pursue training in medicine. He special-

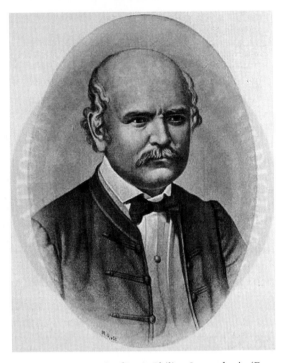

Figure 1-10. Portrait of Ignáz Philipp Semmelweis. (From The National Library of Medicine.)

ized in obstetrics and became interested in a major clinical and public health problem of the day: childbed fever, also known as puerperal fever (the word "puerperal" means related to childbirth or to the period after the birth).

In the early 19th century, childbed fever was a major cause of death among women shortly after childbirth, with mortality rates from childbed fever as high as 25%. Many theories of the cause of childbed fever were popular at the time, including atmospheric toxins, "epidemic constitutions" of some women, putrid air, or solar and magnetic influences. This period was a time of growing interest in pathologic anatomy. Because the cause of childbed fever remained a mystery, great interest arose in correlating the findings at autopsies of women who had died of the disease with the clinical manifestations that characterized them before their deaths.

Semmelweis was placed in charge of the First Obstetrical Clinic of the Allgemeine Krankenhaus [General Hospital] in Vienna in July 1846. At that time there were two obstetrical clinics, the First and the Second. Pregnant women were admitted for childbirth to the First Clinic or to the Second Clinic on an alternating 24-hour basis. The First Clinic was staffed by physicians and medical students and the Second Clinic by midwives. Physicians and medical

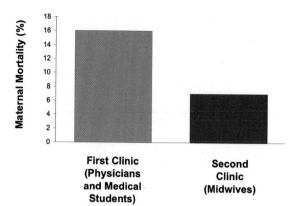

Figure 1-11. Maternal mortality due to childbed fever, First and Second Clinics, General Hospital, Vienna, Austria, 1842. (Adapted from the Centers for Disease Control and Prevention: Hand hygiene in health care settings—Supplemental. www.cdc.gov/handhygiene/download/hand_hygiene_supplement.ppt)

students began their days performing autopsies on women who had died from childbed fever; they then proceeded to provide clinical care for women hospitalized in the First Clinic for childbirth. The midwives staffing the Second Clinic did not perform autopsies. Semmelweis had been impressed by mortality rates in the two clinics in 1842 (Fig. 1-11). Mortality in the First Clinic was more than twice as high as in the Second Clinic—16% compared with 7%.

Semmelweis came to believe that mortality was higher in the First Clinic than in the Second because the physicians and medical students went directly from the autopsies to their patients. Many of the women in labor had multiple examinations by physicians and by medical students learning obstetrics. Often these examinations traumatized the tissues of

the vagina and uterus. Semmelweis suggested that the hands of physicians and medical students were transmitting disease-causing particles from the cadavers to the women who were about to deliver. His suspicions were confirmed in 1847 when his friend and colleague Jakob Kolletschka died from an infection contracted when he was accidentally punctured with a medical student's knife while performing an autopsy. The autopsy on Kolletschka showed pathology very similar to that of the women who were dying from childbed fever. Semmelweis concluded that physicians and medical students were carrying the infection from the autopsy room to the patients in the First Clinic and that this accounted for the high mortality rates from childbed fever in the First Clinic. Mortality rates in the Second Clinic remained low because the midwives who staffed the Second Clinic had no contact with the autopsy room.

Semmelweis therefore developed and implemented a policy for the physicians and medical students in the First Clinic, a policy designed to prevent childbed fever. He required the physicians and medical students in the First Clinic to wash their hands and to brush under their fingernails after they had finished the autopsies and before they came in contact with any of the patients. As seen in Figure 1-12, mortality in the First Clinic dropped from 12.2% to 2.4%, a rate comparable to that seen in the Second Clinic. When Semmelweis was later replaced by an obstetrician who did not subscribe to Semmelweis's theories, and who therefore eliminated the policy of required hand washing, mortality rates from childbed fever rose again in the First Clinic—further evidence supporting a causal relationship.

Unfortunately, for many years Semmelweis refused to present his findings at major meetings or to submit

Figure 1-12. Maternal mortality due to childbed fever, by type of care provider, General Hospital, Vienna, Austria, 1841–1850. (Adapted from Mayhall GC: Hospital Epidemiology and Infection Control, 2nd ed. Philadelphia, Lippincott Williams & Wilkins, 1999.)

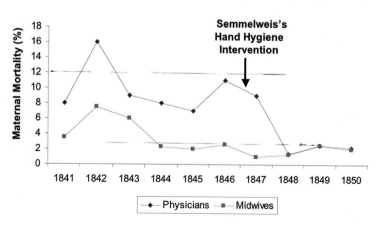

TABLE 1-3. **Compliance with Hand Hygiene among Physicians, by Specialty, at University of Geneva Hospitals**

Physician Specialty	Number of Physicians	Compliance with Hand Hygiene (% of Observations)
Internal medicine	32	87.3
Surgery	25	36.4
Intensive care unit	22	62.6
Pediatrics	21	82.6
Geriatrics	10	71.2
Anesthesiology	15	23.3
Emergency medicine	16	50.0
Other	22	57.2

Data from Pittet D: Hand hygiene among physicians: Performance, beliefs, and perceptions. Ann Intern Med 141(1):1–8, 2004.

written reports of his studies to medical journals. His failure to provide supporting scientific evidence was at least partially responsible for the failure of the medical community to accept his hypothesis of causation of childbed fever and his proposed intervention of hand washing between examinations of patients. Among other factors that fostered resistance to his proposal was the reluctance of physicians to accept the conclusion that by transmitting the agent responsible for childbed fever, they had been inadvertently responsible for the deaths of large numbers of women. In addition, physicians claimed that washing their hands before seeing each patient would be too time-consuming. Another major factor is that Semmelweis was, to say the least, undiplomatic, and had alienated many senior figures in medicine. As a consequence of all of these factors, many years passed before a policy of hand washing was broadly adopted. An excellent biography of Semmelweis by Sherwin Nuland was published in 2003.[3]

The lessons of this story for successful policy-making are still relevant today to the challenge of enhancing both public and professional acceptance of evidence-based prevention policies. These lessons include the need for presenting supporting scientific evidence for a proposed intervention, the need for implementation of the proposed intervention to be perceived as feasible, and the need to lay the necessary groundwork for the policy, including garnering professional as well as community and political support.

Years later, the major cause of childbed fever was recognized to be a streptococcal infection. Semmelweis's major findings and recommendations ultimately had worldwide effects on the practice of medicine. Amazingly, his observations and suggested interventions preceded any knowledge of the germ theory. It is also of interest, however, that although the need for hand washing has now been universally accepted, recent studies have reported that many physicians in hospitals in the United States and in other developed countries still fail to wash their hands as prescribed (Table 1-3).

Edward Jenner and Smallpox

Edward Jenner (Fig. 1-13) was born in 1749 and became very interested in the problem of smallpox, which was a worldwide scourge. For example, in the late 18th century, 400,000 people died from smallpox

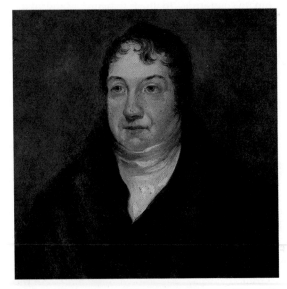

Figure 1-13. Portrait of Edward Jenner. (From the Wellcome Historical Medical Museum and Library, London.)

each year and a third of the survivors became blind as a result of corneal infections. It was known that those who survived smallpox were subsequently immune to the disease and consequently it was a common preventive practice to infect healthy individuals with smallpox by administering to them material taken from smallpox patients, a procedure called *variolation.* However, this was not an optimal method: some variolated individuals died from the resulting smallpox, infected others with smallpox, or developed other infections.

Jenner was interested in finding a better, safer approach to preventing smallpox. He observed, as had other people before him, that dairy maids, the young women whose occupation was milking the cows, developed a mild disease called cowpox. Later, during smallpox outbreaks, the disease appeared not to develop in these young women. In 1768 Jenner heard a claim from a dairy maid, "I can't take the smallpox for I have already had the cowpox." These data were observations and were not based on any rigorous study. But Jenner became convinced that cowpox could protect against smallpox and decided to test his hypothesis.

Figure 1-14 shows a painting by Gaston Melingue of Edward Jenner performing the first vaccination in 1796. (The term "vaccination" is derived from *vacca,*

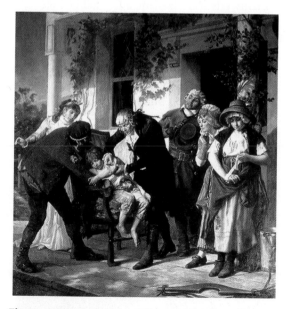

Figure 1-14. Une des premières vaccinations d'Edward Jenner [One of the first vaccinations by Edward Jenner], by Gaston Melingue. (Reproduced by permission of the Bibliothèque de l'Académie Nationale de Médecine, Paris, 2007.)

the Latin word for "cow.") In this painting, a dairy maid, Sarah Nelmes, is bandaging her hand after just having had some cowpox material removed. The cowpox material is being administered by Jenner to an 8-year-old "volunteer," James Phipps. Jenner was so convinced that cowpox would be protective that 6 weeks later, in order to test his conviction, he inoculated the child with material that had just been taken from a smallpox pustule. The child did not contract the disease. We shall not deal in this chapter with the ethical issues and implications of this experiment. (Clearly, Jenner did not have to justify his study before an institutional review board!) In any event, the results of the first vaccination and of what followed were the saving of literally millions of human beings throughout the world from disability and death caused by the scourge of smallpox. The important point is that Jenner knew nothing about viruses and nothing about the biology of the disease. He operated purely on observational data that provided him with the basis for a preventive intervention.

In 1967, the World Health Organization (WHO) began international efforts to eradicate smallpox using vaccinations with vaccinia virus (cowpox). It has been estimated that, until that time, smallpox afflicted 15 million people annually throughout the world, of whom 2 million died and millions of others were left blind or disfigured. In 1980, the WHO certified that smallpox had been eradicated. The smallpox eradication program,[4] directed at the time by Dr. D. A. Henderson (Fig. 1-15), is one of the greatest disease prevention achievements in human history. The WHO estimated that 350 million new cases had been prevented over a 20-year period. However, after the terrorist attacks that killed nearly 3,000 people in the World Trade Center in New York City on September 11, 2001, worldwide concern developed about potential bioterrorism. Ironically, the possibility that smallpox virus might be used for such a purpose reopened issues regarding smallpox and vaccination that many thought had been permanently relegated to history by the successful efforts at eradication of the disease. The magnitude of the smallpox bioterrorism threat, together with issues of vaccinia risk—both to those vaccinated and to those coming in contact with vaccinees, especially in hospital environments—are among many that have had to be addressed. Often, however, only limited or equivocal data are available on these issues to guide the development of relevant public health prevention policy relating to a potential bioterrorism threat of using smallpox as a weapon.

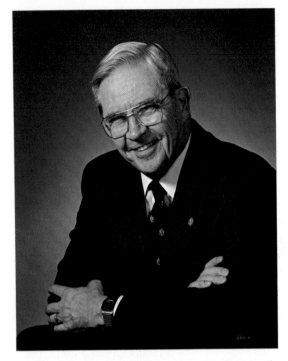

Figure 1-15. Photograph of Dr. D. A. Henderson, who directed the World Health Organization Smallpox Eradication Program.

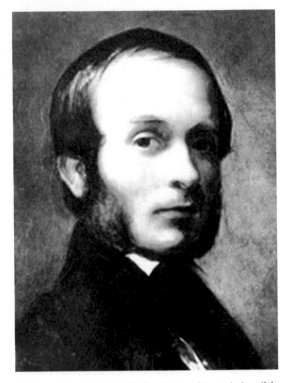

Figure 1-16. Portrait of John Snow. (Portrait in oil by Thomas Jones Barker, 1847, in Zuck D: Snow, Empson and the barkers of Bath. Anaesthesia 56:227–230, 2001.)

John Snow and Cholera

Another example of the translation of epidemiologic observations into public policy immortalized John Snow, whose portrait is seen in Figure 1-16. Snow lived in the 19th century and was well known as the anesthesiologist who administered chloroform to Queen Victoria during childbirth. Snow's true love, however, was the epidemiology of cholera, a disease that was a major problem in England in the middle of the 19th century. In the first week of September 1854, about 600 people living within a few blocks of the Broad Street pump in London died of cholera. At that time, the Registrar General was William Farr. Snow and Farr had a major disagreement about the cause of cholera. Farr adhered to what was called the *miasmatic* theory of disease. According to this theory, which was commonly held at the time, disease was transmitted by a miasm, or cloud, that clung low on the surface of the earth. If this were so, we would expect that people who lived at lower altitudes would be at greater risk of contracting a disease transmitted by this cloud than those living at higher elevations.

Farr collected data to support his hypothesis (Table 1-4). The data are quite consistent with his hypothesis: the lower the elevation, the higher the mortality rate from cholera. Snow did not agree; he believed that cholera was transmitted through contaminated water (Fig. 1-17). In London at that time, a person obtained water by signing up with one of the water supply companies. The intakes for the water companies were in a very polluted part of the Thames River. At one point in time, one of the companies, the Lambeth Company, for technical, non-health-related reasons, shifted its water intake upstream in the Thames to a less polluted part of the river; the other companies did not move the locations of their water intakes. Snow reasoned, therefore, that based on his hypothesis of contaminated water causing cholera, the mortality rate from cholera would be lower in people getting their water from the Lambeth Company than in those obtaining their water from the other companies. He carried out what we call today "shoe-leather epidemiology"—going from house to house, counting all deaths from cholera in each house, and determining which company supplied water to each house.

Snow's findings are shown in Table 1-5. The table shows the number of houses, the number of deaths from cholera, and the deaths per 10,000 houses.

TABLE 1-4. **Deaths from Cholera in 10,000 Inhabitants by Elevation of Residence above Sea Level, London, 1848–1849**	
Elevation above Sea Level (ft)	**Number of Deaths**
<20	120
20–40	65
40–60	34
60–80	27
80–100	22
100–120	17
340–360	8

Data from Farr W: Vital Statistics: A Memorial Volume of Selections from the Reports and Writings of William Farr (edited for the Sanitary Institute of Great Britain by Noel A. Humphreys). London, The Sanitary Institute, 1885.

the death rate was 315 deaths per 10,000 houses. In homes supplied by the Lambeth Company which had relocated its water intake, the rate was only 38 deaths per 10,000 houses. His data were so convincing that they led Farr, the Registrar General, to require the registrar of each district in south London to record which water company supplied each house in which a person died of cholera. Remember that, in Snow's day, the enterotoxic *Vibrio cholerae* was unknown. Nothing was known about the biology of the disease. Snow's conclusion that contaminated water was associated with cholera was based entirely on observational data.[5]

The point is that, although it is extremely important for us to maximize our knowledge of the biology and pathogenesis of disease, it is not always necessary to know every detail of the pathogenic mechanism to be able to prevent a disease. For example, we know that virtually every case of rheumatic fever and rheumatic heart disease follows a streptococcal infection. The *Streptococcus* has been studied and analyzed extensively, but we still do not know how and why it causes rheumatic fever. We do know that after a severe streptococcal infection, as seen in military recruits, rheumatic fever does not develop in 97 of every 100 infected persons. In civilian populations, such as schoolchildren, in whom the infection is less

Although this is not an ideal rate, because a house can contain different numbers of people, it is not a bad approximation. We see that in houses served by the Southwark and Vauxhall Company, which was getting its water from a polluted part of the Thames,

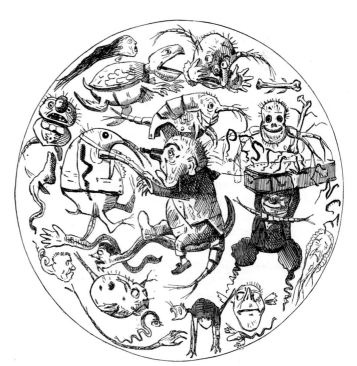

Figure 1-17. A drop of Thames water, as depicted by *Punch* in 1850. (From Extracts from Appendix (A) to the Report of the General Board of Health on the Epidemic Cholera of 1848 and 1849, published by HMSO, London, 1850. Int J Epidemiol 31:900–907, 2002.)

A DROP OF LONDON WATER.

TABLE 1-5. Deaths from Cholera per 10,000 Houses, by Source of Water Supply, London, 1854

Water Supply	Number of Houses	Deaths from Cholera	Deaths per 10,000 Houses
Southwark and Vauxhall Co.	40,046	1,263	315
Lambeth Co.	26,107	98	38
Other districts in London	256,423	1,422	56

Data adapted from Snow J: On the mode of communication of cholera. In Snow on Cholera: A Reprint of Two Papers by John Snow, M.D. New York, The Commonwealth Fund, 1936.

severe, rheumatic fever develops in only 3 of every 1,000 infected school-children, but not in the remaining 997.[6] Why does the disease not develop in those 97 recruits and 997 schoolchildren if they are exposed to the same organism? We do not know. We do not know if the illness is the result of an undetected difference in the organism or if it is caused by a cofactor that may facilitate the adherence of streptococci to epithelial cells. What we do know is that, even without fully understanding the chain of pathogenesis from infection with the *Streptococcus* to rheumatic fever, we can prevent virtually every case of rheumatic fever if we either prevent or promptly and adequately treat streptococcal infections. The absence of biologic knowledge about pathogenesis should not be a hindrance or an excuse for not implementing effective preventive services.

Consider cigarette smoking and lung cancer. We do not know what specific component in cigarettes causes cancer, but we do know that 75% to 80% of cases of lung cancer are caused by smoking. That does not mean that we should not be conducting laboratory research to better understand how cigarettes cause cancer. But again, in parallel with that research, we should be mounting effective community and public health programs based on the observational data available right now.

Figure 1-18 shows mortality data for breast cancer and lung cancer in women in the United States. Breast cancer mortality rate remained relatively constant over several decades but showed evidence of decline in the early years of the 21st century. However, mortality from lung cancer in women has been increasing steadily although it may have begun to stabilize in recent years. Since 1987, more women have died each year from lung cancer than from breast cancer. Thus, we are faced with the tragic picture of a preventable form of cancer, lung cancer,

which results from a personal habit, smoking, as the current leading cause of cancer death in American women.

Furthermore, in 1993, environmental tobacco smoke (secondhand smoke from other people's smoking) was classified as a known human carcinogen by the Environmental Protection Agency, which attributed about 3,000 lung cancer deaths in non-

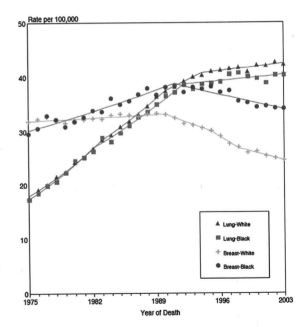

Figure 1-18. Breast versus lung cancer mortality: White females versus black females, United States, 1975–2003, age-adjusted to 2000 standard. (From Ries LAG, Harkins D, Krapcho M, et al (eds): SEER Cancer Statistics Review, 1975–2003, National Cancer Institute. Bethesda, MD. http://seer.cancer.gov/csr/1975_2003/, based on November 2005 SEER data submission, posted to the SEER Web site 2006.)

smoking individuals each year to environmental tobacco smoke.

Although rates of smoking in those older than 18 years of age appear to have decreased in recent years in the United States, a troublesome observation is that, from 1991 to 1997, the prevalence of smoking in high school students increased 32%. Thus, the scourge of smoking remains one of the major unmet prevention challenges for practitioners in both public health and clinical medicine.

CONCLUSION

Prevention and therapy are all too often viewed as mutually exclusive activities, as is shown in Figure 1-19. It is clear, however, that prevention not only is integral to public health, but also is integral to clinical practice. The physician's role is to maintain health as well as to treat disease. But even treatment of disease includes a major component of prevention. Whenever we treat illness we are preventing death, preventing complications in the patient, or preventing a constellation of effects on the patient's family. Thus, much of the dichotomy between therapy and prevention is an illusion. Therapy involves secondary and tertiary prevention, the latter denoting the prevention of complications such as disability. At times it also involves primary prevention. Thus, the entire spectrum of prevention should be viewed as integral to both public health and clinical practice. Epidemi-

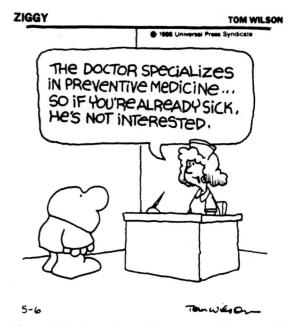

Figure 1-19. Prevention and therapy viewed as mutually exclusive activities. (From Wilson T: Ziggy cartoon. © Universal Press Syndicate, 1986.)

ology is an invaluable tool for providing the rational basis on which effective prevention programs can be planned and implemented and for conducting clinical investigations that contribute to the control of disease and to the amelioration of the human suffering associated with it.

REFERENCES

1. Last JM: A Dictionary of Epidemiology, 4th ed. New York, Oxford University Press, 2000.
2. Rose G: Sick individuals and sick populations. Int J Epidemiol 14:32–38, 1985.
3. Nuland, SB: The Doctors' Plague: Germs, Childbed Fever and the Strange Story of Ignáz Semmelweis. New York, W W Norton, Atlas Books, 2003.
4. Fenner F, Henderson DA, Arita I, et al: Smallpox and Its Eradication. Geneva, World Health Organization, 1988.
5. Johnson S: The Ghost Map: The Story of London's Most Terrifying Epidemic—and How It Changed Science, Cities, and the Modern World. New York, Riverhead Books, 2006.
6. Markowitz M, Gordis L: Rheumatic Fever, 2nd ed. Philadelphia, WB Saunders, 1972.

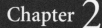
The Dynamics of Disease Transmission

I keep six honest serving-men
(They taught me all I knew);
Their names are What and Why and When
And How and Where and Who.
　　—Rudyard Kipling[1] (1865–1936)

Human disease does not arise in a vacuum. It results from an interaction of the host (a person), the agent (e.g., a bacterium), and the environment (e.g., a contaminated water supply). Although some diseases are largely genetic in origin, virtually all disease results from an interaction of genetic and environmental factors, with the exact balance differing for different diseases. Many of the underlying principles governing the transmission of disease are most clearly demonstrated using communicable diseases as a model. Hence, this chapter primarily uses such diseases as examples in reviewing these principles. However, the concepts discussed are also applicable to diseases that do not appear to be of infectious origin.

Disease has been classically described as the result of an epidemiologic triad shown in Figure 2-1. According to this diagram, it is the product of an interaction of the human host, an infectious or other type of agent, and the environment that promotes the exposure. A vector, such as the mosquito or the deer tick, is often involved. For such an interaction to take place, the host must be susceptible. Human susceptibility is determined by a variety of factors including genetic background and nutritional and immunologic characteristics. The immune status of an individual is determined by many factors including prior experience both with natural infection and with immunization.

The factors that can cause human disease include biologic, physical, and chemical factors as well as other types, such as stress, that may be harder to classify (Table 2-1).

MODES OF TRANSMISSION

Diseases can be transmitted *directly* or *indirectly*. For example, a disease can be transmitted person to person (direct transmission) by means of direct contact. Indirect transmission can occur through a common vehicle such as a contaminated air or water supply, or by a vector such as the mosquito. Some of the modes of transmission are shown in Table 2-2.

Figure 2-2 is a classic photograph showing droplet dispersal after a sneeze. It vividly demonstrates the potential for an individual to infect a large number of people in a brief period of time. As Mims has pointed out:

An infected individual can transmit influenza or the common cold to a score of others in the course of an innocent hour in a crowded room. A venereal infection also must spread progressively from person to person if it is to maintain itself in nature, but it would be a formidable task to transmit venereal infection on such a scale.[2]

Thus, different organisms spread in different ways, and the potential of a given organism for spreading and producing outbreaks depends on the characteristics of the organism, such as its rate of growth and the route by which it is transmitted from one person to another.

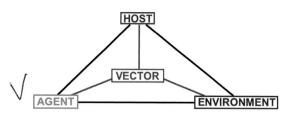

Figure 2-1. The epidemiologic triad of a disease.

TABLE 2-1. **Factors That May Be Associated with Increased Risk of Human Disease**

Host Characteristics	Types of Agents and Examples	Environmental Factors
Age	Biologic	Temperature
Sex	Bacteria, viruses	Humidity
Race	Chemical	Altitude
Religion	Poison, alcohol, smoke	Crowding
Customs	Physical	Housing
Occupation	Trauma, radiation, fire	Neighborhood
Genetic profile	Nutritional	Water
Marital status	Lack, excess	Milk
Family background		Food
Previous diseases		Radiation
Immune status		Air pollution
		Noise

TABLE 2-2. **Modes of Disease Transmission**

1. Direct
   a. Person-to-person contact
2. Indirect
   a. Common vehicle
      (1) Single exposure
      (2) Multiple exposures
      (3) Continuous exposure
   b. Vector

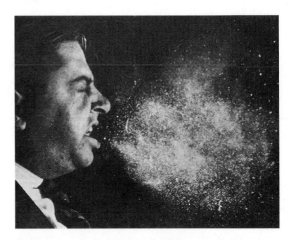

Figure 2-2. Droplet dispersal following a violent sneeze. (Reprinted with permission from Jennison MW: Aerobiology 17:102, 1947. Copyright 1947 American Association for the Advancement of Science.)

Figure 2-3 is a schematic diagram of the human body surfaces as sites of microbial infection and shedding. The alimentary tract can be considered as an open tube that crosses the body, and the respiratory and urogenital systems can be seen as blind inpouchings. Each offers an opportunity for infection. The skin is another important portal of entry for infectious agents, primarily through scratch or injury. Agents that often enter through the skin include streptococci or staphylococci and fungi such as tinea (ringworm). Two points should be made in this regard: First, the skin is not the exclusive portal of entry for many of these agents, and infections can be acquired through more than one route. The same routes also serve as points of entry for noninfectious disease-causing agents. Environmental toxins can be ingested, inspired during respiration, or absorbed directly through the skin. With both infectious and noninfectious conditions, the clinical and epidemiologic characteristics of the condition often relate to the site of the exposure and the portal of entry.

CLINICAL AND SUBCLINICAL DISEASE

It is important to recognize the broad spectrum of disease severity. Figure 2-4 shows the iceberg concept of disease. Just as most of an iceberg is underwater and hidden from view with only its tip visible, so it is with disease: only clinical illness is readily apparent (see Fig. 2-4, *right*). But infections without clinical illness are important, particularly in the web of disease transmission, although they are not visible clinically. In Figure 2-4, the corresponding biologic stages of pathogenesis and disease at the cellular level are seen on the *left*. The iceberg concept is important because it is not sufficient to count only the clinically apparent cases we see; for example,

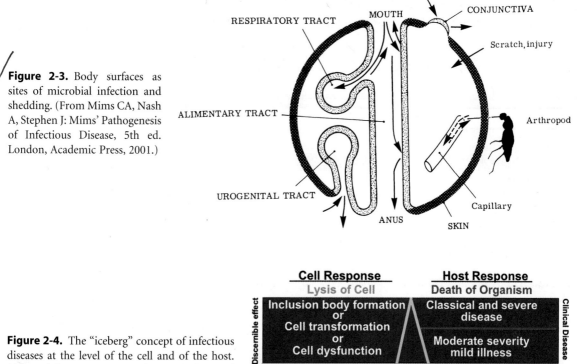

Figure 2-3. Body surfaces as sites of microbial infection and shedding. (From Mims CA, Nash A, Stephen J: Mims' Pathogenesis of Infectious Disease, 5th ed. London, Academic Press, 2001.)

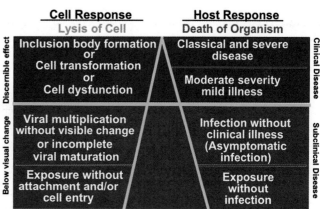

Figure 2-4. The "iceberg" concept of infectious diseases at the level of the cell and of the host. (Adapted from Evans AS, Kaslow RA (eds): Viral Infections of Humans: Epidemiology and Control, 4th ed. New York, Plenum, 1997.)

most cases of polio in prevaccine days were subclinical, but they were still capable of spreading the virus. The epidemiology of polio cannot be explained without a recognition and assessment of the pool of inapparent cases.

Figure 2-5 shows the spectrum of severity for several diseases. Most cases of tuberculosis, for example, are inapparent. However, because inapparent cases can transmit the disease, such cases must be identified to control spread of the disease. In measles, many cases are of moderate severity and only a few are inapparent. At the other extreme, without intervention, rabies has no inapparent cases, and most untreated cases are fatal. Thus, we have a spectrum of severity patterns that varies with the disease. Severity appears to be related to the virulence of the organism (how good the organism is at producing disease) and to the site in the body at which the organism multiplies. All of these factors, as well as such host characteristics as the immune response,

need to be appreciated to understand how disease spreads from one individual to another.

As clinical and biologic knowledge has increased over the years, so has our ability to distinguish different stages of disease. These include clinical and nonclinical disease:

Clinical Disease

Clinical disease is characterized by signs and symptoms.

Nonclinical (Inapparent) Disease

Nonclinical disease may include the following:

1. *Preclinical Disease.* Disease that is not yet clinically apparent, but is destined to progress to clinical disease.
2. *Subclinical Disease.* Disease that is not clinically apparent and is not destined to become clinically apparent. This type of disease is often diagnosed by serologic (antibody) response or culture of the organism.

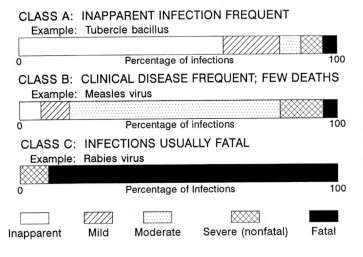

Figure 2-5. Distribution of clinical severity for three classes of infections (not drawn to scale). (Adapted from Mausner JS, Kramer S: Epidemiology: An Introductory Text. Philadelphia, WB Saunders, 1985, p 265.)

3. *Persistent (Chronic) Disease.* A person fails to "shake off" the infection, and it persists for years, at times for life. In recent years, an interesting phenomenon has been the manifestation of symptoms many years after an infection was thought to have been resolved. Some adults who recovered from poliomyelitis in childhood are now reporting severe fatigue and weakness; this has been called post-polio syndrome in adult life. These have thus become cases of clinical disease, albeit somewhat different from the initial illness.

4. *Latent Disease.* An infection with no active multiplication of the agent, as when viral nucleic acid is incorporated into the nucleus of a cell as a provirus. In contrast to persistent infection, only the genetic message is present in the host, not the viable organism.

CARRIER STATUS

In this situation, the individual harbors the organism, but is not infected as measured by serologic studies (no evidence of an antibody response) or by evidence of clinical illness. This person can still infect others, although the infectivity is often lower than with other infections. Carrier status may be of limited duration or may be chronic, lasting for months or years. One of the best-known examples of a long-term carrier was Typhoid Mary, who carried *Salmonella typhi* and died in 1938. Over a period of many years, she worked as a cook in the New York City area, moving from household to household under different names. She was considered to have caused at least 10 typhoid fever outbreaks that included 51 cases and 3 deaths.

ENDEMIC, EPIDEMIC, AND PANDEMIC

Three other terms need to be defined: *endemic, epidemic,* and *pandemic. Endemic* is defined as the habitual presence of a disease within a given geographic area. It may also refer to the usual occurrence of a given disease within such an area. *Epidemic* is defined as the occurrence in a community or region of a group of illnesses of similar nature, clearly in excess of normal expectancy, and derived from a common or from a propagated source (Fig. 2-6). *Pandemic* refers to a worldwide epidemic.

How do we know when we have an excess over what is expected? Indeed, how do we know how much to expect? There is no precise answer to either question. Through ongoing surveillance, we may determine what the usual or expected level may be. With regard to excess, sometimes an "interocular test" may be convincing: the difference is so clear that it hits you between the eyes.

For example, in December 1952, a dense smoke-laden fog (smog) descended on London. From December 6 to 9, the fog was so thick that visibility was reduced to 30 feet in parts of London. Pedestrians had difficulty finding their way, even in familiar neighborhoods. At times, people could not see their own hands and feet. Figure 2-7 shows trends over this time in the mortality rates and in sulfur dioxide (SO_2) level. The SO_2 level serves as a useful indicator of general levels of air pollution. As seen in Figure 2-7, the fog was accompanied by a rapid rise in the mortality rate, clearly exceeding the usual mortality rate. This rate remained elevated for some time after the fog dissipated. More than 4,000 deaths were attributed to the fog. Recently, further analyses have

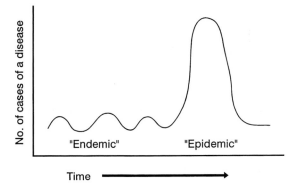

Figure 2-6. Endemic versus epidemic disease.

suggested that about 12,000 excess deaths occurred from December 1952 through February 1953.[3] Many of these deaths occurred in people who were already suffering from chronic lung or cardiovascular disease. The disaster of the London Fog, or the Great Smog, as it became known, led to legislation, including the Clean Air Acts of 1956 and 1968, which banned emissions of black smoke and required residents of urban areas and operators of factories to convert to smokeless fuel.

DISEASE OUTBREAKS

Let us assume that a food becomes contaminated with a microorganism. If an outbreak occurs in the group of people who have eaten the food, it is called a *common-vehicle exposure*, because all the cases that developed were in persons exposed to the food in question. The food may be served only once, for example, at a catered luncheon, resulting in a *single exposure* to the people who eat it, or the food may be served more than once, resulting in *multiple exposures* to people who eat it more than once. When a water supply is contaminated with sewage because of leaky pipes, the contamination can be either *periodic*, causing multiple exposures as a result of changing pressures in the water supply system that may cause intermittent contamination, or *continuous*, in which a constant leak leads to persistent contamination. The epidemiologic picture that is manifested depends on whether the exposure is single, multiple, or continuous.

For purposes of this discussion, we will focus on the *single-exposure, common-vehicle outbreak* because the issues discussed are most clearly seen in this type of outbreak. What are the characteristics of such an outbreak? First, such outbreaks are explosive; there is a sudden and rapid increase in the number of cases of a disease in a population. Second, the cases are limited to people who share the common exposure. This is self-evident, because in the first wave of cases we would not expect the disease to develop in people who were not exposed unless there were another source of the disease in the community. Third, in a food-borne outbreak, cases rarely occur in persons who acquire the disease from a primary case. The reason for the relative rarity of such secondary cases in this type of outbreak is not well understood.

Over recent decades, a growing number of outbreaks of acute gastroenteritis (AGE) have occurred aboard cruise ships. During the first 11 months of 2002, the Centers for Disease Control and Prevention (CDC) received reports of 21 outbreaks of AGE, of which 9 were confirmed by laboratory tests of stool specimens to be associated with noroviruses (from

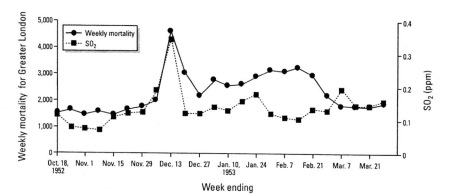

Figure 2-7. Approximate weekly mortality and SO_2 concentrations for Greater London, 1952–1953. (From Bell ML, Davis DL: Reassessment of the lethal London Fog of 1952: Novel indicators of acute and chronic consequences of acute exposure to air pollution. Environ Health Perspect 109[Suppl 3]:389–394, 2001.)

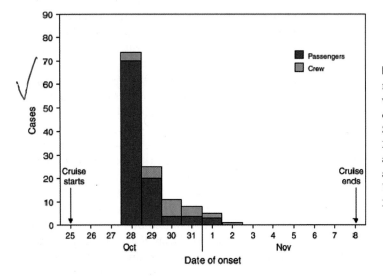

Figure 2-8. Number of passengers and crew members reporting to the ship's infirmary with symptoms of acute gastroenteritis during a 14-day cruise by date of illness onset, Spain to Florida, October 25–November 8, 2002. (From Centers for Disease Control and Prevention: Outbreaks of gastroenteritis associated with noroviruses on cruise ships—United States, 2002. MMWR 51[49]:112–115, 2002.)

the Norwalk virus family). One of these outbreaks is shown in Figure 2-8.[4] On October 25, a cruise ship with 2,882 passengers and 944 crew members left Spain for a 14-day cruise to Florida. On October 28, a total of 70 (2.5%) of the passengers reported to the infirmary with AGE. By November 2, a total of 106 passengers (5%) and 25 (3%) of the crew had reported illnesses. Figure 2-8 shows the rapid rise in the number of cases and the tapering off of the epidemic curve, typical of single-exposure common-vehicle outbreaks. Results of tests on stool specimens from four of six passengers were positive for a strain of norovirus that was different from that observed in previous outbreaks on cruise ships. Ill crew members were quarantined until they were symptom-free for 72 hours, the ship was disinfected, and sanitary practices were reinforced. No additional outbreaks were reported in subsequent cruises on this ship.[4]

DETERMINANTS OF DISEASE OUTBREAKS

The amount of disease in a population depends on a balance between the number of people in that population who are susceptible, and therefore at risk for the disease, and the number of people who are not susceptible, or immune, and therefore not at risk. They may be immune because they have had the disease previously or because they have been immunized. They also may be not susceptible on a genetic basis. Clearly, if the entire population is immune, no epidemic will develop. But the balance is usually struck somewhere in between immunity and susceptibility, and when it moves toward susceptibility, the likelihood of an outbreak increases. This has been

observed particularly in formerly isolated populations who were exposed to disease. For example, in the 19th century, Panum observed that measles occurred in the Faroe Islands in epidemic form when infected individuals entered the isolated and susceptible population.[5] In another example, severe outbreaks of streptococcal sore throats developed when new susceptible recruits arrived at the Great Lakes Naval Station.[6]

HERD IMMUNITY

Herd immunity may be defined as the resistance of a group of people to an attack by a disease to which a large proportion of the members of the group are immune. If a large percentage of the population is immune, the entire population is likely to be protected, not just those who are immune. Why does herd immunity occur? It happens because disease spreads from one person to another in any community. Once a certain proportion of people in the community are immune, the likelihood is small that an infected person will encounter a susceptible person to whom he can transmit the infection; more of his encounters will be with people who are immune. The presence of a large proportion of immune persons in the population lessens the likelihood that a person with the disease will come into contact with a susceptible individual.

Why is the concept of herd immunity so important? When we carry out immunization programs, it may not be necessary to achieve 100% immunization rates to immunize the population successfully. We can achieve highly effective protection by immunizing a large part of the population; the remaining part will be protected because of herd immunity.

For herd immunity to exist, certain conditions must be met. The disease agent must be restricted to a single host species within which transmission occurs, and that transmission must be relatively direct from one member of the host species to another. If we have a reservoir in which the organism can exist outside the human host, herd immunity will not operate because other means of transmission are available. In addition, infections must induce solid immunity. If immunity is only partial, we will not build up a large subpopulation of immune people in the community.

What does this mean? Herd immunity operates if the probability of an infected person encountering every *other individual* in the population (random mixing) is the same. But if a person is infected and all his interactions are with people who are susceptible (i.e., there is no random mixing of the population), he is likely to transmit the disease to other susceptible people. Herd immunity operates optimally when populations are constantly mixing together. This is a theoretical concept because, obviously, populations are never completely randomly mixed. All of us associate with family and friends, for example, more than we do with strangers. However, the degree to which herd immunity is achieved depends on the extent to which the population approaches a random mixing. Thus, we can interrupt the transmission of disease even if not everyone in the population is immune, so long as a critical percentage of the population is immune.

What percentage of a population must be immune for herd immunity to operate? This percentage varies from disease to disease. For example, in the case of measles, which is highly communicable, it has been estimated that 94% of the population must be immune before the chain of transmission is interrupted.

Let us consider poliomyelitis immunization and herd immunity. From 1951 to 1954, an average of 24,220 cases of paralytic poliomyelitis occurred in the United States each year. Two types of vaccine are available. The oral polio vaccine (OPV) not only protects those who are vaccinated, but also protects others in the community through secondary immunity, produced when the vaccinated individual spreads the active vaccine virus to contacts. In effect, the contacts are immunized by the spread of virus from the vaccinated person. If enough people in the community are protected in this way, the chain of transmission is interrupted. However, even inactivated poliovirus vaccine (IPV), which does not produce secondary immunity (does not spread the virus), can produce herd immunity if enough of the population is immunized; even those who are not immunized will be protected because the chain of transmission in the community has been interrupted.

From 1958 to 1961, only IPV was available in the United States. Figure 2-9 shows both the expected number of cases each year if the vaccine had protected only those who received the vaccine and the number of polio cases actually observed. Clearly, the number of cases that occurred was far less than what would have been expected from the direct effects of the vaccine alone. The difference between the two curves represents the effect of herd immunity from the vaccine. Thus, nonimmunized individuals can gain some protection from either the OPV or IPV.

Figure 2-9. Effect of Herd Immunity: expected and observed numbers of paralytic poliomyelitis cases, United States, 1958–1961. (Adapted by permission of American Academy of Pediatrics News. Copyright 1998. From Stickle G: Observed and expected poliomyelitis in the United States, 1958–1961. Am J Public Health 54:1222–1229, 1964.)

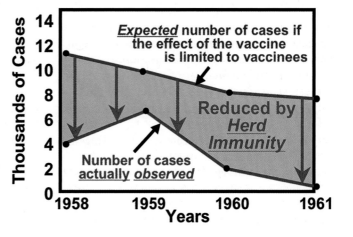

INCUBATION PERIOD

The incubation period is defined as the *interval from receipt of infection to the time of onset of clinical illness.* If you become infected today, the disease with which you are infected may not develop for a number of days or weeks. During this time, the *incubation period*, you feel completely well and show no signs of the disease.

Why doesn't disease develop immediately at the time of infection? What accounts for the incubation period? It may reflect the time needed for the organism to replicate sufficiently until it reaches the critical mass needed for clinical disease to result. It probably also relates to the site in the body at which the organism replicates—whether it replicates superficially, near the skin surface, or deeper in the body. The dose of the infectious agent received at the time of infection may also influence the length of the incubation period. With a large dose, the incubation period may be shorter.

The incubation period is also of historical interest because it is related to what may have been the only medical advance associated with the Black Death in Europe. In 1374, when people were terribly frightened of the Black Death, the Venetian Republic appointed three officials who were to be responsible for inspecting all ships entering the port and for excluding ships that had sick people on board. It was hoped that this intervention would protect the community. In 1377, in the Italian seaport of Ragusa, travelers were detained in an isolated area for 30 days (*trentini giorni*) after arrival to see whether infection developed. This period was found to be insufficient, and the period of detention was lengthened to 40 days (*quarante giorni*). This is the origin of the word *quarantine.*

How long would we want to isolate a person? We would want to isolate a person until he or she is no longer infectious to others. When a person is clinically ill, we generally have a clear sign of potential infectiousness. An important problem arises *before* the person becomes clinically ill—that is, during the incubation period. If we knew when he or she became infected and also knew the general length of the incubation period for the disease, we would want to isolate the infected person during this period to prevent the communication of the disease to others. In most situations, however, we do not know that a person has been infected, and we may not know until signs of clinical disease become manifest.

This leads to an important question: Is it worthwhile to quarantine—isolate—a patient, such as a child with chickenpox? The problem is that, during at least part of the incubation period, when a person is still free of clinical illness, he or she can transmit the disease to others. Thus, we have people who are not (yet) clinically ill, but who have been infected and are able to transmit the disease. For many common childhood diseases, by the time clinical disease develops in the child, he or she has already transmitted the disease to others. Therefore, isolating such a person at the point at which he or she becomes clinically ill will not necessarily be effective. On the other hand, isolation can be very valuable. In February 2003 a serious respiratory illness was first reported in Asia (having occurred in 2002) and was termed *severe acute respiratory syndrome* (SARS). The disease is characterized by fever over 38°C, headache, overall discomfort, and, after 2 to 7 days, development of cough and difficulty in breathing in some patients. The cause of SARS has been shown to be infection with a previously unrecognized human coronavirus, called SARS-associated coronavirus.

SARS appears to spread by close, person-to-person contact. Because modern travel, particularly air travel, facilitates rapid and extensive spread of disease, within a few months the illness had spread to more than two dozen countries in North America, South America, Europe, and Asia. However, by late July 2003, no new cases were being reported and the outbreak was considered contained. However, the possibility remains that SARS outbreaks will occur again in the future.

The World Health Organization reported that worldwide, 8,437 people became ill with SARS during the November 2002 to July 2003 outbreak and of those, 813 died (Table 2-3). The differences in case-fatality among different countries are at least partially attributable to differences in completeness of reporting and to international variations in defining and diagnosing SARS. A major contributor to control of the epidemic was probably the strong measures implemented early for isolating probable SARS cases and for reducing interpersonal contacts of travelers with a history of travel to highly affected areas.

Different diseases have different incubation periods. A precise incubation period does not exist for a given disease; rather, a range of incubation periods is characteristic for that disease. Figure 2-10 shows the range of incubation periods for several diseases. In general, the length of the incubation period is characteristic of the infective organism.

TABLE 2-3. Probable Cases of Severe Acute Respiratory Syndrome (SARS), SARS-Related Deaths, and SARS Case-Fatality, by Country, November 1, 2002–July 11, 2003

Country	Cumulative Number of Cases	Number of Deaths	Case-Fatality (%)
Canada	250	38	15.2
China	5,327	348	6.5
China, Hong Kong	1,755	298	17.0
Singapore	206	32	15.5
Taiwan	671	84	12.5
United States	75	0	0.0
Vietnam	63	5	7.9
All other countries	90	8	8.9
All countries	8,437	813	9.6

Data from SarsNet-Isolates, Activity, http://rhone.b3e.jussieu.fr/sarsnet/www/activity.html, July 19, 2003.

The incubation period for infectious diseases has its analogue in noninfectious diseases. Thus, even when an individual is exposed to a carcinogen or other toxin, the disease is often manifest only after months or years. For example, mesotheliomas resulting from asbestos exposure may occur 20 to 30 years after the exposure.

Figure 2-11 is a graphic representation of an outbreak of *Salmonella typhimurium* at a medical conference in Wales in 1986. Each bar represents the number of cases of disease developing at a certain point in time after the exposure; the number of hours since exposure is shown along the horizontal axis. If we draw a line connecting the tops of the bars it is

called the *epidemic curve*, which is defined as the distribution of the times of onset of the disease. In a *single-exposure, common-vehicle epidemic,* the epidemic curve represents the distribution of the incubation periods. This should be intuitively apparent: if the infection took place at one point in time, the interval from that point to the onset of each case is the incubation period in that person.

As seen in Figure 2-11, there was a rapid, explosive rise in the number of cases within the first 16 hours, which suggests a single-exposure, common-vehicle epidemic. In fact, this pattern is the classic epidemic curve for a single-exposure common-vehicle outbreak (Fig. 2-12, *left*). The reason for this configura-

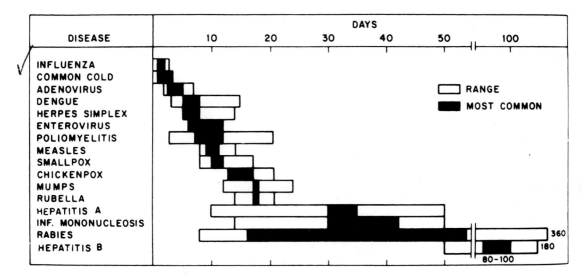

Figure 2-10. Incubation periods of viral diseases. (From Evans AS, Kaslow RA [eds]: Viral Infections of Humans: Epidemiology and Control, 4th ed. New York, Plenum, 1997.)

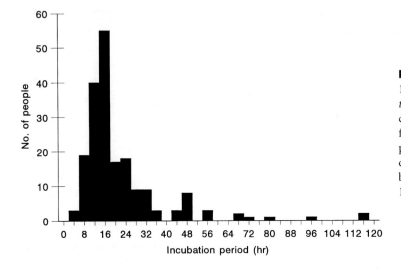

Figure 2-11. Incubation periods for 191 delegates affected by a *Salmonella typhimurium* outbreak at a medical conference in Wales, 1986. (Adapted from Glynn JR, Palmer SR: Incuba-tion period, severity of disease, and infecting dose: Evidence from a Salmonella out-break. Am J Epidemiol 136:1369–1377, 1992.)

tion is not known. But it has an interesting property: if the curve is plotted against the logarithm of time rather than against time, the curve becomes a normal curve (see Fig. 2-12, *right*). If plotted on log-normal graph paper, we obtain a straight line, and estimation of the median incubation period is facilitated.

The three critical variables in investigating an outbreak or epidemic are: (1) When did the exposure take place? (2) When did the disease begin? and (3) What was the incubation period for the disease? If we know any two of these, we can calculate the third.

ATTACK RATE

An attack rate is defined as:

$$\frac{\text{Number of people at risk in whom a certain illness develops}}{\text{Total number of people at risk}}$$

The attack rate is similar to the incidence rate, which is also used for less acute diseases. The attack rate (or the incidence rate) is useful for comparing the risk of disease in groups with different exposures. The attack rate can be specific for a given exposure. For example, the attack rate in people who ate a certain food is called a *food-specific attack rate*. It is calculated by:

$$\frac{\text{Number of people who ate a certain food and became ill}}{\text{Total number of people who ate that food}}$$

In general, *time* is not explicitly specified in an attack rate; given what is usually known about how long after an exposure most cases develop, the time period is implicit in the attack rate. Examples of calculating attack rates are seen in Table 2-5 (p. 34).

A person who acquires the disease from that exposure (e.g., from a contaminated food) is called a

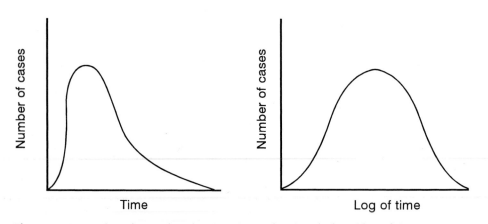

Figure 2-12. Number of cases plotted against time and against the logarithm of time.

primary case. A person who acquires the disease from exposure to a primary case is called a *secondary case*. The *secondary attack rate* is therefore defined as the attack rate in susceptible people who have been exposed to a primary case. It is a good measure of person-to-person spread of disease after the disease has been introduced into a population, and it can be thought of as a ripple moving out from the primary case. We often calculate the secondary attack rate in family members of the index case.

The secondary attack rate also has application in noninfectious diseases when family members are examined to determine the extent to which a disease clusters among first-degree relatives of an index case, which may yield a clue regarding the relative contributions of genetic and environmental factors to the cause of a disease.

EXPLORING THE OCCURRENCE OF DISEASE

The concepts outlined in this chapter form the basis for exploring the occurrence of disease. When a disease appears to have occurred at more than an endemic level, and we wish to investigate its occurrence, we ask:

Who was attacked by the disease?
When did the disease occur?
Where did the cases arise?
It is well known that disease risk is affected by all of these factors.

Who

The characteristics of the human host are clearly related to disease risk. Factors such as sex, age, and race have a major effect.

Gonorrhea

As shown in Figure 2-13, rates of gonorrhea have been higher in men than in women, and this sex dif-ference is observed at least as far back as 1960 (not shown in this graph). Because women are more likely to be asymptomatic, the disease in women has probably been underreported. Rates have been decreasing in both men and women over the past few decades, and in recent years, the sex difference has largely disappeared, possibly as a result of increased screening in women. However, despite the declines in rates, neither male nor female rates reached the level of the national objective in the United States, that of the Healthy People Year 2010 target, shown by the dotted line. Indeed, since 1997, rates in both men and women have increased slightly.

Pertussis

In 2004, the incidence rate of reported pertussis in the United States increased for the third year in a row. The rate reached 8.9 cases per 100,000 population, more than twice that reported in 2003. In 1994, the rate was 1.8. The number of cases in 2004 was the highest reported since 1959. Although childhood pertussis vaccine coverage levels are high in the United States, pertussis continues to cause morbidity. Some of this increase may result from improved diagnostics, as well as recognition and reporting of cases. As seen in Figure 2-14, the lowest rates for pertussis in the United States were observed from 1974 to 1981. Interestingly, since 1993, the number of cases reported after each epidemic year has not returned to the baseline of the pre-epidemic year.

Pertussis occurrence is clearly related to age (Fig. 2-15). Although, the *number* of reported cases was highest in children ages 10 to 14 (as seen in Fig. 2-15), the highest *rate* of pertussis was in infants less than 6 months of age (136.5 per 100,000 population) (not shown in Fig. 2-15). Among older infants aged 6 to 11 months, the rate was 31.8 per 100,000. Two thirds of pertussis cases in the United States are now seen in adolescents and adults. Although the specific cause

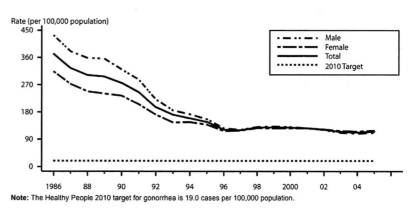

Figure 2-13. Gonorrhea, reported cases per 100,000 by sex, United States, 1986–2005, and the Healthy People Year 2010 target. (From Centers for Disease Control and Prevention: STD Surveillance, National Profile—Gonorrhea, 2005. www.cdc.gov/std/stats05/figures/fig12.htm.)

Note: The Healthy People 2010 target for gonorrhea is 19.0 cases per 100,000 population.

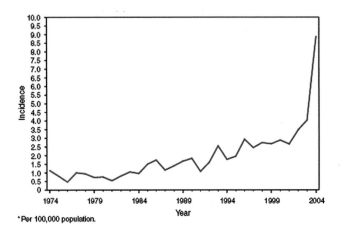

Figure 2-14. Pertussis (whooping cough), reported cases per 100,000 population by year, United States, 1974–2004. (From Centers for Disease Control and Prevention: Summary of notifiable diseases, United States: 2004. MMWR 53[53]:1–79, 2006.)

of this phenomenon is unknown, it could result from a waning of protection 5 to 10 years after pertussis immunization.

When

Certain diseases occur with a certain periodicity. For example, aseptic meningitis peaks yearly (Fig. 2-16). Often, there is a seasonal pattern to the temporal variation. For example, diarrheal disease is most common during the summer months, and respiratory disease is most common during the winter months. The question of *when* is also addressed by examining trends in disease incidence over time. For example, in the United States, both incidence of, and

deaths from, acquired immunodeficiency syndrome (AIDS) increased for many years, but began to decline in 1996, largely as a result of new therapy and health education efforts.

Where

Disease is not randomly distributed in time or place. For example, Figure 2-17 shows the geographic distribution of Lyme disease in the United States, by county, in 2005. There is a clear clustering of cases along the Northeast coast, in the north-central part of the country, and in the Pacific coast region. The states in which established enzootic cycles of *Borrelia burgdorferi*, the causative agent, have been reported

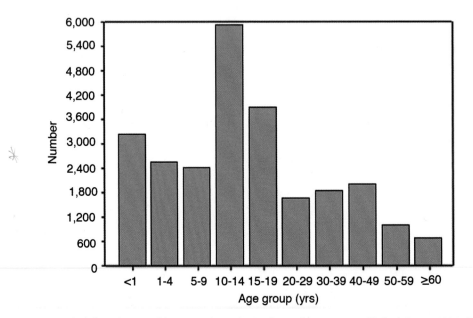

Figure 2-15. Pertussis (whooping cough), reported numbers of cases by age group, United States, 2004. (From Centers for Disease Control and Prevention: Summary of notifiable diseases, United States: 2004. MMWR 53[53]:1–79, 2006.)

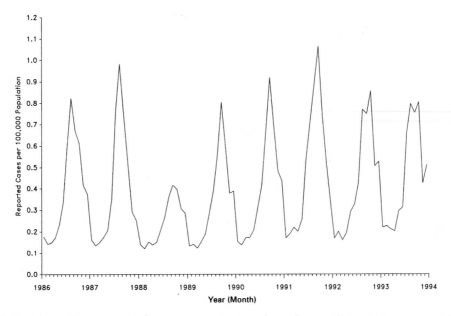

Figure 2-16. Aseptic meningitis, reported cases per 100,000 population by month, United States, 1986–1993. (From Centers for Disease Control and Prevention: Summary of notifiable diseases, United States: 1993. MMWR 42:22, 1994.)

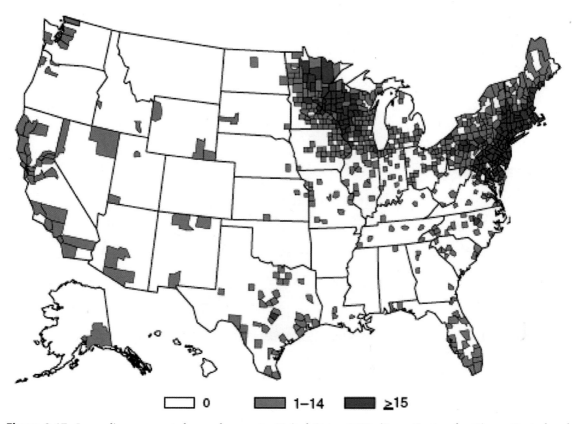

Figure 2-17. Lyme disease, reported cases by county, United States, 2005. (From Centers for Disease Control and Prevention: Summary of notifiable diseases, United States, 2005. MMWR 54[53]:2–92, 2007.)

accounted for 94% of the cases. The distribution of the disease closely parallels that of the deer tick vector.

A dramatic example of spread of disease is seen with West Nile virus (WNV) in the United States.[7] WNV was first isolated and identified in 1937 in the West Nile region of Uganda, and for many years, it was found only in the Eastern hemisphere. The basic cycle of the disease is bird-mosquito-bird. Mosquitoes become infected when they bite infected birds. When mosquitoes that bite both birds and humans become infected, they pose a threat to people. Most human infections are subclinical, but approximately 1 of 150 infections in recent years has resulted in meningitis or encephalitis. The risk of neurologic disease is significantly increased in people older than 50 years of age. Other symptoms include fever, nausea and vomiting, rash, headache, and muscle weakness. The case-fatality can be as high as 14%. Advancing age is a major risk factor for death from WNV, with one study reporting death nine times as frequently in older compared with younger patients. Treatment is supportive, and prevention is largely addressed through mosquito control and the use of insect repellents. Tracking the distribution of the disease depends 'on surveillance for human cases, and on monitoring birds and animals for the disease and deaths from the disease.

WNV was first identified in New York City in 1999. Figure 2-18 shows the rapid spread of WNV across the United States from 1999 to 2002. In 2002, human cases were reported from 619 counties in 37 states and the District of Columbia. Of the 3,389 cases of WNV-associated disease reported, 2,354 patients (69%) had West Nile meningoencephalitis. Looking at data from the 2002 outbreak of WNV meningoencephalitis in Figure 2-19, we see that the epidemic peaked in August, with the peak occurring 1 week earlier in the south (gray bars) than in the north (blue bars). Nine percent of people who developed West Nile meningoencephalitis died. Figure 2-20 shows the picture for 2006 and the number of cases reported by state. Much remains to be learned about this disease to facilitate treatment, prevention, and control.

OUTBREAK INVESTIGATION

The characteristics just discussed are the central issues in virtually all outbreak investigations. The steps for investigating an outbreak follow this general pattern (Table 2-4).

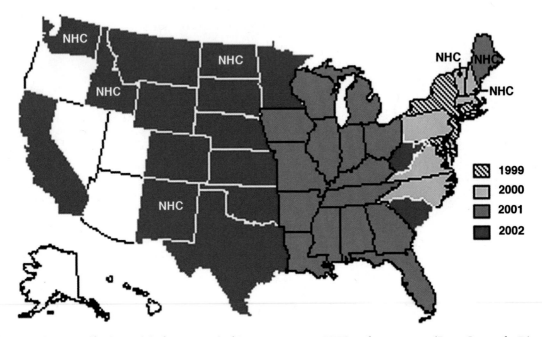

Figure 2-18. West Nile virus activity by state, United States, 1999–2002. NHC, no human cases. (From Centers for Disease Control and Prevention: Provisional surveillance summary of the West Nile Virus epidemic, United States, January–November, 2002. MMWR 51[50]:1129–1133, 2002.)

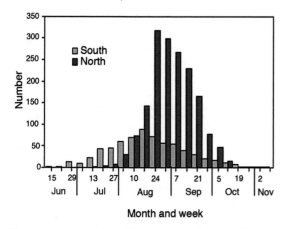

Figure 2-19. Number of human West Nile meningoencephalitis cases, by location and week and month of illness onset, United States, June–November 2002. (From Centers for Disease Control and Prevention: Provisional surveillance summary of the West Nile Virus epidemic, United States, January–November, 2002. MMWR 51[50]:1129–1133, 2002.)

Cross-Tabulation

When confronted with several possible causal agents as is often the case in a food-borne disease outbreak, a very helpful method for determining which of the possible agents is likely to be the cause is called *cross-tabulation*. This is illustrated by an outbreak of foodborne streptococcal disease in a Florida jail reported some years ago by the CDC.[8]

In August 1974, an outbreak of group A β-hemolytic streptococcal pharyngitis affected 325 of 690 inmates. On a questionnaire administered to 185 randomly selected inmates, 47% reported a sore throat between August 16 and August 22. Based on a second questionnaire, food-specific attack rates for items that were served to randomly selected inmates showed a significant association between two food items and the risk of developing a sore throat: beverage and egg salad served at lunch on August 16 (Table 2-5).

In Table 2-5, for each of the suspected exposures (beverage and egg salad), the attack rate was calculated for those who ate or drank the item (were exposed) and those who did not eat or drink the item (were not exposed). For both the beverage and the egg salad, attack rates are clearly higher among those who ate or drank the item than among those who did not. However, this table does not permit us to determine whether the beverage or the egg salad accounted for the outbreak.

In order to answer this question, we use the technique of cross-tabulation. In Table 2-6, we again examine the attack rates in those who ate egg salad

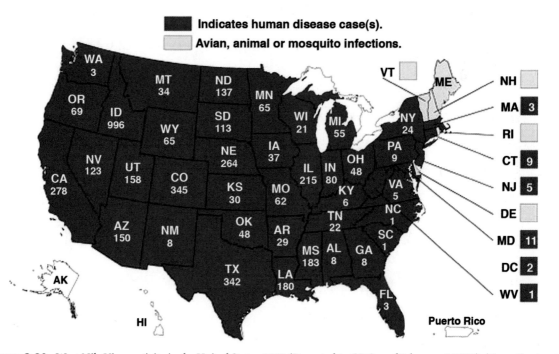

Figure 2-20. West Nile Virus activity in the United States, 2006 (Reported to CDC as of February 6, 2007). (From Centers for Disease Control and Prevention: West Nile Virus: Statistics, Surveillance and Control. www.cdc.gov/ncidod/dvbid/westnile/Mapsactivity/surv&control06Maps.htm.)

TABLE 2-4. Steps in Investigating an Acute Outbreak

Investigating an acute outbreak may be primarily deductive (i.e., reasoning from premises or propositions proved previously) or inductive (i.e., reasoning from particular facts to a general conclusion), or it may be a combination of both.

Important considerations in investigating an acute outbreak of infectious diseases include determining that an outbreak has in fact occurred and defining the extent of the population at risk, determining the measure of spread and reservoir, and characterizing the agent.

Steps commonly used are listed below, but depending on the outbreak, the exact order may differ.

1. *Define the outbreak and validate the existence of an outbreak*
   a. Define the "numerator" (cases)
      (1) Clinical features: is the disease known?
      (2) What are its serologic or cultural aspects?
      (3) Are the causes partially understood?
   b. Define the "denominator": What is the population at risk of developing disease?
   c. Determine whether the observed number of cases clearly exceeds the expected number
   d. Calculate the attack rates
2. *Examine the distribution of cases by the following:*
   a. Time ⎫ Look for time–place interactions
   b. Place ⎭
3. *Look for combinations (interactions) of relevant variables*
4. *Develop hypotheses based on the following:*
   a. Existing knowledge (if any) of the disease
   b. Analogy to diseases of known etiology
   c. Findings from investigation of the outbreak
5. *Test hypotheses*
   a. Further analyze existing data (case-control studies)
   b. Refine hypotheses and collect additional data that may be needed
6. *Recommend control measures*
   a. Control of current outbreak
   b. Prevention of future similar outbreaks
7. *Prepare a written report of the investigation and the findings*
8. *Communicate findings to those involved in policy development and implementation and to the public*

TABLE 2-5. Food-Specific Attack Rates for Items Consumed August 16, 1974, Dade County Jail, Miami

	ATE			DID NOT EAT			
Item Consumed	Sick	Total	% Sick (Attack Rate)	Sick	Total	% Sick (Attack Rate)	P
Beverage	179	264	67.8	22	50	44.0	<.010
Egg salad sandwiches	176	226	77.9	27	73	37.0	<.001

From Centers for Disease Control and Prevention: Outbreak of foodborne streptococcal disease. MMWR 23:365, 1974.

TABLE 2-6. Cross-Table Analysis for Egg Salad and Beverage Consumed August 16, 1974, Dade County Jail, Miami

	ATE EGG SALAD				DID NOT EAT EGG SALAD			
	Sick	Well	Total	% Sick (Attack Rate)	Sick	Well	Total	% Sick (Attack Rate)
Drank beverage	152	49	201	75.6	19	53	72	26.4
Did not drink beverage	12	3	15	80.0	7	21	28	25.0

From Centers for Disease Control and Prevention: Outbreak of foodborne streptococcal disease. MMWR 23:365, 1974.

compared with those who did not, but this time we do so separately for those who drank the beverage and for those who did not.

Looking at the data by columns, we see that both among those who ate egg salad and among those who did not, drinking the beverage did not increase the incidence of streptococcal illness (75.6% vs. 80% and 26.4% vs. 25%, respectively). However, looking at the data in the table horizontally, we see that eating the egg salad significantly increased the attack rate of the illness, both in those who drank the beverage (75.6% vs. 26.4%) and in those who did not (80% vs. 25%). Thus, the egg salad is clearly implicated.

This example demonstrates the use of cross-tabulation in a food-borne outbreak of an infectious disease, but the method has broad applicability to any condition in which multiple etiologic factors are suspected. It is discussed further in Chapter 15.

CONCLUSION

This chapter reviewed some basic concepts that underlie the epidemiologic approach to acute communicable diseases. Many of these concepts apply equally well to nonacute diseases that at this time do not appear to be infectious in origin. Moreover, for an increasing number of chronic diseases originally thought to be noninfectious, infection seems to play some role. Thus, hepatitis B infection is a major cause of primary liver cancer. Papillomaviruses have been implicated in cervical cancer, and Epstein-Barr virus has been implicated in Hodgkin disease. The boundary between the epidemiology of infectious and noninfectious diseases has blurred in many areas. In addition, even for diseases that are not infectious in origin, the patterns of spread share many of the same dynamics, and the methodologic issues in studying them are similar. Many of these issues are discussed in detail in Section II.

REFERENCES

1. Kipling R: Just-So Stories: The Elephant's Child, 1902. Reprinted by Everyman's Library Children's Classics. New York, Alfred A Knopf, 1992, p 79.
2. Mims CA: The Pathogenesis of Infectious Disease, 3rd ed. London, Academic Press, 1987.
3. Bell ML, Davis DL: Reassessment of the lethal London Fog of 1952: Novel indicators of acute and chronic consequences of acute exposure to air pollution. Environ Health Perspect 109(Suppl 3):389–394, 2001.
4. Centers for Disease Control and Prevention: Outbreaks of gastroenteritis associated with noroviruses on cruise ships, United States, 2002. MMWR 51:1112–1115, 2002.
5. Panum PL: Observations Made During the Epidemic of Measles on the Faroe Islands in the Year 1846. New York, Delta Omega Society, Distributed by the American Public Health Association, 1940.
6. Frank PF, Stollerman GH, Miller LF: Protection of a military population from rheumatic fever. JAMA 193:775, 1965.
7. Petersen LR, Marfin AA: West Nile virus: A primer for the clinician. Ann Intern Med 137:173–179, 2002.
8. Outbreak of foodborne streptococcal disease. MMWR 23:365, 1974.

REVIEW QUESTIONS FOR CHAPTER 2

1. *Endemic* means that a disease
   a. Occurs clearly in excess of normal expectancy
   b. Is habitually present in human populations
   c. Affects a large number of countries simultaneously
   d. Exhibits a seasonal pattern
   e. Is prevalent among animals

Questions 2 and 3 are based on the information given below:

The first table shows the total number of persons who ate each of two specified food items that were possibly infective with group A streptococci. The second table (p. 36) shows the number of sick persons (with acute sore throat) who ate each of the various specified combinations of the food items.

Total Number of Persons Who Ate Each Specified Combination of Food Items		
	Ate Tuna	**Did Not Eat Tuna**
Ate egg salad	75	100
Did not eat egg salad	200	50

Total Number of Persons Who Ate Each Specified Combination of Food Items and Who Later Became Sick (with Acute Sore Throats)		
	Ate Tuna	**Did Not Eat Tuna**
Ate egg salad	60	75
Did not eat egg salad	70	15

2. What is the sore throat attack rate in persons who ate both egg salad and tuna?
   a. 60/75
   b. 70/200
   c. 60/135
   d. 60/275
   e. None of the above

3. According to the results shown in the preceding tables, which of the following food items (or combination of food items) is most likely to be infective?
   a. Tuna only
   b. Egg salad only
   c. Neither tuna nor egg salad
   d. Both tuna and egg salad
   e. Cannot be calculated from the data given

4. In the study of an outbreak of an infectious disease, plotting an epidemic curve is useful because:
   a. It helps to determine what type of outbreak (e.g., single-source, person-to-person) has occurred
   b. It shows whether herd immunity has occurred
   c. It helps to determine the median incubation period
   d. *a* and *c*
   e. *a, b,* and *c*

5. Which of the following is characteristic of a single-exposure, common-vehicle outbreak?
   a. Frequent secondary cases
   b. Increasing severity with increasing age
   c. Explosive
   d. Cases include both people who have been exposed and those who were not exposed
   e. All of the above

Chapter 3

Measuring the Occurrence of Disease: I. Morbidity

We owe all the great advances in knowledge to those who endeavor to find out how much there is of anything.
—James Maxwell, physicist (1831–1879)

If you can measure that of which you speak, and can express it by a number, you know something of your subject, but if you cannot measure it, your knowledge is meager and unsatisfactory.
—William Thomson, Lord Kelvin, engineer, mathematician, and physicist (1824–1907)

In Chapter 2, we discussed how diseases are transmitted. It is clear from that discussion that in order to examine the transmission of disease in human populations, we need to be able to measure the frequency of both disease occurrence and deaths from the disease. In this chapter, we will therefore discuss how we use rates to express the extent of morbidity resulting from a disease, and in the next chapter (see Chapter 4), we will turn to expressing the extent of mortality in quantitative terms.

Let us begin this discussion by considering the development and course of a disease in an individual over a period of time.

Figure 3-1A shows the progression of disease in a population as reflected by the levels of illness and medical care. The outside rectangle represents the total population, and the smaller rectangles represent progressively smaller subsets, from sick to hospitalized patients. As a person becomes ill, he moves from the outside rectangle to the progressively smaller rectangles in the diagram as shown by the curved arrows. As seen in Figure 3-1B, deaths occur in all of these rectangles as shown by the small straight arrows, but the death rate is proportionately greater in groups with more severe illness.

Figure 3-2A shows the timeline for the development of a disease in an individual. An individual is healthy (i.e., without disease), and at some point, biologic onset of a disease occurs. The person is often unaware of the point in time when the disease begins. Later, symptoms develop and lead the patient to seek medical care. In certain situations, hospitalization may be required, either for diagnosis or for treatment, or for both. In any case, at some point a diagnosis is made and treatment is initiated. One of several outcomes can then result: cure, control of the disease, disability, or death.

What sources of data can be used to obtain information about the person's illness? For the period of the illness that necessitates hospitalization, medical and hospital records are useful (Fig. 3-2B). If hospitalization is not required, physicians' records may be the best source. If we want information about the illness even before medical care was sought, we may have to obtain this information from the patient, using a questionnaire or an interview. Not shown in this figure are the records of health insurers, which at times can provide very useful information.

The source of data from which cases are identified clearly influences the rates that we calculate for expressing the frequency of disease. For example, hospital records will not include data about patients who obtained care only in physicians' offices. Consequently, when we see rates for the frequency of occurrence of a certain disease, we must identify the sources of the cases and determine how the cases were identified. When we interpret the rates and compare them to rates reported in other populations and at other times, we must take into consideration the characteristics of the sources from which the data were obtained.

Occurrence of disease can be measured using rates or proportions. *Rates* tell us how fast the disease is occurring in a population; *proportions* tell us what

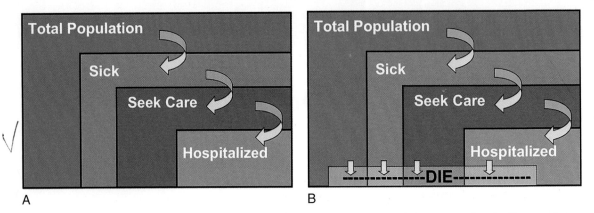

Figure 3-1. A, The population: Progression from health to varying degrees of disease severity. **B**, The population: progression from health to varying degrees of disease severity and the occurrence of deaths in each group. (Adapted from White KL, Williams TF, Greenberg BG: The ecology of medical care. N Engl J Med 265:885–892, 1961.)

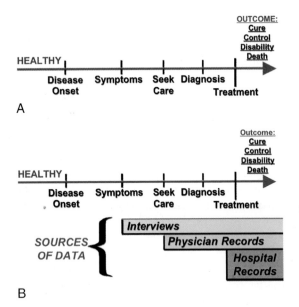

Figure 3-2. A, The natural history of disease. **B**, The natural history of disease and some sources of data relating to each interval.

fraction of the population is affected. Let us turn to how we use rates and proportions for expressing the extent of disease in a community or other population. In this chapter we discuss measures of illness or morbidity; measures of mortality are discussed in Chapter 4.

MEASURES OF MORBIDITY

Incidence Rate

The incidence rate of a disease is defined as the number of new cases of a disease that occur during

a specified period of time in a population at risk for developing the disease.

Incidence rate per 1,000 =

$$\frac{\substack{\text{No. of new cases of a disease occurring}\\ \text{in the population during}\\ \text{a specified period of time}}}{\substack{\text{No. of persons who are at risk of}\\ \text{developing the disease during}\\ \text{that period of time}}} \times 1,000$$

In this rate, the result has been multiplied by 1,000 so that we can express the incidence per 1,000 persons. The choice of 1,000 is completely arbitrary—we could have used 10,000, 1 million, or any other figure.

The critical element in defining incidence rate is *NEW* cases of disease. Incidence rate is a measure of events—the disease is identified in a person who develops the disease and did not have the disease previously. Because the incidence rate is a measure of events (i.e., transition from a nondiseased to a diseased state), the incidence rate is a measure of risk. This risk can be looked at in any population group, such as a particular age group, males or females, an occupational group, or a group that has been exposed to a certain environmental agent, such as radiation or a chemical toxin.

The denominator of an incidence rate represents the number of people who are at risk for developing the disease. For an incidence rate to be meaningful, any individual who is included in the denominator must have the potential to become part of the group that is counted in the numerator. Thus, if we are calculating incidence of uterine cancer, the denominator must include only women, because men would not have the potential to become part of the group that is counted by the numerator, that is, men are not at risk for developing uterine cancer. Although this point seems obvious, it is not always so clear, and we shall return to this issue later in the discussion.

Another important issue regarding the denominator is the issue of time. Incidence measures can use two types of denominators: people at risk who are observed throughout a defined time period; or, when all people are not observed for the full time period, person-time (or units of time when each person is observed). Let us consider each of these approaches.

People at Risk Who Are Observed throughout a Defined Time Period

In the first type of denominator for incidence rate, we specify a period of time, and we must know that all of the individuals in the group represented by the denominator have been followed up for *that entire period*. The choice of time period is arbitrary: We could calculate incidence in 1 week, incidence in 1 month, incidence rate in 1 year, incidence rate in 5 years, and so on. The important point is that whatever time period is used in the calculation must be clearly specified, and all individuals included in the calculation must have been observed (at risk) for the entire period. The incidence rate calculated using a period of time during which all of the individuals in the population are considered to be at risk for the outcome is also called *cumulative incidence*, which is a measure of risk.

When All People Are Not Observed for the Full Time Period, Person-Time, or Units of Time When Each Person Is Observed

Often, however, every individual in the denominator has not been followed for the full time specified for a variety of reasons, including loss to follow-up or death from a cause other than that being studied. When different individuals are observed for different lengths of time, we calculate an incidence rate (also called an incidence density), in which the denominator consists of the sum of the units of time that each individual was at risk and was observed. This is called person-time and is often expressed in terms of person-months or person-years of observation.

Let us consider person-years: One person at risk who is observed for one year = one person-year. One person at risk observed for 5 years = 5 person-years. But 5 people at risk, each of whom is observed for only 1 year, also = 5 person-years.

Let us assume we have a 5-year study and 5 people have been observed for the entire period (as indicated by the arrow for each in Fig. 3-3). In each of

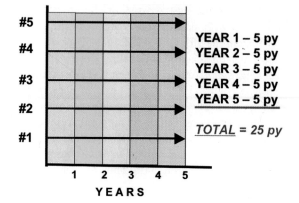

Figure 3-3. When all the people in the population being studied are observed for the entire period: Person-years of observation.

the 5 years of the study, all 5 participants are observed, so that we have 5 person-years (py) of observation in each of the 5 years, for a total of 25 person-years of observation in the entire study.

Now let us consider the situation where all 5 people at risk are not observed for the entire 5 years of the study but are observed for different lengths of time (Fig. 3-4A). In this diagram, the two arrows represent 2 people who were observed for all 5 years. The timelines for the 3 other people end with a red "x" which indicates the point at which the observation of each individual ended, either because the event of interest occurred, or the person was lost to follow-up, or other problems.

How do we calculate the total number of person-years observed in this study? Let us look at the first year of the study (Fig. 3-4B). All 5 people were observed during the first year, so we have 5 person-years of observation in the first year (Fig. 3-4C).

Now look at the second year of the study (Fig. 3-4D). Note that participant #2 was only observed for the first year, so that in the second year we have only 4 participants who contributed 4 person-years to the study (Fig. 3-4E).

Looking at the third year of the study, we see that participant #3 was only observed for the first 2 years of the study (Fig. 3-4F). Therefore, only 3 participants were observed in the third year generating 3 person-years of observation during the third year (Fig. 3-4G). These participants were also all observed for the fourth year of the study (Fig. 3-4H) and they again contributed 3 person-years of observation during the fourth year of the study (Fig. 3-4I).

Finally, let us look at the fifth year of the study (Fig. 3-4J). We see that participant #5 was only observed for the first 4 years of the study. As a result, only 2 participants remained and were observed in the fifth year of the study. They contributed 2 person-years of observation during the fifth year (Fig. 3-4K). As seen in Figure 3-4L, we therefore had 5 + 4 + 3 + 3 + 2 person-years of observation during the entire 5-year study, yielding a total of 17 person-years of observation. (This compares with 25 person-years of observation if all 5 participants had been observed throughout the entire 5 years of the study, as seen in Figure 3-3.) Thus, *if people at risk*

are observed for different periods of time, the incidence rate is:

Incidence rate per 1,000 =

$$\frac{\begin{array}{c}\text{Number of NEW cases of a disease}\\ \text{occurring in a population during a}\\ \text{specified period of time}\end{array}}{\begin{array}{c}\text{Total person-time (The sum of the}\\ \text{time periods of observation of each}\\ \text{person who has been observed for all or}\\ \text{part of the entire time period)}\end{array}} \times 1{,}000$$

Person-time is discussed further in Chapter 6.

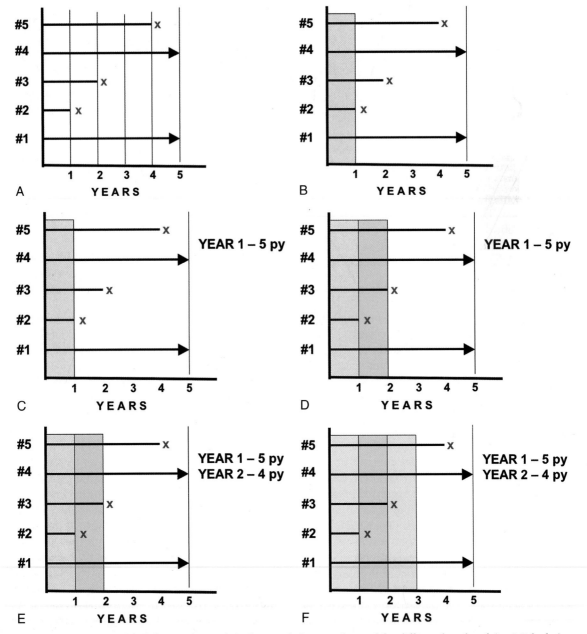

Figure 3-4. A–L, But what if the people at risk in the population are observed for different lengths of time? Calculation of person-time as person-years observed.

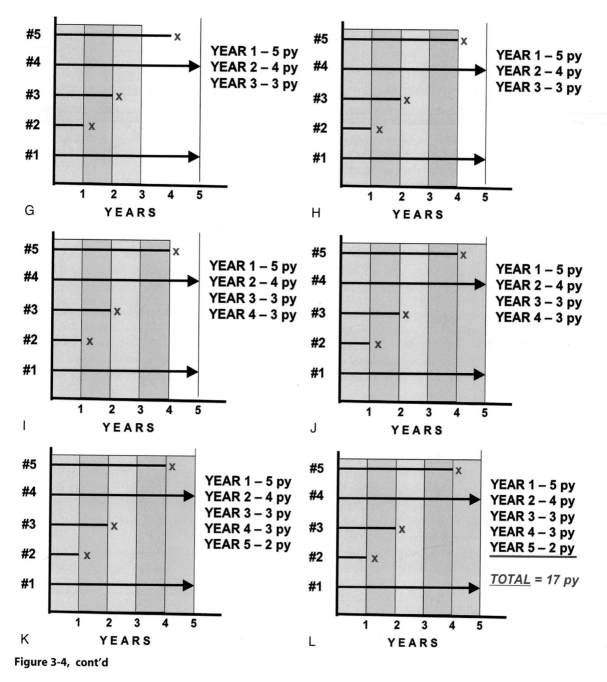

Figure 3-4, cont'd

Attack Rate

Occasionally, time may be specified implicitly rather than explicitly. For example, in Chapter 2 we discussed investigating a food-borne disease outbreak, in which we speak of an *attack rate* which is defined as the number of people exposed to a suspect food who became ill, divided by the number of people who were exposed to that food. The attack rate does not explicitly specify the time interval because

for many food-borne disease outbreaks we know that most cases occur within a few hours or a few days after the exposure. Consequently, cases that develop months later are not considered part of the same outbreak. However, in many situations, current knowledge of the biology and natural history of the disease does not clearly define a time frame, and so the time must be stated explicitly. A further consideration is that attack rate is not truly a rate but a proportion. A food-borne attack rate actually tells us the *proportion* of all people who ate a certain food who became ill.

Identifying New Cases in Order to Calculate Incidence

Practically speaking, when we wish to calculate incidence, how do we identify all new cases in a population during a specified time period? In certain situations it may be possible to monitor an entire population over time with tests that can detect newly developed cases of a disease. However, often this is not possible and instead a population is identified and screened for the disease at baseline (prevalent cases defined in the next section) (Fig. 3-5). Those who do not have the disease are followed for the specified time, for example, 1 year, and they are then rescreened (Fig. 3-6). Any cases that are identified clearly developed during the 1-year period since those followed were free of disease at the beginning of the year. Thus these cases are new or incident cases and serve as the numerator for the incidence rate.

Although in most situations it is necessary to express incidence by specifying a denominator, at times, the number of cases alone may be informative. For example, Figure 3-7 shows the number of expected and observed cases of tuberculosis reported in the United States from 1980 to 1992. (Note that the vertical axis is a logarithmic scale.) The smallest number of cases ever reported in a year in the United States (since reporting began) was in 1985. The number had declined from 1980 to 1985, and the figure shows the number of cases that would have been expected had the decline continued. However, the decline suddenly stopped in 1985. From 1985 to

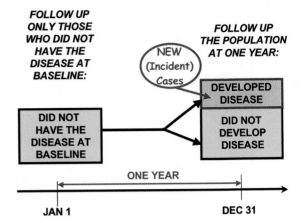

Figure 3-6. Identifying newly detected cases of a disease. Step 2: Follow-up and rescreening at 1 year to identify cases that developed during the year.

1992, the reported number of cases of tuberculosis increased by 20%; had the projected decline continued, approximately 51,700 fewer cases would have been expected. Much of the increase in tuberculosis seen here was associated with simultaneous infection with human immunodeficiency virus (HIV). However, even before acquired immunodeficiency syndrome (AIDS) and HIV were recognized as major public health problems, tuberculosis had remained a serious, but often neglected, problem, particularly in certain urban areas of the United States. We see that even a graph that plots numbers of cases without a denominator can be very helpful when there is no reason to suspect a significant change in the denominator during a given time period.

In general, however, our goal in calculating incidence is to be able to do so with the information

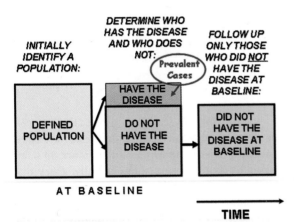

Figure 3-5. Identifying newly detected cases of a disease. Step 1: Screening for prevalent cases at baseline.

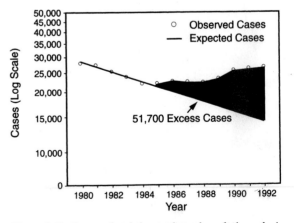

Figure 3-7. Expected and observed number of tuberculosis cases, United States, 1980–1992. (From Centers for Disease Control and Prevention: MMWR 42:696, 1993.)

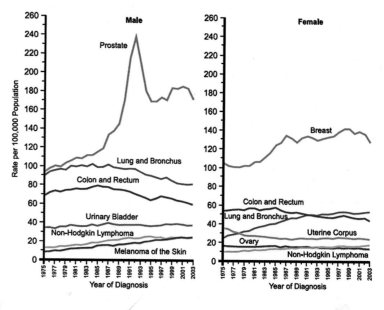

Figure 3-8. Annual age-adjusted cancer incidence rates among males and females for selected cancers, United States, 1975–2003. (From Surveillance, Epidemiology, and End Result [SEER] Program. Delay-Adjusted Incidence Database: "SEER incidence delay-adjusted rates, 9 registries, 1975–2003." National Cancer Institute, released April 2006.)

needed for both the numerator and denominator so that valid comparisons can be made. Figure 3-8 presents data on cancer incidence in the United States for males (left) and females (right) from 1975 to 2003. As seen here, lung cancer incidence has been declining in men and leveling off in women. After marked rises in incidence for many years, prostate cancer in men has been declining since 2001. Breast cancer in women is also characterized by recent declines. After having been level for a number of years, colon and rectal cancers have been decreasing in both men and women.

Prevalence

Prevalence is defined as the number of affected persons present in the population at a specific time divided by the number of persons in the population at that time, that is, what proportion of the population is affected by the disease at that time?

Prevalence per $1,000 =$

$$\frac{\text{No. of cases of a disease present in the population at a specified time}}{\text{No. of persons in the population at that specified time}} \times 1,000$$

For example, if we are interested in knowing the prevalence of arthritis in a certain community on a certain date, we might visit every household in that community and, using interviews or physical examinations, determine how many people have arthritis on that day. This number becomes the numerator for prevalence. The denominator is the population in the community on that date.

What is the difference between *incidence* and *prevalence*? Prevalence can be viewed as a snapshot or a slice through the population at a point in time at which we determine who has the disease and who does not. But in so doing, we are not determining when the disease developed. Some individuals may have developed arthritis yesterday, some last week, some last year, and some 10 or 20 years ago. Thus, when we survey a community to estimate the prevalence of a disease, we generally do not take into account the duration of the disease. Consequently, the numerator of prevalence includes a mix of people with different durations of disease, and as a result we do not have a measure of risk. If we wish to measure risk, we must use incidence, because in contrast to prevalence, it includes only new cases or events and a specified time period during which those events occurred.

In the medical and public health literature, the word prevalence is often used in two ways:

Point prevalence. Prevalence of the disease at a certain point in time—this is the use of the term *prevalence* that we have just discussed.

Period prevalence. How many people have had the disease at any point during a certain time period? The time period referred to may be arbitrarily selected, such as a month, a single calendar year, or a 5-year period. Some people may have developed the disease during that period, and others may have had the disease before and died or been cured during that period. The important point is that every person represented by the

TABLE 3-1.	Examples of Point and Period Prevalence and Cumulative Incidence in Interview Studies of Asthma	
Interview Question		**Type of Measure**
"Do you currently have asthma?"		Point prevalence
"Have you had asthma during the last [n] years?"		Period prevalence
"Have you ever had asthma?"		Cumulative incidence

numerator had the disease at some time during the period specified.

The two types of prevalence, as well as cumulative incidence, are illustrated in Table 3-1 using questions regarding asthma.

Returning to point prevalence, practically speaking, it is virtually impossible to survey an entire city on a single day. Therefore, although conceptually we are thinking in terms of a single point in time, in reality, the survey would take much longer. When we see the word prevalence used without any modifier, it generally refers to point prevalence, and for the rest of this chapter, we will use prevalence to mean point prevalence.

Let us consider incidence and prevalence. Figure 3-9 shows five cases of a disease in a community in 2008. The first case of the disease occurred in 2007, and the patient died in 2008.

The second case developed in 2008 and continued into 2009. The third case was a person who became ill in 2008 and was cured in 2008. The fourth case occurred in 2007, and the patient was cured in 2008. The fifth case occurred in 2007 and continued through 2008 and into 2009.

For this example, we will consider only the cases (numerators) and will ignore the denominators. In this example, what is the numerator for incidence in 2008? We know that incidence counts only new cases, and because two of the five cases developed in 2008, the numerator for incidence in 2008 is 2.

What about the numerator for point prevalence in 2008? This depends on when we do our prevalence survey (Fig. 3-10). If we do the survey in May, the numerator will be 5. If we do the survey in July, the numerator will also be 4. If we do the survey in September, however, the numerator will be 3, and if we do it in December, the numerator will be 2. Thus, the prevalence will depend on the point during the year at which the survey is performed.

Figures 3-11 through 3-14 show the relationship between incidence and prevalence. A flask is shown that represents a community (Fig. 3-11), and the beads in the flask represent the prevalent cases of a disease in the community. How can we add to or increase the prevalence? As seen in Figure 3-12, we can do so through incidence—by the addition of new cases. What if we could drain beads from the flask and lower the prevalence? How might this be accomplished? As seen in Figure 3-13, it could occur through either death or cure. Clearly, these two outcomes represent a major difference to a patient, but with regard to prevalence, cure and death have the same effect: they reduce the number of diseased persons in the population and thus lower prevalence. Therefore, what exists is the dynamic situation shown in Figure 3-14. A continual addition of new cases (incidence) is increasing the prevalence, while death and/or cure is decreasing the prevalence.

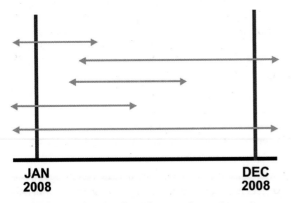

Figure 3-9. Example of incidence and prevalence: I.

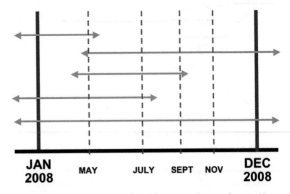

Figure 3-10. Example of incidence and prevalence: II.

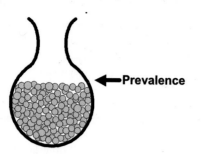

Figure 3-11. Relationship between incidence and prevalence: I.

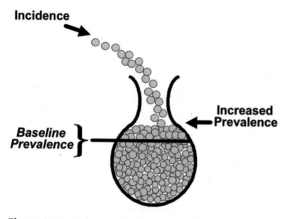

Figure 3-12. Relationship between incidence and prevalence: II.

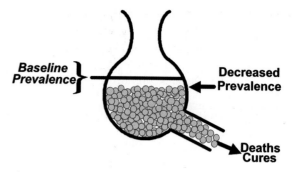

Figure 3-13. Relationship between incidence and prevalence: III.

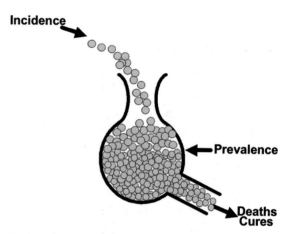

Figure 3-14. Relationship between incidence and prevalence: IV.

This effect of lowering prevalence through either death or cure underlies an important issue in public health and clinical medicine. For example, when insulin first became available, what happened to the prevalence of diabetes? The prevalence increased because diabetes was not cured, but was only controlled. Many patients with diabetes who formerly would have died now survived; therefore, the prevalence increased. This seeming paradox is often the case with public health programs: a new measure is introduced that enhances survival or detects the disease in more people, and the net effect is an apparent increase in prevalence. It may be difficult to convince some people that a program is successful if the prevalence of the disease that is the target of the program actually increases. However, this clearly occurs when death is prevented and the disease is not cured.

We have said that prevalence is not a measure of risk. If so, why bother to estimate prevalence? Prevalence is an important and useful measure of the burden of disease in a community. For example, how many people in the community have arthritis? This information might help us to determine, for example, how many clinics are needed, what types of rehabilitation services are needed, and how many and what types of health professionals are needed. Prevalence is therefore valuable for planning health services. When we use prevalence, we also want to make future projections and anticipate the changes that are likely to take place in the disease burden. However, if we want to look at the cause, or etiology, of disease, we must explore the relationship between an exposure and the risk of disease, and to do this, we need incidence rates.

Nevertheless, prevalence data may at times be very useful—they may be suggestive if not confirmatory in studies of the etiology of certain diseases. For example, asthma is a disease of children for which incidence is difficult to measure because the exact time of the beginning of the disease (its inception) is often hard both to define and to ascertain. For this reason, when we are interested in time trends and geographic distribution of asthma, prevalence is the measure most frequently used. Information on prevalence of asthma is often obtained from self-reports such as interviews or questionnaires. Figure 3-15 shows current asthma prevalence in children up to 17 years of age, by state in the United States for 2001–2005. Current asthma prevalence was based on two questions: "Has a doctor or other health professional ever told you that (child's name) had asthma?" and "Does (child's name) still have asthma?" Overall, prevalence was highest in the northeastern states. The explanation for this observation is not entirely clear. Although adverse climate and polluted air may be implicated, other factors may also play a role in the high asthma prevalence in the northeast, such as more complete ascertainment of cases in the medical care system and higher asthma prevalence in Puerto Rican children who are concentrated in this region.

Another example of the value of prevalence data is seen in Figure 3-16. One of the most significant and challenging public health problems today in the United States and in other developed countries is the dramatically increasing prevalence of obesity. Obesity is associated with significant morbidity and mortality and is a risk factor for diseases such as hypertension, type 2 diabetes, coronary disease, and stroke. In this figure, prevalence of obesity by state is shown for each of four years: 1990, 1995, 2000, and 2005. The trend over time is grim: In 1990, all reporting states reported obesity prevalence data below 15%. By 2005, all but four states had prevalence estimates above 20%; 17 states reported a prevalence of obesity equal to or greater than 25% and three of these states (Louisiana, Mississippi, and West Virginia) reported obesity prevalence over 30%.

One limitation of these data is that they are based on self-reported heights and weights given by respondents by telephone. In this study, the participants were classified according to their body mass index (BMI), which is defined as a person's weight in kilograms divided by the square of the person's height in meters (BMI = weight (kg)/height^2[meters^2]). A BMI of 25 or greater is categorized as overweight and a BMI of 30 or greater as obese. Survey respondents,

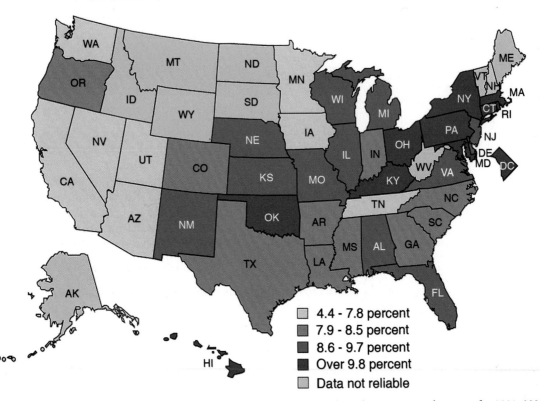

Figure 3-15. Current asthma prevalence in children ages 0 to 17 years of age, by state, annual average for 2001–2005. (From Akinbami LJ: The state of childhood asthma, United States, 1980–2005. Advance data from vital and health statistics, No. 381, Hyattsville, MD, National Center for Health Statistics, 2006.)

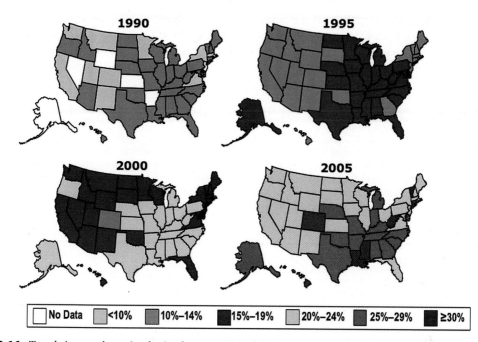

Figure 3-16. Trends in prevalence in obesity, by state, United States, 1990, 1995, 2000, and 2005 based on self reported height and weight. Obesity was defined by BMI (body mass index ≥ 30, or ~30 lbs overweight for a 5′ 4″ person). (Adapted from Centers for Disease Control and Prevention, based in part on data from the Behavioral Risk Factor Surveillance System, www.cdc.gov/nccdphp/dnpa/obesity/trend/maps/index.htm. Also see CDC: State-specific prevalence of obesity among adults, United States, 2005. MMWR 55[36]:985–988, 2006.)

especially in telephone surveys, have been reported to understate their weights, overstate their heights, or both, leading to an artificially low BMI. The result is an underestimation of obesity prevalence based on BMI so that the true prevalence of obesity by state is probably higher than that seen in Figure 3-16. Given the trends described above and seen in Figure 3-16, an enormous public health effort and commitment will be needed to reverse this steadily worsening public health problem.

Table 3-2 lists some possible sources of morbidity statistics. Each has its limitations, primarily because most of these sources are not established for research purposes. Therefore, they may be characterized by incomplete or ambiguous data and, at times, may only refer to a highly selected population that may not be representative of the population to which we would like to generalize the findings.

Problems with Incidence and Prevalence Measurements
Problems with Numerators

The first problem is defining who has the disease. One example demonstrates this problem; rheumatoid arthritis (RA) is often a difficult disease to diagnose, and when such a diagnostic difficulty arises, expert groups are often convened to develop sets of

TABLE 3-2. Some Sources of Morbidity Statistics

1. Disease reporting—communicable diseases, cancer registries
2. Data accumulated as a by-product of insurance and prepaid medical care plans
   a. Group health and accident insurance
   b. Prepaid medical care plans
   c. State disability insurance plans
   d. Life insurance companies
   e. Hospital insurance plans—Blue Cross
   f. Railroad Retirement Board
3. Tax-financed public assistance and medical care plans
   a. Public assistance, aid to the blind, aid to the disabled
   b. State or federal medical care plans
   c. Armed Forces
   d. Veterans Administration
4. Hospitals and clinics
5. Absenteeism records—industry and schools
6. Pre-employment and periodic physical examinations in industry and schools
7. Case-finding programs
8. Records of military personnel
9. Morbidity surveys on population samples (e.g., National Health Survey, National Cancer Surveys)

TABLE 3-3. Criteria for Rheumatoid Arthritis*

American Rheumatism Association Criteria	New York Criteria
1. Morning stiffness 2. Joint tenderness or pain on motion 3. Soft-tissue swelling of one joint 4. Soft-tissue swelling of a second joint (within 3 months) 5. Soft-tissue swelling of symmetrical joints (excludes distal interphalangeal joint) 6. Subcutaneous nodules 7. X-ray changes 8. Serum positive for rheumatoid factors	1. History of episode of three painful limb joints[†] 2. Swelling, limitation, subluxation, or ankylosis of three limb joints (must include a hand, wrist, or foot and symmetry of one joint pair and must exclude distal interphalangeal joints, fifth proximal interphalangeal joints, first metatarsophalangeal joints, and hips) 3. X-ray changes (erosions) 4. Serum positive for rheumatoid factors

*A score of three or four points indicates "probable" rheumatoid arthritis; five or more points indicates "definite" rheumatoid arthritis.
[†]Count each joint group (e.g., proximal interphalangeal joints) as one joint, scoring each side separately.
From O'Sullivan JB, Cathcart ES: The prevalence of rheumatoid arthritis. Ann Intern Med 76:573, 1972.

diagnostic criteria. Two sets of diagnostic criteria for RA are those of the New York Rheumatism Association and the American Rheumatism Association (Table 3-3). Figure 3-17 shows the results of a survey conducted in Sudbury, Massachusetts, using both sets of criteria. We see that the prevalence estimate is significantly affected by the set of criteria that is used.

More recently, a cohort of 1,879 men and women 65 years of age and older who were enrolled in the Canadian Study of Health and Aging (CSHA) were examined.[1] The proportion who were given a diagnosis of dementia using six commonly used classification systems was calculated. Depending on which diagnostic system was used, the proportion of subjects with dementia varied from 3.1% to 29.1% (Fig. 3-18). This marked variation in prevalence estimates has important potential implications both for research and for the provision of appropriate health services. When the results of any morbidity survey are reported, it is essential that the precise definition used for a case be clearly specified. The decision as to which definition to use is not always simple. Often it will largely depend on the specific purpose for which a given survey has been conducted.

The next issue relating to numerators is that of ascertaining which persons should be included in the numerator. How do we find the cases? We can use regularly available data, or as discussed earlier in this chapter, we can conduct a study specifically designed to gather data for estimating incidence or prevalence. In many such studies the data are obtained from interviews, and some of the problems with interview data are listed in Table 3-4.

Problems with Denominators

Many factors affect the denominators used. Selective undercounting of certain groups in the population may occur. For example, young men in ethnic minority groups have been missed in many counts of the population. Frequently, we wish to determine whether a certain group has a higher-than-expected risk of disease so that appropriate preventive measures can be directed to that group. We are therefore interested

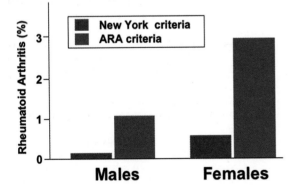

Figure 3-17. Percent of population with a diagnosis of rheumatoid arthritis. New York criteria versus American Rheumatism Association (ARA) criteria, Sudbury, Massachusetts, 1964. (Adapted from O'Sullivan JB, Cathcart ES: The prevalence of rheumatoid arthritis: Follow-up evaluation of the effect of criteria on rates in Sudbury, Massachusetts. Ann Intern Med 76:573–577, 1972.)

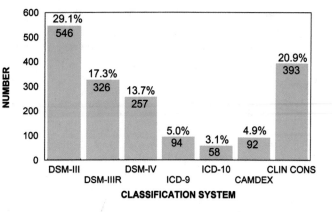

Figure 3-18. Number of people with and prevalence (%) of dementia in the Canadian Study of Health and Aging cohort (*n* = 1,879) as diagnosed by different classification systems. The various abbreviations refer to commonly used diagnostic manuals for medical conditions. (Data from Erkinjuntti T, Østbye T, Steenhuis R, Hachinski V: The effect of different diagnostic criteria on the prevalence of dementia. N Engl J Med 337:1667–1774, 1997.)

in the rates of disease for different ethnic groups rather than just for the population as a whole. However, there are different ways to classify people by ethnic group, such as by language, country of origin, heritage, or parental ethnic group. When different studies use different definitions, comparison of the results is difficult. What is most important in any study is that the working definition be clearly stated so that the reader can judge whether the results are truly comparable.

In an earlier section we stated that for a rate to make sense, everyone in the group represented by the denominator must have the potential to enter the group that is represented by the numerator. The issue is not a simple one. For example, hysterectomy is one of the most commonly performed surgical procedures in the United States. This raises a question about uterine cancer rates. For if we include women who have had hysterectomies in the denominator, clearly they are not at risk for developing uterine

cancer. Figure 3-19 shows uterine cancer incidence rates from Alameda County, California; both uncorrected rates and rates corrected for hysterectomy are presented. We see that the corrected rates are higher. Why? Because in the corrected rates women who have had hysterectomies are removed from the denominator. Consequently, the denominator gets smaller and the rate increases. However, in this case the trend over time is not significantly changed whether we use corrected or uncorrected rates.

Problems with Hospital Data

Data from hospital records are one of the most important sources of information in epidemiologic studies. However, Table 3-5 lists some of the problems that arise in using hospital data for research purposes. First, hospital admissions are selective. They may be selective on the basis of personal characteristics, severity of disease, associated medical conditions, and admissions policies that vary from

---

TABLE 3-4. Possible Sources of Error in Interview Surveys

1. The respondent may have the disease, but may have no symptoms and may not be aware of the disease.
2. The respondent may have the disease and may have had symptoms, but may not have had medical attention and therefore may not know the name of the disease.
3. The respondent may have the disease and may have had medical attention, but the diagnosis may not have been made or conveyed to the person or the person may have misunderstood.
4. The respondent may not accurately recall an episode of illness or events and exposures related to the illness.
5. The respondent may be involved in litigation about the illness and may choose not to respond or may alter his or her response.
6. The respondent may provide the information, but the interviewer may not record it or may record it incorrectly.
7. The interviewer may not ask the question he or she is supposed to ask or may ask it incorrectly.
8. The interviewer may be biased by knowing the hypothesis being tested and may probe more intensively in one group of respondents than in another.
9. Problems of selection bias may occur, possibly including significant nonresponse rates.

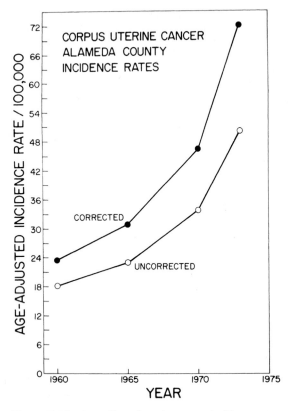

Figure 3-19. Age-adjusted uterine cancer incidence rates, corrected and uncorrected by hysterectomy status, Alameda County, California. (From Lyon JL, Gardner JW: The rising frequency of hysterectomy: Its effect on uterine cancer rates. Am J Epidemiol 105:439–443, 1977.)

hospital to hospital. Second, hospital records are not designed for research but rather for patient care. Records may be incomplete, illegible, or missing. The diagnostic quality of the records of hospitals, physicians, and clinical services may differ. Thus, if we

---

TABLE 3-5. **Some Limitations of Hospital Data**

1. Hospital admissions are selective in relation to
   a. Personal characteristics
   b. Severity of disease
   c. Associated conditions
   d. Admission policies
2. Hospital records are not designed for research. They may be:
   a. Incomplete, illegible, or missing
   b. Variable in diagnostic quality
3. Population(s) at risk (denominator) is (are) generally not defined

---

TABLE 3-6. **Some Notes Dictated by Physicians for Inclusion in Patients' Medical Records**

"Patient has two teenage children, but no other abnormalities."
"On the second day the knee was better and on the third day it had completely disappeared."
"Patient was alert and unresponsive."
"When she fainted, her eyes rolled around the room."
"Rectal examination revealed a normal size thyroid."
"By the time he was admitted, his rapid heart had stopped, and he was feeling better."

---

want to aggregate patients from different hospitals, we may have problems of comparability. Third, if we wish to calculate rates, we have a problem defining denominators, because most hospitals do not have defined catchment areas—that is, areas that require that all persons in those areas who are hospitalized be admitted to a particular hospital, and that none from outside the catchment area be admitted to that hospital.

On a lighter note, Table 3-6 lists some notes that were dictated by physicians for inclusion in their patients' medical records.

Relationship Between Incidence and Prevalence

We have said that incidence is a measure of risk and that prevalence is not, because it does not take into account the duration of the disease. However, there is an important relationship between incidence and prevalence: in a steady-state situation, in which the rates are not changing and in-migration equals out-migration, the following equation applies:

$$\text{Prevalence} = \text{Incidence} \times \text{Duration of disease}$$

This is demonstrated in the following hypothetical example. Using chest x-rays, 2,000 persons are screened for tuberculosis: 1,000 are upper-income individuals from Hitown and 1,000 are lower-income individuals from Lotown (Table 3-7). X-ray findings are positive in 100 of the Hitown people and in 60 of the Lotown people. Can we therefore conclude that the risk of tuberculosis is higher in Hitown people than in Lotown people? Clearly, we cannot, for what we are measuring with a chest x-ray is the point prevalence of disease—we do not know how long any of the people with positive x-rays have had their

TABLE 3-7. **Hypothetical Example of Chest X-Ray Screening: I. Populations Screened and Numbers with Positive X-Rays**	
Screened Population	**Number with Positive X-Ray**
1,000 Hitown	100
1,000 Lotown	60

TABLE 3-8. **Hypothetical Example of Chest X-Ray Screening: II. Point Prevalence**		
Screened Population	**Number with Positive X-Ray**	**Point Prevalence per 1,000 Population**
1,000 Hitown	100	100
1,000 Lotown	60	60

disease (Table 3-8). We could in fact consider a hypothetical scenario that might explain the higher prevalence in Hitown people that is not related to any higher risk in Hitown people (Table 3-9). We have said that prevalence = incidence × duration. Let us assume that Lotown people have a much higher risk (incidence) of tuberculosis than Hitown people— 20 cases/year in Lotown people compared with 4 cases/year in Hitown people. But for a variety of reasons, such as poorer access to medical care and poor nutritional status, Lotown people survive with their disease, on average, for only 3 years, whereas Hitown people survive, on average, for 25 years. In this example, therefore, there is a higher prevalence in Hitown people than in Lotown people not because

the risk of disease is higher in Hitown people, but because affected Hitown people survive longer; the prevalence of disease (incidence × duration) is therefore higher in Hitown people than in Lotown people.

Figure 3-20 shows the percent of all births in New Zealand that were extramarital from 1962 to 1979. Much concern was expressed because of the apparent steady rise in extramarital births. However, as seen in Figure 3-21, there had really been no increase in the rate of extramarital births; there had been a decline in total births that was largely accounted for by a decline in births to married women. The extramarital births, as a result, accounted for a greater percent of all births, even though the rate of extramarital births had not increased.

This example makes two points: First, a proportion is not a rate, and we shall return to this point in our discussion of mortality. Second, birth can be viewed as an event, just as the development of disease is an event, and appropriate rates can be computed. In discussing babies born with malformations, some people prefer to speak of the prevalence of malformations at birth rather than the incidence of malformations at birth, because the malformation was clearly present (but often unrecognized), even before birth. Furthermore, because some proportion of cases with malformations abort before birth, any estimate of the frequency of malformations at birth is probably a significant underestimate of the true incidence. Hence, the term "prevalence at birth" is often used.

Figure 3-22 shows breast cancer incidence rates in women by age and the distribution of breast cancer in women by age. Ignore the bar graph for the moment, and consider the line curve. The pattern is one of continually increasing incidence with age, with a change in the slope of the curve between ages 45 and 50 years. This change is observed in many countries. It has been suggested that something happens near the time of menopause, and that

TABLE 3-9. **Hypothetical Example of Chest X-Ray Screening: III. Prevalence, Incidence, and Duration**			
Screened Population	**Point Prevalence per 1,000**	**Incidence (Occurrences/yr)**	**Duration (yrs)**
Hitown	100	4	25
Lotown	60	20	3
	Prevalence = Incidence × Duration		

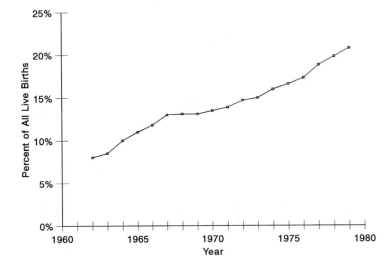

Figure 3-20. Percentage of births that were extramarital in New Zealand, 1962–1979, based on data from the Department of Statistics. (Adapted from Benfield J, Kjellstrom T: New Zealand ex-nuptial births and domestic purposes benefits in a different perspective. N Z Nurs J 74:28–31, 1981.)

premenopausal and postmenopausal breast cancer may be different diseases. Note that, even in old age, the incidence or risk of breast cancer continues to rise.

Now let us look at the histogram—the distribution of breast cancer cases by age. If the incidence is increasing so dramatically with age, why are only fewer than 5% of the cases occurring in the oldest age group of women? The answer is that there are very few women alive in that age group, so that even though they have the highest risk of breast cancer, the group is so small that they contribute only a small proportion of the total number of breast cancer cases seen at all ages. The fact that so few cases of breast cancer are seen in this age group has contributed to a false public impression that the risk of breast cancer is low in this group and that mammography is therefore not important in the elderly. This is a serious

misperception. The need to change public thinking on this issue is a major public health challenge. We therefore see the importance of recognizing the distinction between the distribution of disease or the proportion of cases, and the incidence rate or risk of the disease.

Spot Maps

One approach to examining geographic or spatial differences in incidence is to plot the cases on a map, with each point representing a case. Figure 3-23 shows a spot map for rheumatic fever in Baltimore from 1960 to 1964. Rheumatic fever was frequently observed in this period, and as seen on the map, the cases clustered in the inner city, consistent with the often-made observation that rheumatic fever is strongly associated with low socioeconomic status. It

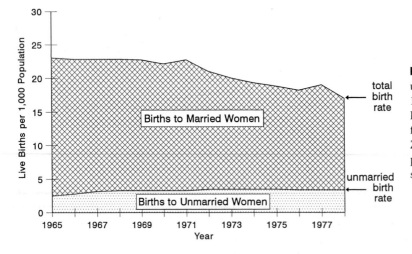

Figure 3-21. Births to married and unmarried women in New Zealand, 1965–1978, based on data from the Department of Statistics. (Adapted from Benfield J, Kjellstrom T: New Zealand ex-nuptial births and domestic purposes benefits in a different perspective. N Z Nurs J 74:28–31, 1981.)

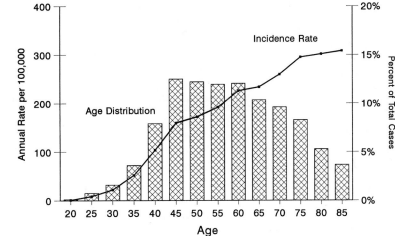

Figure 3-22. Breast cancer incidence rates in white women and distribution of cases by age. (Data from Cutler SJ, Young Jr JL: Third National Cancer Survey: Incidence data. Natl Cancer Inst Monogr 41, 1975.)

should be pointed out that such a clustering seen on a spot map does not demonstrate a higher incidence in the area of the cluster. For if the population also clusters in this area, the rate in the area of the cluster may be no different from that elsewhere in the city. However, a spot map may offer important clues to disease etiology that can then be pursued with more rigorous studies.

Figure 3-24 shows such a spot map for 1977 to 1981. By this time, rheumatic fever had become

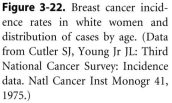

Figure 3-23. Spot map of residence distribution of patients with rheumatic fever, ages 5 to 19 years, hospitalized for first attacks, Baltimore, 1960–1964. (Reprinted from Gordis L, Lilienfeld A, Rodriguez R: Studies in the epidemiology and preventability of rheumatic fever: I. Demographic factors and the incidence of acute attacks. J Chronic Dis 21:645–654, 1969. Copyright 1969, with kind permission from Elsevier Science Ltd.)

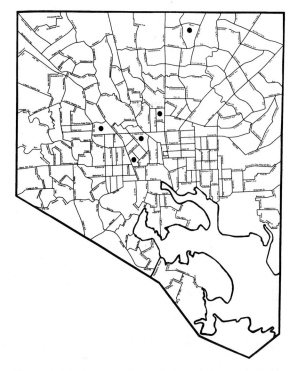

Figure 3-24. Spot map for patients with rheumatic fever, ages 5 to 19 years, hospitalized for first attacks in Baltimore, 1977–1981. (Reproduced with permission. From Gordis L: The virtual disappearance of rheumatic fever in the United States: Lessons in the rise and fall of disease. Circulation 72:1155–1162, 1985. Copyright 1985, American Heart Association.)

almost nonexistent in Baltimore, although there had not been any concerted program specifically aimed at eradicating the disease.

Clustering, the phenomenon shown by spot maps, is often reported. Residents of a community may report apparent clusters of cancer deaths in children. For example, in Woburn, Massachusetts, a cluster of cases of childhood leukemia was reported and attributed to industrial contamination.[2] This cluster led to action in the courts.[3] However, many apparent clusters are due only to chance, and an important epidemiologic challenge is to investigate such groups of cases and rule out an environmental etiology for what appears to be a greater-than-expected proximity of cases of a disease in time and space.

SURVEILLANCE

Surveillance is a fundamental role of public health. Surveillance may be carried out to monitor changes in disease frequency or to monitor changes in prevalence of risk factors. Much of our information about morbidity and mortality from disease comes from programs of systematic disease surveillance. Surveillance is most frequently conducted for infectious diseases, but in recent years it has become increasingly important in monitoring changes in other types of conditions such as congenital malformations, cancer, asthma, and chemical poisoning and for injuries and illnesses after natural disasters such as hurricanes or earthquakes. Surveillance is also used to monitor for completeness of vaccination coverage and protection of a population and for the prevalence of drug-resistant organisms such as drug-resistant tuberculosis and malaria.

The Centers for Disease Control and Prevention (CDC) defined epidemiologic surveillance as the "ongoing systematic collection, analysis, and interpretation of health data essential to the planning, implementation, and evaluation of public health practice closely integrated with the timely dissemination of these data to those who need to know."[4]

An important element of this as well as other definitions of surveillance is providing decision-makers with guidance for developing and implementing the best strategies for programs for disease prevention and control. In order to enable countries or states to develop coordinated public health approaches, mechanisms for information exchange are essential. Consequently, standardized definitions of disease and diagnostic criteria are needed that can be applied in different countries. The forms used for reporting must also be standardized.

Surveillance can be of two types: *passive* or *active*. *Passive surveillance* denotes surveillance in which either available data on reportable diseases are used or reporting is mandated or requested with the responsibility for the reporting often falling on the health care provider or district health officer. The completeness and quality of the data reported thus largely depend on this individual and his or her staff who often take on this role without additional funds or resources. As a result, under-reporting and lack of completeness of reporting are likely; to minimize this problem, the reporting instruments must be simple and brief. When passive reporting is used, local outbreaks may be missed because the relatively small number of cases often ascertained (numerator for incidence) become diluted within a large denominator of a total population of a province or country. However, a passive reporting system is relatively inexpensive and relatively easy to develop initially. In addition, as many countries have systems of passive reporting for a number of reportable diseases that are generally infectious, passive reporting allows for inter-national comparisons that can identify areas that urgently need assistance in confirming new cases and in providing appropriate interventions for control and treatment.

Active surveillance denotes a system in which project staff make periodic field visits to health care facilities such as clinics and hospitals to identify new cases of a disease or diseases or deaths from the disease that have occurred (case finding). Active surveillance may involve interviewing physicians and patients, reviewing medical records, and, in developing countries and rural areas, surveying villages and towns to detect cases either on a routine basis or after an index case has been reported. Reporting is generally more accurate when it is active than when it is passive because active surveillance is conducted by individuals who have been specifically employed to carry out this responsibility. This is in contrast to passive surveillance in which those expected to report new cases are often overburdened by their primary responsibilities of providing health care and administering health services. For them, filing reports is an additional burden that they often view as peripheral to their main responsibilities. With active reporting, local outbreaks are generally identified. However, active reporting is more expensive to maintain than passive reporting and is often more difficult to develop initially.

Surveillance in developing countries may present additional problems. For example, areas in need of surveillance may be difficult to reach, and it may be difficult to maintain communication from such areas to the central authorities who must make policy decisions and allocate the resources necessary for follow-up and disease control and prevention. Furthermore, definitions of disease used in developed countries may at times be inappropriate or unusable in developing countries because of a lack of the laboratory and other sophisticated resources needed for full diagnostic evaluation of suspected cases. The result may therefore be an under-reporting of observed clinical cases.

Surveillance is of great value in many settings. Figure 3-25 shows trends in incidence of thyroid cancer in children in Belarus, Ukraine, and Russia from 1986 to 1994 following the explosion in the Chernobyl reactor.[5] The highest incidence rates were found in the most contaminated areas—Gomel in southern Belarus and parts of northern Ukraine. However, a problem in interpreting such data is the possibility that the observed increase could be due to intensive screening following the accident, which could have identified tumors that would otherwise not have been detected. However, there is now general agreement that the observed increase in thyroid cancer in children and adolescents in areas exposed to Chernobyl fallout is, in fact, real.

Surveillance may also be carried out to assess changes in levels of environmental risk factors for disease. For example, monitoring levels of particulate air pollution or atmospheric radiation may be conducted, particularly after an accident has been reported, such as the explosion at the Three Mile Island nuclear reactor. Such monitoring may give an early warning about a possible rise in rates of disease associated with that environmental agent. Thus, surveillance for changes in either disease rates or levels of environmental risk factors may serve as a measure of the severity of the accident and point to possible directions for reducing such hazards in the future.

QUALITY OF LIFE

Most diseases have a major impact on the afflicted individual above and beyond mortality. Diseases that may not be lethal may be associated with considerable suffering and disability. For this reason, it is also important to consider the impact of a disease as measured by its effect on a person's quality of life, even though such measures are not, in fact, measures of disease occurrence. For example, it is possible to examine the extent to which patients with arthritis are compromised by the illness in carrying out activities of daily living. Although considerable controversy exists about which quality-of-life measures are most appropriate and valid, there is general agreement that such measures can be reasonably used to plan short-term treatment programs for groups of patients. Such patients can be evaluated over a period of months to determine the effects of the treatment on their self-reported quality of life. Quality-of-life measures have also been used for establishing priorities for scarce health care resources. Although prioritization of health care resources is often primarily based on mortality data, quality of life must also be taken into account for this purpose because many

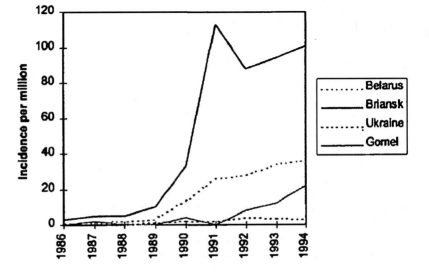

Figure 3-25. Trends of incidence of childhood thyroid cancer in Belarus, Ukraine and Russia, 1986–1994. (From Bard D, Verger P, Hubert P: Chernobyl, 10 years after: Health consequences. Epidemiol Rev 19:187–204, 1997.)

diseases are chronic and non-life-threatening. Patients may place different weights on different quality-of-life measures depending on differences in personality, cultural background, education, and moral and ethical values. As a result, measuring quality of life and developing valid indices that are useful for obtaining comparative data in different patients and in different populations remain major challenges.

CONCLUSION

In this chapter, we have reviewed different approaches to measuring morbidity. We have seen that a rate involves specification of a numerator, a denominator of people at risk, and time—either explicitly or implicitly. We have discussed the importance of these morbidity indices in surveillance for human disease, which is one of the major uses of epidemiology. In the next chapter, we will turn to measures of mortality. In Chapter 5, we discuss how we use screening and diagnostic tests to identify individuals who are ill (who are included in the numerator) and distinguish them from those in the population who are not ill. In Chapter 18, we discuss how epidemiology is used for evaluating screening programs.

--- **REFERENCES** ---

1. Erkinjuntti T, Østbye T, Steenhuis R, Hachinski V: The effect of different diagnostic criteria on the prevalence of dementia. N Engl J Med 337:1667, 1997.
2. Lagakos SW, Wessen BJ, Zelen M: An analysis of contaminated well water and health effects in Woburn, Massachusetts. J Am Stat Assoc 81:583, 1986.
3. Harr J: A Civil Action. New York, Random House, 1995.
4. Thacker S, Berkelman RL: Public health surveillance in the United States. Epidemiol Rev 10:164, 1988.
5. Bard D, Verger P, Hubert P: Chernobyl, 10 years after: Health consequences. Epidemiol Rev 19:187, 1997.

REVIEW QUESTIONS FOR CHAPTER 3

1. At an initial examination in Oxford, Mass., migraine headache was found in 5 of 1,000 men aged 30 to 35 years and in 10 of 1,000 women aged 30 to 35 years. The inference that women have a two times greater risk of developing migraine headache than do men in this age group is:
   a. correct
   b. incorrect, because a ratio has been used to compare male and female rates
   c. incorrect, because of failure to recognize the effect of age in the two groups
   d. incorrect, because no data for a comparison or control group are given
   e. incorrect, because of failure to distinguish between incidence and prevalence

2. A prevalence survey conducted from January 1 through December 31, 2003, identified 1,000 cases of schizophrenia in a city of 2 million persons. The incidence rate of schizophrenia in this population is 5/100,000 persons each year. What percent of the 1,000 cases were newly diagnosed in 2003?

3. Which of the following is an advantage of active surveillance?
   a. requires less project staff
   b. is relatively inexpensive to employ
   c. more accurate due to reduced reporting burden for health care providers
   d. relies on different disease definitions to account for all cases
   e. reporting systems can be developed quickly

4. What would be the effect on age-specific incidence rates if women with hysterectomies were excluded from the denominator of calculations, assuming that there are some women in each age group who have had hysterectomies?
   a. the rates would remain the same
   b. the rates would tend to decrease
   c. the rates would tend to increase
   d. the rates would increase in older groups and decrease in younger groups
   e. it cannot be determined whether the rates would increase or decrease

5. A survey was conducted among the nonhospitalized adult population of the United States during 1988 through 1991. The results from this survey are shown below.

Age Group	Persons with Hypertension (%)
18–29 years	4
30–39 years	10
40–49 years	22
50–59 years	43
60–69 years	54
70 and older	64

The researchers stated that there was an age-related increase in the risk of hypertension in this population. You conclude that the researchers' interpretation:

a. is correct

b. is incorrect because it was not based on rates

c. is incorrect because incidence rates do not describe risk

d. is incorrect because prevalence is used

e. is incorrect because the calculations are not age-adjusted

Questions 6 and 7 use the information below:

Population of the city of Atlantis on March 30, 2003 = 183,000

No. of new active cases of TB occurring between January 1 and June 30, 2003 = 26

No. of active TB cases according to the city register on June 30, 2003 = 264

6. The incidence rate of active cases of TB for the 6-month period was:

   a. 7 per 100,000 population

   b. 14 per 100,000 population

   c. 26 per 100,000 population

   d. 28 per 100,000 population

   e. 130 per 100,000 population

7. The prevalence rate of active TB as of June 30, 2003, was:

   a. 14 per 100,000 population

   b. 130 per 100,000 population

   c. 144 per 100,000 population

   d. 264 per 100,000 population

   e. none of the above

Chapter 4

Measuring the Occurrence of Disease: II. Mortality

You do not die from being born, nor from having lived, nor from old age. You die from something. . . . There is no such thing as a natural death: Nothing that happens to a man is ever natural, since his presence calls the world into question. All men must die: but for every man his death is an accident and, even if he knows it and consents to it, an unjustifiable violation.

—Simone de Beauvoir, writing of her mother's death, in *A Very Easy Death*[1]

Mortality is of great interest for several reasons. First of all, death is the ultimate experience that every human being is destined to have. Death is clearly of tremendous importance to each person including questions of when and how death will occur and whether there is any way to delay it. From the standpoint of studying disease occurrence, expressing mortality in quantitative terms can pinpoint differences in the risk of dying from a disease between people in different geographic areas and subgroups in the population. Mortality rates can serve as measures of disease severity, and can help us to determine whether the treatment for a disease has become more effective over time. In addition, given the problem that often arises in identifying new cases of a disease, mortality rates may serve as surrogates for incidence rates when the disease being studied is a severe and lethal one. This chapter will address the quantitative expression of mortality and the uses of such measures in epidemiologic studies.

MEASURES OF MORTALITY

Figure 4-1 shows the number of cancer deaths up to the year 2000 in the United States. Clearly, the *number* of people dying from cancer is seen increasing significantly through the year 2000, but from this graph, we cannot say that the *risk* of dying from cancer is increasing, because the only data that we have in this graph are numbers of deaths (numerators); we do not have denominators (populations at risk). If, for example, the size of the U.S. population is also increasing at the same rate, the risk of dying from cancer does not change.

For this reason, if we wish to address the risk of dying, we must deal with rates. Figure 4-2 shows mortality rates for several types of cancer in men from 1930 to 2003. The most dramatic increase is in deaths from lung cancer. This increase is clearly of epidemic proportions and, tragically, lung cancer is a preventable cause of death. Fortunately, since the mid 1990s, lung cancer mortality has declined, paralleling earlier decreases in smoking among men. Other cancers are also of interest. Mortality from prostate cancer also peaked in the mid 1990s, and has declined since. Cancers of the colon and rectum have declined over many years. The rate of death from stomach cancer has declined dramatically since 1930, although the precise explanation is not known. It has been suggested that the decline may be the result of the increased availability of refrigeration, which decreased the need to smoke foods and thereby decreased human exposure to carcinogens produced in the smoking process. Another possible cause is improved hygiene, which may have reduced the incidence of *Helicobacter pylori* infections which have been implicated in the etiology (or cause) of stomach cancer.

Figure 4-3 shows a similar presentation for cancer mortality in women for the period 1930 to 2003. Breast cancer mortality remained at essentially the same level for many years but has declined since the early 1990s until 2003. It would be desirable to study changes in the incidence of breast cancer. Such a study is difficult, however, because with aggressive public education campaigns encouraging women to have mammograms and perform breast self-examination, many breast cancers may be detected

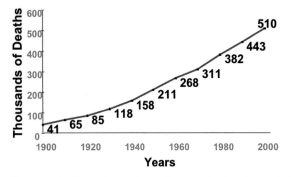

Figure 4-1. Trend in numbers of cancer deaths observed in the United States in the early and mid 20th century and forecast to the year 2000. (Data from the American Cancer Society.)

today that might have gone undetected years ago. Nevertheless, available evidence suggests that the true incidence of breast cancer in women may have increased for many years and decreased from 2001 to 2003.

Uterine cancer mortality has declined, perhaps because of earlier detection and diagnosis. Lung cancer mortality in women has increased, and lung cancer has exceeded breast cancer as a cause of death in women. Lung cancer is now the leading cause of cancer death in women. It is a tragedy that an almost completely preventable cause of cancer that is precipitated by a lifestyle habit, cigarette smoking, which has been voluntarily adopted by many women, is the main cause of cancer death in women in the United States.

We may be particularly interested in mortality relating to age. Figure 4-4 shows death rates from cancer and from heart disease for people younger than 85 and for those 85 or older. Cancer is the leading cause of death in men and women younger than 85 years, but above age 85, heart disease clearly exceeds cancer as a cause of death.

Figure 4-5 shows the causes of death worldwide for children younger than 5 years. Six causes accounted for 73% of the 10.6 million deaths each year: pneumonia, diarrhea, malaria, neonatal pneumonia or sepsis, preterm delivery, and asphyxia at birth. Over half of all child deaths under 5 years were accounted for by the four communicable disease categories.

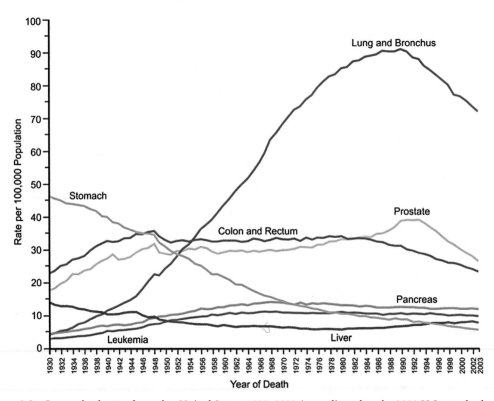

Figure 4-2. Cancer death rates for males, United States, 1930–2003 (age-adjusted to the 2000 U.S. standard population). (From Jemal A, Siegel R, Ward E, et al: Cancer statistics, 2007. CA Cancer J Clin 57:43–66, 2007.)

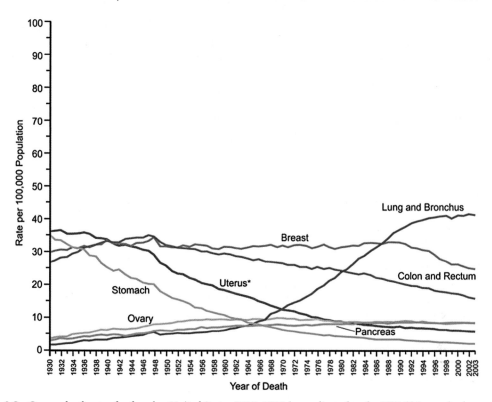

Figure 4-3. Cancer death rates for females, United States, 1930–2003 (age-adjusted to the 2000 U.S. standard population). *Uterine cancer rates are for uterine cervix and corpus combined. (From Jemal A, Siegel R, Ward E, et al: Cancer statistics, 2007. CA Cancer J Clin 57:43–66, 2007.)

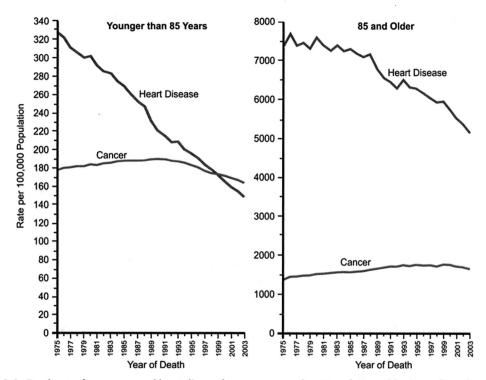

Figure 4-4. Death rates from cancer and heart disease for ages younger than 85 and 85 or older (age-adjusted to the 2000 U.S. standard population). (From Jemal A, Siegel R, Ward E, et al: Cancer statistics, 2007. CA Cancer J Clin 57:43–66, 2007. Based on data from U.S. Mortality Public Use Data Tapes, 1960 to 2003, National Center for Health Statistics, Centers for Disease Control and Prevention, 2006.)

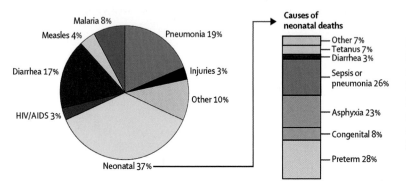

Figure 4-5. Major causes of death in children younger than age 5 years and in neonates (yearly average for 2000–2003). (From Bryce J, Boschi-Pinto C, Shibuya K, Black RE: WHO estimates of the causes of death in children. Lancet 365:1147–1152, 2005.)

Mortality Rates

How is mortality expressed in quantitative terms? Let us examine some types of mortality rates. The first is the annual death rate, or mortality rate, from all causes:

Annual mortality rate for all causes
(per 1,000 population) =

$$\frac{\text{Total no. of deaths from all causes in 1 year}}{\text{No. of persons in the population at midyear}} \times 1,000$$

Note that because the population changes over time, the number of persons in the population at midyear is generally used as an approximation.

The same principles mentioned in the discussion of morbidity apply to mortality: for a mortality rate to make sense, anyone in the group represented by the denominator must have the potential to enter the group represented by the numerator.

We may not always be interested in a rate for the entire population; perhaps we are interested only in a certain age group, in men or in women, or in one ethnic group. Thus, if we are interested in mortality in children younger than 10 years, we can calculate a rate specifically for that group:

Annual mortality rate from all causes
for children younger than 10 years of age
(per 1,000 population) =

$$\frac{\substack{\text{No. of deaths from all causes in one year} \\ \text{in children younger than 10 years of age}}}{\substack{\text{No. of children in the population} \\ \text{younger than 10 years of age at midyear}}} \times 1,000$$

Note that in putting a restriction, on age, for example, the same restriction must apply to *both* the numerator and the denominator, so that every person in the denominator group will be at risk for entering the numerator group. When a restriction is placed on a rate, it is called a *specific rate*. This, then, is an *age-specific mortality rate*.

We could also place a restriction on a rate by specifying a diagnosis, and thus limit the rate to deaths from a certain disease, that is, a *disease-specific* or a *cause-specific rate*. For example, if we are interested in mortality from lung cancer, we would calculate it in the following manner:

Annual mortality rate from lung cancer
(per 1,000 population) =

$$\frac{\text{No. of deaths from lung cancer in one year}}{\text{No. of persons in the population at midyear}} \times 1,000$$

We can also place restrictions on more than one characteristic simultaneously, for example, age and cause of death, as follows:

Annual mortality rate from leukemia
in children younger than 10 years of age
(per 1,000 population) =

$$\frac{\substack{\text{No. of deaths from leukemia in one year} \\ \text{in children younger than 10 years of age}}}{\substack{\text{No. of children in the population} \\ \text{younger than 10 years of age at midyear}}} \times 1,000$$

Time must also be specified in any mortality rate. Mortality can be calculated over 1 year, 5 years, or longer. The period selected is arbitrary, but it must be specified precisely.

Case-Fatality Rates

We must distinguish between a *mortality rate* and a *case-fatality rate*. A case-fatality rate is calculated as follows:

Case-fatality rate (percent) =

$$\frac{\substack{\text{No. of individuals dying during a} \\ \text{specified period of time after disease} \\ \text{onset or diagnosis}}}{\text{No. of individuals with the specified disease}} \times 100$$

In other words, what percentage of *people diagnosed as having a certain disease* die within a certain time after diagnosis? What is the difference between case-fatality rate and mortality rate? In the mortality rate, the denominator represents the entire population at risk of dying from the disease, including both those who have the disease and those who do not

---

TABLE 4-1. Comparison of Mortality Rate and Case-Fatality Rate

Assume a population of 100,000 people of whom 20 are sick with disease X, and in 1 year, 18 of the 20 die from disease X

The mortality rate in that year as a result of disease $X = \dfrac{18}{100,000} = 0.00018$, or 0.018%

The case-fatality rate as a result of $X = \dfrac{18}{20} = 0.9$, or 90%

---

have the disease (but who are at risk of developing the disease). In the case-fatality rate, however, the denominator is limited to those who already have the disease. Thus, case-fatality is a measure of the severity of the disease. It can also be used to measure any benefits of a new therapy: as therapy improves, the case-fatality rate would be expected to decline.

The numerator of a case-fatality rate should ideally be restricted to deaths *from that disease*. However, it is not always easy to distinguish between deaths from that disease and deaths from other causes. For example, an alcoholic person may die in a car accident; the death may or may not be related to alcohol intake.

Let us look at a hypothetical example to clarify the difference between mortality and case-fatality (Table 4-1).

Assume that in a population of 100,000 persons, 20 have disease X. In one year, 18 people die from that

disease. The mortality is very low (.018%) because the disease is rare; however, once a person has the disease, the chances of his or her dying are great (90%).

Proportionate Mortality

Another measure of mortality is proportionate mortality, which is not a rate. The proportionate mortality from cardiovascular disease in the United States in 1999 is defined as follows:

Proportionate mortality from cardiovascular diseases in the U.S. in 1999 (percent) =

$$\dfrac{\text{No. of deaths from cardiovascular diseases in the U.S. in 1999}}{\text{Total deaths in the U.S. in 1999}} \times 100$$

In other words, of all deaths in the United States, what *proportion* was caused by cardiovascular disease? Figure 4-6 shows proportionate mortality from heart

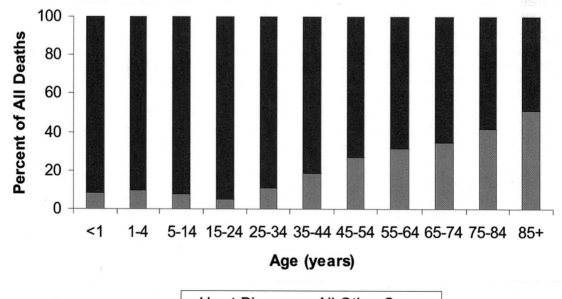

Figure 4-6. Deaths from heart disease as a percentage of deaths from all causes, by age group, United States, 2001. (From National Institutes of Health. National Heart, Lung, and Blood Institute. Morbidity and Mortality: 2004 Chart Book on Cardiovascular, Lung, and Blood Diseases. US Department of Health and Human Services, Washington, DC, 2004.)

TABLE 4-2. **Comparison of Mortality Rate and Proportionate Mortality: I. Deaths from Heart Disease in Two Communities**

	Community A	Community B
Mortality rate from all causes	30/1,000	15/1,000
Proportionate mortality from heart disease	10%	20%
Mortality rate from heart disease	3/1,000	3/1,000

disease by age group. In each age group, the full bar represents all deaths (100%), and deaths from heart disease are indicated by the blue portion. We see that the *proportion* of deaths from heart disease increases with age. However, this does not tell us that the *risk* of death from heart disease is also increasing. This is demonstrated in the following examples.

Table 4-2 shows all deaths and deaths from heart disease in two communities, A and B. All-cause mortality in community A is twice that in community B. When we look at proportionate mortality, we find that 10% of the deaths in community A and 20% of the deaths in community B are due to heart disease. Does this tell us that the risk of dying from heart disease is twice as high in community B as it is in A? The answer is no. For when the mortality rates from heart disease are calculated (10% of 30/1,000 and 20% of 15/1,000), we find that the mortality rates are identical.

If we observe a change in proportionate mortality from a certain disease over time, the change may be due not to changes in mortality from that disease, but to changes in the mortality of some other disease. Let us consider a hypothetical example: In Table 4-3, we see mortality rates from heart disease, cancer, and other causes in a population in an early period and a later period. First compare the mortality rates in the two time periods: Mortality from heart disease doubled over time (from 40/1,000 to 80/1,000), but mortality rates from cancer and from all other causes (20/1,000) did not change. However, if we now examine the proportionate mortality from each cause, we see that the proportionate mortality from cancer and from other causes has decreased in the population, but only because the proportionate mortality from heart disease has increased. Thus, if the proportion of one segment of the mortality "pie" increases, there will necessarily be a decrease in the proportion of some other segment (Fig. 4-7). Another view of this is seen in Figure 4-8.

As seen in the example in Table 4-4, if all-cause mortality rates differ, cause-specific mortality rates can differ significantly, even when the proportionate mortality is the same. Thus, these examples show that, although proportionate mortality can give us a quick look at the major causes of death, it cannot tell us the risk of dying from a disease. For that, we need a mortality rate.

Years of Potential Life Lost

In recent years, another mortality index, years of potential life lost (YPLL), has been increasingly used for setting health priorities. YPLL is a measure of premature mortality, or early death. YPLL recognizes

TABLE 4-3. **Hypothetical Example of Mortality Rates and Proportionate Mortality in Two Periods**

Cause of Death	EARLY PERIOD		LATER PERIOD	
	Mortality Rate	**Proportionate Mortality**	**Mortality Rate**	**Proportionate Mortality**
Heart disease	40/1,000	50%	80/1,000	66.7%
Cancer	20/1,000	25%	20/1,000	16.7%
All other causes	20/1,000	25%	20/1,000	16.7%
All deaths	80/1,000	100%	120/1,000	100%

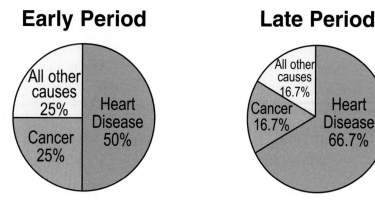

Figure 4-7. Hypothetical example of proportionate mortality: Changes in proportionate mortality from heart disease, cancer, and other causes from the early period to the late period.

that death occurring in the same person at a younger age clearly involves a greater loss of future productive years than death occurring at an older age. Two steps are involved in this calculation: In the first step, for each cause, each deceased person's age at death is subtracted from a predetermined age at death. In the United States, this predetermined "standard" age is usually 65 years. Thus, an infant dying at 1 year of age has lost 64 years of life (65 − 1), but a person dying at 50 years of age has lost 15 years of life (65 − 50). Thus, the younger the age at which death occurs, the more years of potential life are lost. In the second step, the "years of potential life lost" for each individual are then added together to yield the total YPLL for the specific cause of death. When looking at reports that use YPLL, it is important to note what assumptions the author has made, including what predetermined standard age has been selected.

Figure 4-9 shows the years of potential life lost in the United States before age 65 years in 2004. The top bar shows the total YPLL from all causes (100%), and the bars below show the individual YPLL from each leading cause of death, with the percentage of YPLL

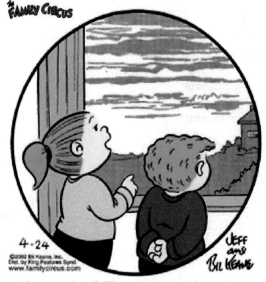

"Know what? The days get longer at the same time the nights get shorter."

Figure 4-8. Understanding proportionate mortality. (© Bill Keane, Inc. Reprinted with Special Permission of King Features Syndicate.)

TABLE 4-4. **Comparison of Mortality Rate and Proportionate Mortality: II. Deaths from Heart Disease in Two Communities**

	Community A	Community B
Mortality rate from all causes	20/1,000	10/1,000
Proportionate mortality from heart disease	30%	30%
Mortality rate from heart disease	6/1,000	3/1,000

Cause of Death	YPLL	Percent	
All Causes	11,612,630		100.0%
Unintentional Injury	2,219,044		19.1%
Malignant Neoplasms	1,877,690		16.2%
Heart Disease	1,413,158		12.2%
Perinatal Period	922,191		7.9%
Suicide	687,395		5.9%
Homicide	565,979		4.9%
Congenital Anomalies	486,853		4.2%
HIV	261,784		2.3%
Cerebrovascular	245,074		2.1%
Liver Disease	231,132		2.0%
All Others	2,702,330		25.2%

Figure 4-9. Years of potential life lost (YPLL) before age 65, all races, both sexes, all deaths, United States, 2004. (Adapted from Centers for Disease Control and Prevention. National Center for Injury Prevention and Control. Years of Potential Life Lost [YPLL] Reports, 1999–2004, webapp.cdc.gov/sasweb/ncipc/ypll10.html.)

from all causes for which it accounts. We see that the greatest single source of YPLL was unintentional injury, which in the same year, was the fifth leading cause of death by its mortality rate (see Fig. 1-2). The discrepancy between the ranking of death from unintentional injury by its YPLL and by its mortality rate results from the fact that injury is the leading cause of death up to age 34 years and, therefore, it accounts for a large proportion of years of potential life lost.

Figure 4-10 shows YPLL before age 65 years for children and adults younger than 20 years of age. We see that the YPLL from injuries exceeds the effect of YPLL from congenital malformations and prematurity combined. Thus, if we want to have an impact on YPLL in children and young adults, we should address the causes of injuries, half of which are related to motor vehicles.

Table 4-5 shows a ranking of causes of death in the United States for 1989 and 1990 by YPLL, together with cause-specific mortality rates. By cause-specific mortality, human immunodeficiency virus (HIV) infection ranked tenth, but by YPLL, it ranked sixth. This reflects the fact that a large proportion of HIV-related deaths occur in young persons.

YPLL can assist in three important public health functions: establishing research and resource priorities, surveillance of temporal trends in premature mortality, and evaluating the effectiveness of program interventions.[2]

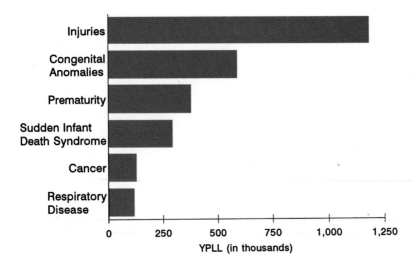

Figure 4-10. Years of potential life lost (YPLL) before age 65 years among children younger than 20 years from injuries and other diseases, United States, 1986. (Adapted from Centers for Disease Control and Prevention: Fatal injuries to children: United States, 1986. MMWR 39: 442–451, 1990.)

TABLE 4-5. Estimated Years of Potential Life Lost (YPLL) Before Age 65 Years and Mortality Rates per 100,000 Persons, by Cause of Death, United States, 1989 and 1990

Cause of Death (ICD-9 Codes)	YPLL for Persons Dying in 1989	YPLL for Persons Dying in 1990	Cause-Specific Crude Death Rate, 1990
All causes (total)	12,339,045	12,083,228	861.9
Unintentional injuries (E800–E949)	2,235,335	2,147,094	37.3
Malignant neoplasms (140–208)	1,832,039	1,839,900	201.7
Suicide/homicide (E950–E978)	1,402,524	1,520,780	22.5
Diseases of the heart (390–398, 402, 404–429)	1,411,399	1,349,027	289.0
Congenital anomalies (740–759)	660,346	644,651	5.3
Human immunodeficiency virus infection (042–044)	585,992	644,245	9.6
Prematurity (765, 769)	487,749	415,638	2.5
Sudden infant death syndrome (798)	363,393	347,713	2.2
Cerebrovascular disease (430–438)	237,898	244,366	57.9
Chronic liver disease and cirrhosis (571)	233,472	212,707	10.2
Pneumonia/influenza (480–487)	184,832	165,534	31.3
Diabetes mellitus (250)	145,501	143,250	19.5
Chronic obstructive pulmonary disease (490–496)	135,507	127,464	35.5

Data from Centers for Disease Control and Prevention: MMWR 41:314, 1992.

Why Look at Mortality?

Mortality is clearly an index of the severity of a disease from both clinical and public health standpoints, but mortality can also be used as an index of the risk of disease, as shown in Figures 4-2 and 4-3. However, when a disease is mild and not fatal, mortality is not a good index of incidence. A mortality rate is a good reflection of the incidence rate under two conditions: First, when the case-fatality rate is high (as in untreated rabies), and second, when the duration of disease (survival) is short. Under these conditions, mortality is a good measure of incidence, and thus a measure of the risk of disease. For example, cancer of the pancreas is a highly lethal disease: death generally occurs within a few months of diagnosis, and long-term survival is rare. Thus, unfortunately, mortality from pancreatic cancer is a good surrogate for incidence of the disease.

Figures 4-11 and 4-12 show mortality trends in the United States from 1982 to 2000 for the leading

Figure 4-11. Annual death rates (per 100,000 population) for the leading causes of death among men 25 to 44 years old, by year, 1987–2002. (For 1982 to 1986, estimates were made because an International Classification of Diseases [ICD]-9 code for HIV did not yet exist. For 1999–2000, deaths were classified according to ICD-10; for 1987–1998, ICD-10 rules were retroactively applied to deaths that were previously coded according to ICD-9 rules.) (Drawn from data prepared by Richard M. Selik, MD, Division of HIV/AIDS Prevention, Centers for Disease Control and Prevention, 2003. www.cdc.gov/hiv/graphics/mortalit.htm.)

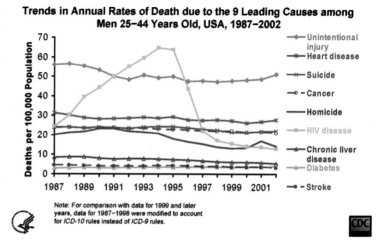

Trends in Annual Rates of Death due to the 9 Leading Causes among Men 25–44 Years Old, USA, 1987–2002

Note: For comparison with data for 1999 and later years, data for 1987–1998 were modified to account for ICD-10 rules instead of ICD-9 rules.

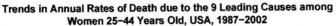

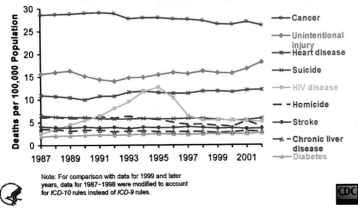

Trends in Annual Rates of Death due to the 9 Leading Causes among Women 25–44 Years Old, USA, 1987–2002

Note: For comparison with data for 1999 and later years, data for 1987–1998 were modified to account for *ICD-10* rules instead of *ICD-9* rules.

Figure 4-12. Annual death rates (per 100,000 population) for leading causes of death among women 25 to 44 years old, by year, 1987–2002. (See also Fig. 4-11.) (Drawn from data prepared by Richard M. Selik, MD, Division of HIV/AIDS Prevention, Centers for Disease Control and Prevention, 2003. www.cdc.gov/hiv/graphics/mortalit.htm.)

causes of death in men and in women, respectively, ages 25 to 44 years. Mortality from HIV infection increased rapidly in both sexes from 1982 to 1995, but decreased dramatically from 1995 to 1997, largely because of newly introduced, highly active antiretroviral therapy as well as lifestyle changes resulting from public health education. Mortality in people aged 25 to 44 years continued to drop at a slower rate through 2000. With the drop in mortality and the lengthening of the life span of many people with AIDS, the prevalence of the disease has increased significantly.

A comparison of mortality and incidence is seen in Figures 4-13 and 4-14. Figure 4-13 shows ectopic pregnancy rates by year in the United States from 1970 to 1987. During this period, the rate per 1,000 reported pregnancies increased almost fourfold. This increase

has been attributed to improved diagnosis and to increased frequency of pelvic inflammatory disease resulting from sexually transmitted diseases. As seen in Figure 4-14, however, death rates from ectopic pregnancy decreased markedly during the same time period, perhaps as a result of earlier detection and increasingly prompt medical and surgical intervention.

Figure 4-15 presents interesting data on time trends in incidence and mortality from breast cancer in black women and white women in the United States. Compare the time trends in incidence and mortality. What do these curves tell us about new cases of breast cancer over time and survival from breast cancer? Compare the experiences of black women and white women in regard to both inci-dence and mortality. How can we describe the differences, and what could be some of the possible explanations?

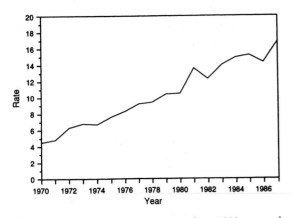

Figure 4-13. Ectopic pregnancy rates (per 1,000 reported pregnancies), by year, United States, 1970–1987. (From Centers for Disease Control and Prevention: MMWR 39:401, 1990.)

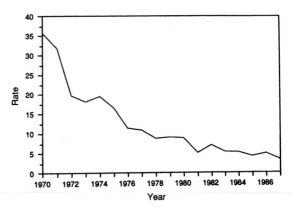

Figure 4-14. Ectopic pregnancy death rates (per 10,000 ectopic pregnancies), by year, United States, 1970–1987. (From Centers for Disease Control and Prevention: MMWR 39:403, 1990.)

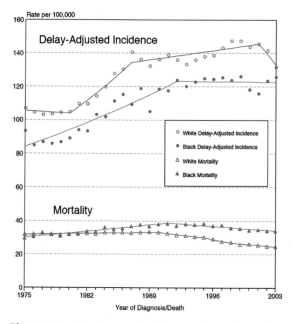

Figure 4-15. Breast cancer incidence and mortality: white women versus black women. (From Ries LAG, Harkins D, Krapcho M, et al [eds]: Breast cancer delay-adjusted incidence and mortality: White females vs. black females, 1975–2003. SEER Cancer Statistics Review, 1975–2003, National Cancer Institute, Bethesda, MD, 2006.)

A final example relates to reports in recent years that the incidence of thyroid cancer in the United States has been increasing. One of two possible explanations is likely. The first explanation is that these reports reflect a true increase in incidence that has resulted from increases in prevalence of risk factors for the disease. The second explanation is that the reported increased incidence is only an increase in *apparent* incidence. It does not reflect any true increase in new cases but rather an increase in the detection and diagnosis of subclinical cases, because new diagnostic methods permit us to identify small and asymptomatic thyroid cancers that could not be detected previously.

In order to distinguish between these two possible explanations, Davies and Welch studied changes in incidence and mortality from thyroid cancer in the United States from 1973 to 2002. Figure 4-16 shows that during the period of the study, the *incidence rate* of thyroid cancer more than doubled but during the same period, *mortality* from thyroid cancer remained virtually unchanged.

Thyroid cancer is characterized by different histologic types, as seen in Figure 4-17: at one extreme, papillary carcinoma has the best prognosis and at the opposite extreme, poorly differentiated types—medullary and anaplastic—are generally the most aggressive with poorest prognoses. The authors found that the increase in incidence of thyroid cancer was almost entirely due to an increase in the incidence of papillary cancer (Fig. 4-18). Within the papillary cancers, most of the increase in this incidence was accounted for by the smallest size tumors (Fig. 4-19). Thus, the authors found that 87% of the increase in thyroid cancer incidence over a 30-year period was accounted for by an increase in the smallest sized papillary cancers, tumors that have the best prognosis. A number of earlier studies have shown a high prevalence of previously unrecognized, asymptomatic small papillary cancers at autopsy.

If the increase in incidence is due to a true increase in occurrence of the disease, it would be likely to be reflected in increased incidence of all histologic types. If, on the other hand, the increased incidence is due to the availability of more refined diagnostic methods, we would expect to see an increase in the incidence of small tumors as the authors found in their study.

Figure 4-16. Thyroid cancer incidence and mortality, United States, 1973–2002. (From Davies L, Welch HG: Increasing incidence of thyroid cancer in the United States, 1973–2002. JAMA 295:2164–2167, 2006.)

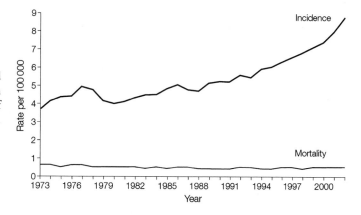

HISTOLOGIC TYPE   PROGNOSIS.

Papillary

Follicular

**Poorly differentiated
(medullary/anaplastic)**

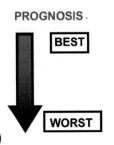

BEST

WORST

Figure 4-17. Histologic types of thyroid cancer and their prognoses.

This is also consistent with the observation that overall thyroid cancer mortality was stable.

Problems with Mortality Data

Most of our information about deaths comes from death certificates. A death certificate is shown in

Figure 4-20. By international agreement, deaths are coded according to the *underlying cause*. The underlying cause of death is defined as "the disease or injury which initiated the train of morbid events leading directly or indirectly to death or the circumstances of the accident or violence which produced the fatal injury."[3] Thus, the death certificate from which Figure 4-21 is taken would be coded as a death from chronic ischemic heart disease, the underlying cause, which is always found on the lowest line used in part I of item 23 of the certificate. The underlying cause of death therefore "excludes information pertaining to the immediate cause of death, contributory causes and those causes that intervene between the underlying and immediate causes of death."[4] As pointed out by Savage and coworkers,[5] the total contribution of a given cause of death may not be reflected in the mortality data as generally reported;

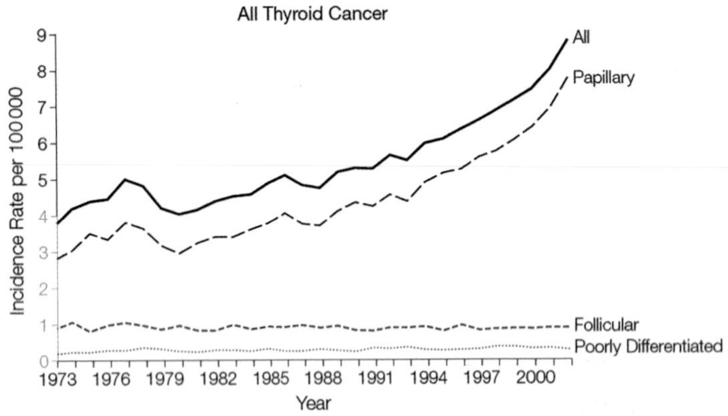

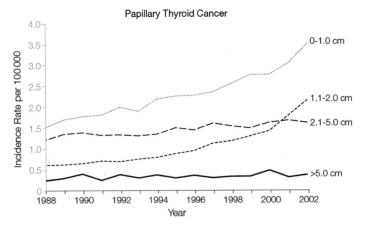

Figure 4-18. Trends in incidence of thyroid cancer by histologic type, United States, 1973–2002. (From Davies L, Welch HG: Increasing incidence of thyroid cancer in the United States, 1973–2002. JAMA 295:2164–2167, 2006.)

Figure 4-19. Trends in incidence of papillary tumors of the thyroid, by size, United States, 1988–2002. (From Davies L, Welch HG: Increasing incidence of thyroid cancer in the United States, 1973–2002. JAMA 295:2164–2167, 2006).

1 - FOR STATE REGISTRAR

STATE OF MARYLAND / DEPARTMENT OF HEALTH AND MENTAL HYGIENE
CERTIFICATE OF DEATH   REG. NO.

TO BE COMPLETED BY FUNERAL DIRECTOR

| 1. DECEDENT'S NAME *(First, Middle, Last)* | | | | 2. DATE OF DEATH MONTH   DAY   YEAR | | 3. TIME OF DEATH M |

| 4. SOCIAL SECURITY NUMBER | 5. SEX 1 ☐ M 2 ☐ F | 6. AGE *(In yrs. last birthday)* YRS. | IF UNDER 1 YEAR MONTHS DAYS | IF UNDER 24 HRS. HOURS MIN. | 7. DATE OF BIRTH *(Month, Day, Year)* | 8. BIRTHPLACE *(State or Foreign Country)* |

| 9a. FACILITY NAME *(If not institution, give street and number)* | 9b. CITY, TOWN OR LOCATION OF DEATH | 9c. COUNTY OF DEATH |

RESIDENCE OF DECEDENT

| 10a. STATE | 10b. COUNTY | 10c. CITY, TOWN OR LOCATION | 10d. INSIDE CITY LIMITS? 1 ☐ YES 2 ☐ NO |

| 10e. STREET AND NUMBER | 10f. ZIP CODE | 10g. CITIZEN OF WHAT COUNTRY? |

| 11. MARITAL STATUS 1 ☐ Never Married   2 ☐ Married 3 ☐ Widowed   4 ☐ Divorced | 12. WAS DECEDENT EVER IN U.S. ARMED FORCES?   1 ☐ YES   2 ☐ NO IF YES, GIVE WAR OR DATES | 13. WAS DECEDENT OF HISPANIC ORIGIN? (Specify Yes or No— If yes, specify Cuban, Mexican, Puerto Rican, etc.) 1 ☐ YES 2 ☐ NO   Specify: | 14. RACE — American Indian, Black, White, etc. Specify: |

| 15. DECEDENT'S EDUCATION *(Specify only highest grade completed)* Elementary/Secondary (0-12)   College (1-4 or 5 +) | 16a. DECEDENT'S USUAL OCCUPATION *(Give kind of work done during most of working life. Do NOT use retired.)* | 16b. KIND OF BUSINESS/INDUSTRY |

| 17. FATHER'S NAME *(First, Middle, Last)* | 18. MOTHER'S NAME *(First, Middle, Maiden Surname)* |

| 19a. INFORMANT'S NAME *(Type/Print)* | 19b. MAILING ADDRESS *(Street and Number or Rural Route Number, City or Town, State, Zip Code)* |

| 20a. METHOD OF DISPOSITION 1 ☐ Burial 2 ☐ Cremation 3 ☐ Removal from State 4 ☐ Donation 5 ☐ Other (Specify) _____ | 20b. PLACE AND DATE OF DISPOSITION *(Name of cemetery, crematory or other place)* | DATE | 20c. LOCATION — City or Town, State |

| 21. SIGNATURE OF FUNERAL SERVICE LICENSEE ▶ | 22. NAME AND ADDRESS OF FACILITY |

TO BE COMPLETED BY PHYSICIAN: MEDICAL CERTIFICATION

23. PART I. Enter the diseases, or complications that caused the death. Do not enter the mode of dying, such as cardiac or respiratory arrest, shock, or heart failure. List only one cause on each line.   Approximate Interval Between Onset and Death

IMMEDIATE CAUSE (Final disease or condition resulting in death) ➡   a. ____
    DUE TO (OR AS A CONSEQUENCE OF):

Sequentially list conditions, if any, leading to immediate cause. Enter UNDERLYING CAUSE (Disease or injury that initiated events resulting in death) LAST
    b. ____
    DUE TO (OR AS A CONSEQUENCE OF):
    c. ____
    DUE TO (OR AS A CONSEQUENCE OF):
    d. ____

PART II. Other significant conditions contributing to death but not resulting in the underlying cause given in Part I.

24a. WAS AN AUTOPSY PERFORMED? 1 ☐ YES 2 ☐ NO

24b. WERE AUTOPSY FINDINGS AVAILABLE PRIOR TO COMPLETION OF CAUSE OF DEATH? 1 ☐ YES 2 ☐ NO

DID TOBACCO USE CONTRIBUTE TO CAUSE OF DEATH   YES ☐ NO ☐ UNCERTAIN ☐

| 25. WAS CASE REFERRED TO MEDICAL EXAMINER? 1 ☐ YES 2 ☐ NO | 26. PLACE OF DEATH (Check only one) HOSPITAL: 1 ☐ Inpatient 2 ☐ ER/Outpatient 3 ☐ DOA   OTHER: 4 ☐ Nursing Home 5 ☐ Residence 6 ☐ Other (Specify) |

| 27. MANNER OF DEATH 1 ☐ Natural   5 ☐ Pending Investigation 2 ☐ Accident 3 ☐ Suicide   6 ☐ Could not be determined 4 ☐ Homicide | 28a. DATE OF INJURY *(Month, Day, Year)* | 28b. TIME OF INJURY M | 28c. INJURY AT WORK? 1 ☐ YES 2 ☐ NO | 28d. DESCRIBE HOW INJURY OCCURED |
| | 28e. PLACE OF INJURY — At home, farm, street, factory, office building, etc. (Specify) | | | 28f. LOCATION *(Street and Number or Rural Route Number, City or Town, State)* |

29a. CERTIFIER *(Check only one)*   1 ☐ CERTIFYING PHYSICIAN: To the best of my knowledge, death occurred at the time, date and place, and due to the cause(s) and manner as stated.
2 ☐ MEDICAL EXAMINER: On the basis of examination and/or investigation, in my opinion, death occured at the time, date and place, and due to the cause(s) and manner as stated.

| 29b. SIGNATURE AND TITLE OF CERTIFIER | 29c. LICENSE NUMBER | 29d. DATE SIGNED *(Month, Day, Year)* ▶ |

| 30. NAME AND ADDRESS OF PERSON WHO COMPLETED CAUSE OF DEATH (ITEM 27) *(Type, Print)* |

| 31. DATE FILED *(Month, Day, Year)* | 32. REGISTRAR'S SIGNATURE |

DHMH-16 Rev 1/89

Figure 4-20. Death certificate for the state of Maryland. (Courtesy of the State of Maryland Department of Health and Mental Hygiene.)

23. PART I. Enter the diseases, or complications that caused the death. Do not enter the mode of dying, such as cardiac or respiratory arrest, shock, or heart failure. List only one cause on each line.	Approximate Interval Between Onset and Death
IMMEDIATE CAUSE (Final disease or condition resulting in death) → a. **Rupture of myocardium** DUE TO (OR AS A CONSEQUENCE OF):	Mins.
Sequentially list conditions, if any, leading to immediate cause. Enter UNDERLYING CAUSE (Disease or Injury that initiated events resulting in death) LAST b. **Acute myocardial infarction** DUE TO (OR AS A CONSEQUENCE OF):	6 days
c. **Chronic ischemic heart disease** DUE TO (OR AS A CONSEQUENCE OF):	5 years
d.	

PART II. Other significant conditions contributing to death but not resulting in the underlying cause given in Part I. **Diabetes, Chronic obstructive pulmonary disease, smoking**	24a. WAS AN AUTOPSY PERFORMED? 1 ☒ YES 2 ☐ NO	24b. WERE AUTOPSY FINDINGS AVAILABLE PRIOR TO COMPLETION OF CAUSE OF DEATH? 1 ☒ YES 2 ☐ NO
DID TOBACCO USE CONTRIBUTE TO CAUSE OF DEATH YES ☒ NO ☐ UNCERTAIN ☐		

Figure 4-21. Example of a completed cause-of-death section on a death certificate, including immediate and underlying causes and other significant conditions.

this may apply to a greater extent in some diseases than in others.

Countries and regions vary greatly in the quality of the data provided on their death certificates. Studies of validity of death certificates compared with hospital and autopsy records generally find higher validity for certain diseases, such as cancers, than for others.

Deaths are coded according to the International Classification of Diseases (ICD), now in its tenth revision. Because coding categories and regulations change from one revision to another, any study of time trends in mortality that spans more than one revision must examine the possibility that observed changes could be due entirely or in part to changes in the ICD. In 1949, mortality rates from diabetes showed a dramatic decline in both men and women (Fig. 4-22). However, any euphoria that these data might have caused was short-lived; analysis of this drop indicated that it occurred at a time of change from the 7th revision to the 8th revision of the ICD. Prior to 1949, the policy was that any death certificate that included mention of diabetes anywhere be coded as a death from diabetes. After 1949, only death certificates on which the underlying cause of death was listed as diabetes were coded as a death from diabetes. Hence, the decline seen in Figure 4-22 was artifactual. Whenever we see a time trend of an increase or a decrease in mortality, the first question we must ask is, "Is it real?" Specifically, when we look at trends in mortality over time, we must ask whether any changes took place in how death certificates were coded during the period being examined and whether these changes could have contributed to changes observed in mortality during the same period.

Changes in the definition of disease can also have a significant effect on the number of cases of the disease that are reported or that are reported and subsequently classified as meeting the diagnostic cri-

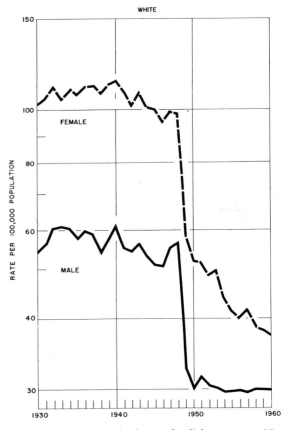

Figure 4-22. Drop in death rates for diabetes among 55- to 64-year-old men and women, United States, 1930–1960, due to changes in ICD coding. (From US Public Health Service publication No. 1000, series 3, No. 1. Washington, DC, U.S. Government Printing Office, 1964.)

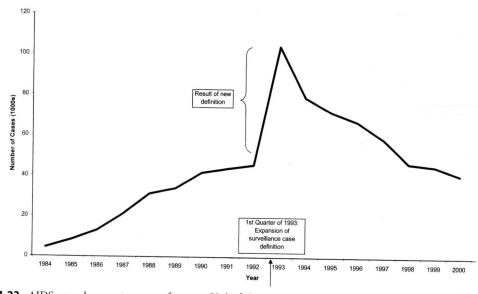

Figure 4-23. AIDS cases by quarter year of report, United States, 1984–2000. (From Centers for Disease Control and Prevention. Summary of notifiable diseases, United States, 2000. MMWR 49:86, 2000; and Centers for Disease Control and Prevention: Summary of notifiable diseases, United States, 1993. MMWR 45:68, 1993.)

teria for the disease. In early 1993, a new definition of AIDS was introduced; as shown in Figure 4-23, this change resulted in a rapid rise in the number of reported cases. With the new definition, even after the initial peak, the number of reported cases remained higher than it had been for several years.

In discussing morbidity in Chapter 3, we said that everyone in the group represented by the denominator must be at risk to enter the group represented by the numerator, and we looked at uterine cancer incidence rates as an example. The same principle regarding numerator and denominator applies to mortality rates. Figure 4-24 shows a similar set of observations for mortality rates from uterine cancer. Once again, correcting for hysterectomy reduces the number of women in the denominator and thus increases the mortality rate. In a lighter vein, Table 4-6 lists some causes of death that were listed on death certificates early in the 20th century.

COMPARING MORTALITY IN DIFFERENT POPULATIONS

An important use of mortality data is to compare two or more populations, or one population in different time periods. Such populations may differ in regard to many characteristics that affect mortality, of which age distribution is the most important. In fact, age is the single most important predictor of mortality. Therefore, methods have been devel-

oped for comparing mortality in such populations while effectively holding constant characteristics such as age.

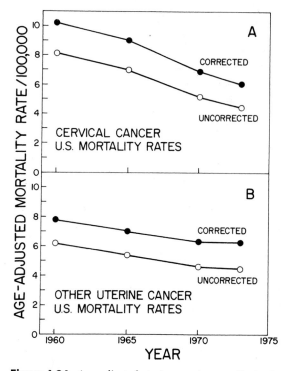

Figure 4-24. Age-adjusted uterine cancer mortality rates, corrected and uncorrected by hysterectomy status, Alameda County, California. (From Lyon JL, Gardner JW: The rising frequency of hysterectomy: Its effect on uterine cancer rates. Am J Epidemiol 105:439–443, 1977.)

TABLE 4-6. Some Causes of Death That Were Reported on Death Certificates in the Early 1900s

"Died suddenly without the aid of a physician"
"A mother died in infancy"
"Deceased had never been fatally sick"
"Died suddenly, nothing serious"
"Went to bed feeling well, but woke up dead"

TABLE 4-7. Crude Mortality Rates by Race, Baltimore City, 1965

Race	Mortality per 1,000 Population
White	14.3
Black	10.2

Table 4-7 shows data that exemplify the problem. Mortality rates for white and black residents of Baltimore in 1965 are given. The data may seem surprising because we would expect rates to have been higher for blacks, given the problems associated with poorer living conditions and less access to medical care, particularly at that time. When we look at Table 4-8, we see the data from Table 4-7 on the left, but now we have added data for each age-specific stratum (layer) of the population. Interestingly, although in each age-specific group, mortality is higher in blacks than in whites, the overall mortality (also called *crude* or *unadjusted mortality*) is higher in whites than in blacks. Why is this so? This is a reflection of the fact that in both whites and blacks, mortality increases markedly in the oldest age groups; older age is the major contributor to mortality. However, the white population in this example is older than the black population, and in 1965, there were few blacks in the oldest age groups. Thus, in whites, the overall mortality is heavily weighted by high rates in the oldest age groups. The overall (or crude) mortality rate in whites is increased by the greater number of deaths in the large subgroup of older whites, but the overall mortality rate in blacks is not increased as much because there are fewer deaths in the smaller number of blacks in the older age groups. Clearly, the crude mortality reflects both differences in the force of mortality, and differences in the age composition of the population. Let us look at two approaches for dealing with this problem: direct and indirect age adjustment.

Direct Age Adjustment

Tables 4-9 through 4-11 show a hypothetical example of direct age adjustment. Table 4-9 shows mortality in a population in two different periods. The mortality rate is considerably higher in the later period. These data are supplemented with age-specific data in Table 4-10. Here, we see three age groups, and age-specific mortality for the later period is lower in each group. How, then, is it possible to account for the higher overall mortality in the later period in this example?

The answer lies in the changing age structure of the population. Mortality is highest in the oldest age groups, and during the later period, the size of the oldest group doubled from 100,000 to 200,000, whereas the number of young people declined substantially, from 500,000 to 300,000. We would like to eliminate this age difference and, in effect, ask: If the age composition of the populations were the same, would there be any differences in mortality between the early period and the later period?

In *direct age-adjustment*, a standard population is used in order to eliminate the effects of any differ-

---

TABLE 4-8. Death Rates by Age and Race, Baltimore City, 1965

		DEATH RATES BY AGE PER 1,000 POPULATION					
Race	All Ages	<1 yr	1–4 yr	5–17 yr	18–44 yr	45–64 yr	>65 yr
White	14.3	23.9	0.7	0.4	2.5	15.2	69.3
Black	10.2	31.3	1.6	0.6	4.8	22.6	75.9

From Department of Biostatistics: Annual Vital Statistics Report for Maryland, 1965. Baltimore, Maryland State Department of Health, 1965.

TABLE 4-9. A Hypothetical Example of Direct Age Adjustment: I. Comparison of Total Death Rates in a Population at Two Different Times

EARLY PERIOD			LATER PERIOD		
Population	Number of Deaths	Death Rate per 100,000	Population	Number of Deaths	Death Rate per 100,000
900,000	862	96	900,000	1,130	126

TABLE 4-10. A Hypothetical Example of Direct Age Adjustment: II. Comparison of Age-Specific Death Rates in Two Different Time Periods

	EARLY PERIOD			LATER PERIOD		
Age Group (yr)	Population	Number of Deaths	Death Rates per 100,000	Population	Number of Deaths	Death Rates per 100,000
All ages	900,000	862	96	900,000	1,130	126
30–49	500,000	60	12	300,000	30	10
50–69	300,000	396	132	400,000	400	100
70+	100,000	406	406	200,000	700	350

TABLE 4-11. A Hypothetical Example of Direct Age Adjustment: III. Carrying Out an Age Adjustment Using the Total of the Two Populations as the Standard

Age Group (yr)	Standard Population	"Early" Age-specific Mortality Rates per 100,000	Expected Number of Deaths Using "Early" Rates	"Later" Age-specific Mortality Rates per 100,000	Expected Number of Deaths Using "Later" Rates
All ages	1,800,000				
30–49	800,000	12	96	10	80
50–69	700,000	132	924	100	700
70+	300,000	406	1,218	350	1,050
Total number of deaths expected in the standard population:			2,238		1,830
Age-adjusted rates:		"Early" $= \dfrac{2,238}{1,800,000} = 124.3$		"Later" $= \dfrac{1,830}{1,800,000} = 101.7$	

ences in age between two or more populations being compared (Table 4-11). A hypothetical "standard" population is created to which we apply both the age-specific mortality rates from the early period and the age-specific mortality rates from the later period. By applying mortality rates from both periods to a single standard population, we eliminate any possi-

bility that observed differences could be a result of age differences in the population. (In this example, we have created a standard by adding the populations from the early and the later periods, but any population could have been used.)

By applying each age-specific mortality rate to the population in each age group of the standard population, we derive the expected number of deaths that would have occurred had those rates been applied. We can then calculate the total number of deaths expected in the standard population had the age-specific rates of the early period applied and the total number of deaths expected in the standard population had the age-specific rates of the later period applied. Dividing each of these two total expected numbers of deaths by the standard population, we can calculate an expected mortality rate in the standard population if it had had the mortality experience of the early period and the expected mortality rate for the standard population if it had had the mortality experience for the later period. These are called *age-adjusted rates*, and they appropriately reflect the decline seen in the age-specific rates. Differences in age-composition of the population are no longer a factor.

In this example the rates have been adjusted for age, but adjustment can be carried out for any characteristic such as sex, socioeconomic status, or race, and techniques are also available to adjust for multiple variables simultaneously.

Let us look at an example of direct age adjustment using real data.[6] When mortality in the United States and in Mexico was compared for 1995 to 1997, the crude mortality rate for all ages in the United States was 8.7 per 1,000 population and in Mexico only 4.7 per 1,000 population. But for each age group, the age-specific mortality rate was higher in Mexico than in the United States (aside from the over 65 group in which the rates were similar). Could the considerably higher crude mortality rate in the United States be due to the fact that there is a difference in the age distributions of the two populations, in that the U.S. population has a greater proportion of older individuals than does the population in Mexico?

In order to eliminate the possibility that the differences in mortality between the United States and Mexico could have been due to differences in the age structure of the two populations, we need to control for age. Therefore, we select a standard population and apply both the age-specific mortality rates from the United States and from Mexico to the same standard population. As seen in Table 4-12, when we examine the age-adjusted rates using the mortality rates from the United States and from Mexico, we find that the age-adjusted rate in the United States is 5.7 per 1,000, lower than that in Mexico (6.4/1,000). Thus, the higher crude rate observed in the United States was due to the older age of the U.S. population.

TABLE 4-12. An Example of Direct Age Adjustment: Comparison of Age-adjusted Mortality Rates in Mexico and in the United States, 1995–1997

Age Group (yr)	Standard Population	Age-specific Mexico Mortality Rates per 100,000	Expected Numbers of Deaths Using Mexico Rates	Age-specific United States Mortality Rates per 100,000	Expected Numbers of Deaths Using United States Rates
All ages	100,000				
<1	2,400	1,693.2	41	737.8	18
1–4	9,600	112.5	11	38.5	4
5–14	19,000	36.2	7	21.7	4
15–24	17,000	102.9	17	90.3	15
25–44	26,000	209.6	55	176.4	46
45–64	19,000	841.1	160	702.3	133
65+	7,000	4,967.4	<u>348</u>	5,062.6	<u>354</u>
Total numbers of deaths expected in the standard population			639		574

Age-adjusted rates:

$$\text{Mexico} = \frac{639}{100,000} = \frac{6.39}{1,000}$$

$$\text{United States} = \frac{574}{100,000} = \frac{5.74}{1,000}$$

From Analysis Group, Pan American Health Organization Special Program for Health Analysis: Standardization: A classic epidemiological method for the comparison of rates. Epidemiol Bull 232(3):9–12, 2002.

Although age-adjusted rates can be very useful in making comparisons, the first step in examining and analyzing comparative mortality data should always be to carefully examine the age-specific rates for any interesting differences or changes. These may be hidden by the age-adjusted rates, and they may be lost if we proceed immediately to age adjustment.

Age-adjusted rates are hypothetical because they involve applying actual age-specific rates to a hypothetical standard population. They do not reflect the true mortality risk of a "real" population because the numerical value of an age-adjusted death rate depends on the standard population used. Selection of such a population is somewhat arbitrary because there is no "correct" standard population, but it is generally accepted that the "standard" should not be markedly different from the populations that are being compared with regard to age or whatever the variable is for which the adjustment is being made. In the United States, for more than 50 years, the 1940 U.S. population was regularly used as the standard population for age adjustment for most purposes, but in recent years, this population was increasingly considered outdated and incompatible with the older age structure of the U.S. population. Beginning with 1999 mortality statistics, the U.S. population in the year 2000 replaced the 1940 population as the standard population for adjustment.

The change in standard population to the year 2000 U.S. population will have some significant effects.[7] For example, there will be increases in age-adjusted mortality rates for causes in which risk increases significantly with age. For example, age-adjusted death from cerebrovascular diseases (stroke) is 26.7 deaths per 100,000 using the 1940 standard, but it is 63.9 per 100,000 using the 2000 standard. Cancer mortality will increase using the 2000 population standard compared to when an earlier population is used as a standard because more people are surviving into older ages, when many of the leading types of cancer are more common. Rates for heart disease, chronic obstructive lung disease, diabetes, kidney disease, and Alzheimer's disease will be similarly affected because age-specific death rates for all these conditions are higher in older age groups.

Age-adjusted rates of cancer are higher in blacks compared to whites in the United States, but the differential between blacks and whites will be less with the 2000 population standard than with the earlier standard population. Thus, the change to the year 2000 U.S. population as the standard complicates comparisons of age-adjusted rates before and after 1999 because many of the rates before 1999 were calculated using the 1940 standard population, but the rates from 1999 and on are being calculated using the year 2000 population as the new standard.

Indirect Age Adjustment (Standardized Mortality Ratios)

Indirect age adjustment is often used when numbers of deaths for each age-specific stratum are not available. It is also used to study mortality in an occupationally exposed population: Do people who work in a certain industry, such as mining or construction, have a higher mortality than people of the same age in the general population? Is an additional risk associated with that occupation?

To answer the question of whether a population of miners has a higher mortality than we would expect in a similar population that is not engaged in mining, the age-specific rates for such a known population, such as all men of the same age, are applied to each age group in the population of interest. This will yield the number of deaths expected in each age group in the population of interest, if this population had had the mortality experience of the known population. Thus, for each age group, the number of deaths *expected* is calculated, and these numbers are totaled. The numbers of deaths that were actually *observed* in that population are also calculated and totaled. The ratio of the total number of deaths actually observed to the total number of deaths expected, if the population of interest had had the mortality experience of the known population, is then calculated. This ratio is called the *standardized mortality ratio (SMR)*.

The SMR is defined as follows:

$$SMR = \frac{\text{Observed no. of deaths per year}}{\text{Expected no. of deaths per year}}$$

Let us look at the example in Table 4-13. In a population of 534,533 white male miners, 436 deaths from tuberculosis occurred in 1950. Is this mortality experience from tuberculosis greater than, less than, or about the same as that expected in white men of the same ages in the general population? For each age-specific group of white miners, we take the age-specific mortality rate from the general population (expected) and ask, "How many deaths would we expect in these white miners if they had the same mortality experience as white men in the same age group in the general population?" These data are listed in column 3. Column 4 shows the actual number of deaths observed in the miners.

TABLE 4-13. Computation of a Standardized Mortality Ratio (SMR) for Tuberculosis, All Forms (TBC), for White Miners Ages 20 to 59 Years, United States, 1950

Age (yr)	Estimated Population for White Miners	Death Rate (per 100,000) for TBC in Males in the General Population	Expected Deaths from TBC in White Miners if They Had the Same Risk as the General Population	Observed Deaths from TBC in White Miners
	(1)	(2)	(3) = (1) × (2)	(4)
20–24	74,598	12.26	9.14	10
25–29	85,077	16.12	13.71	20
30–34	80,845	21.54	17.41	22
35–44	148,870	33.96	50.55	98
45–54	102,649	56.82	58.32	174
55–59	42,494	75.23	31.96	112
Totals	534,533		181.09	436

$$SMR = \frac{\text{Observed deaths for an occupation} - \text{cause} - \text{race group}}{\text{Expected deaths for an occupation} - \text{cause} - \text{race group}} \times 100$$

$$SMR\,(\text{for } 20-59\text{-yr-olds}) = \frac{436}{181.09} \times 100 = 241$$

Adapted from Vital Statistics: Special Reports. Washington, DC, Department of Health, Education, and Welfare, vol 53(5), 1963.

The SMR is calculated by totaling the observed number of deaths (436) and dividing it by the expected number of deaths (181.09), which yields a result of 2.41. Multiplication by 100 is often done to yield results without decimals. If this were done in this case, the SMR would be 241. An SMR of 100 indicates that the observed number of deaths is the same as the expected number of deaths. An SMR greater than 100 indicates that the observed number of deaths exceeds the expected number, and an SMR less than 100 indicates that the observed number of deaths is less than the expected number.

The Cohort Effect

Table 4-14 shows age-specific death rates from tuberculosis per 100,000 persons in Massachusetts from 1880 to 1930. (For this discussion, we will ignore children ages 0 to 4 years, because tuberculosis in this age group is a somewhat different phenomenon.) If, for example, we then read *down* the column in the

TABLE 4-14. Age-specific Death Rates per 100,000 from Tuberculosis (All Forms), Males, Massachusetts, 1880–1930

Age (yr)	YEAR					
	1880	1890	1900	1910	1920	1930
0–4	760	578	309	309	108	41
5–9	43	49	31	21	24	11
10–19	126	115	90	63	49	21
20–29	444	361	288	207	149	81
30–39	378	368	296	253	164	115
40–49	364	336	253	253	175	118
50–59	366	325	267	252	171	127
60–69	475	346	304	246	172	95
70+	672	396	343	163	127	95

Data from Frost WH: The age selection for mortality from tuberculosis in successive decades. J Hyg 30:91–96, 1939.

TABLE 4-15. **Age-specific Death Rates per 100,000 from Tuberculosis (All Forms), Males, Massachusetts, 1880–1930**

| Age (yr) | YEAR | | | | | |
	1880	1890	1900	1910	1920	1930
0–4	760	578	309	309	108	41
5–9	43	49	31	21	24	11
10–19	126	115	90	63	49	21
20–29	444	361	288	207	149	81
30–39	378	368	296	253	164	115
40–49	364	336	253	253	175	118
50–59	366	325	267	252	171	127
60–69	475	346	304	246	172	95
70+	672	396	343	163	127	95

Data from Frost WH: The age selection for mortality from tuberculosis in successive decades. J Hyg 30:91–96, 1939.

table (the data for a given calendar year) for 1910, it appears that tuberculosis mortality peaks when people reach their 30s or 40s and then declines with advancing age. Such a view of the data, by year, is called a *cross-sectional view*.

Actually, however, the picture of tuberculosis risk is somewhat different (Table 4-15). A person who was 10 to 19 years of age in 1880 was 20 to 29 years of age in 1890, and 30 to 39 years of age in 1900. In other words, persons who were born in a certain year are moving through time together. We can now examine the mortality over time of the same cohort (i.e., a group of people who share the same experience), born in the same 10-year period. Looking at people who were 0 to 9 years of age in 1880 and following them over time, as indicated by the boxes in the table, it is apparent that peak mortality actually occurred at a younger age than it would seem to have occurred from the cross-sectional view of the data. When we examine changes in mortality over time, we should always ask whether any apparent changes that are observed could be the result of such a cohort effect.

Interpreting Observed Changes in Mortality

If we find a difference in mortality over time or between populations—either an increase or a decrease—it may be artifactual or real. If it is an artifact, the artifact could result from problems with either the numerator or the denominator (Table 4-16). However, if we conclude that the change is real, what could be the possible explanation? Some possibilities are seen in Table 4-17.

Projecting the Future Burden of Disease

An interesting and valuable use of current data to predict the future impact of disease was a comprehensive assessment of current mortality and disability from diseases, injuries, and risk factors for all

TABLE 4-16. **Possible Explanations of Trends or Differences in Mortality: I. Artifactual**

1. Numerator	Errors in diagnosis
	Errors in age
	Changes in coding rules
	Changes in classification
2. Denominator	Errors in counting population
	Errors in classifying by demographic characteristics (e.g., age, race, sex)
	Differences in percentages of populations at risk

TABLE 4-17. **Possible Explanations of Trends or Differences in Mortality: II. Real**

Change in survivorship without change in incidence
Change in incidence
Change in age composition of the population(s)
Combination of the above factors

regions of the world in 1990, which was projected to the year 2020. The study, entitled the Global Burden of Disease, attempted to quantify not only deaths but also the impact of premature death and disability on a population and to combine these into a single index to express the overall "burden of disease."[8] The index that was developed for this study is the Disability-Adjusted Life Year (DALY), which is the years of life lost to premature death and years lived with a disability of specified severity and duration. Thus, a DALY is 1 lost year of healthy life.

The results showed that 5 of the 10 leading causes of disability in 1990 were psychiatric conditions; psychiatric and neurologic conditions accounted for 28% of all years lived with disability of known severity and duration, compared with 1.4% of all deaths and 1.1% of years of life lost. Figure 4-25 shows the 10 leading causes of disease burden in girls and women ages 15 to 44 years in both developed and developing countries in 1990. Again, the importance of noncommunicable diseases, such as mental conditions and injuries, is dramatically evident.

In 1999, the disease burden was not equitably distributed. Michaud et al. pointed out that the sub-Saharan African population, which represents 10% of the world's population, accounts for 26% of the total DALYs.[9] As seen in Table 4-18, the top 10 causes of disease burden were responsible for 46% of all DALYs. Five of the top 10 causes primarily affect children younger than 5 years of age. Three of the top 10 (unipolar major depression, ischemic heart disease, and cerebrovascular disease) are chronic conditions. This table shows the value of using a measure such as DALYs to assess the burden of disease, a measure that is not limited to either morbidity or mortality, but is weighted by both.

With the aging of the population worldwide, an "epidemiologic transition" is taking place so that, by 2020, noncommunicable diseases are likely to account for 70% of all deaths in developing countries, compared with less than half of deaths today. As projected in Figure 4-26, by 2020, the disease burden due to communicable diseases, maternal and perinatal conditions, and nutritional deficiencies (group I) is expected to decrease dramatically. The burden due to group II (noncommunicable diseases) is expected to increase sharply, as will the burden from injuries (group III). Also by 2020, the burden of disease attributable to tobacco is expected to exceed that caused by any single disease—clearly a strong call for public health action. Although there is no universal agreement on the methodology or applicability of a single measure of disease burden such as the DALY, this study is an excellent demonstration of an attempt at worldwide surveillance designed to develop such a measure to permit valid regional comparisons and future projections so that appropriate interventions can be developed.

CONCLUSION

This chapter has reviewed some approaches to quantitatively measuring and expressing human mortality. We will turn next to questions about the numerators of morbidity rates: How do we identify people who have a disease and distinguish them from those who do not, and how do we evaluate the quality of the diagnostic and screening tests that are used to separate these individuals and populations? These questions are addressed in Chapter 5.

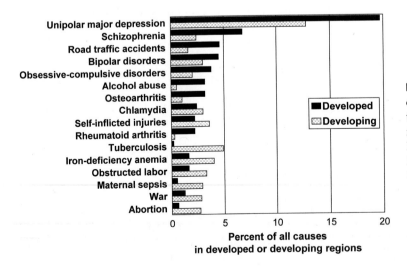

Figure 4-25. The ten leading causes of disease burden for women ages 15 to 44 in developed and developing regions, 1990. (From Murray CJL, Lopez AD: The Global Burden of Disease. Cambridge, MA, Harvard University Press, 1996.)

TABLE 4-18. **Leading Causes of Disability-adjusted Life Years (DALYs) for the World in 1999**

Rank	Cause	DALYs (thousands)	Total DALYs (%)	Deaths (thousands)
	All conditions	1,438,154	100	55,965
1	Lower respiratory tract infections	96,682	6.72	3,963
2	Human immunodeficiency virus (HIV)	89,819	6.25	2,673
3	Conditions arising during the perinatal period	89,508	6.22	2,356
4	Diarrheal diseases	72,083	5.01	2,213
5	Unipolar major depression	59,030	4.10	1
6	Ischemic heart disease	58,981	4.10	7,089
7	Vaccine-preventable diseases	54,638	3.80	1,554
8	Cerebrovascular diseases	49,858	3.47	5,544
9	Malaria	44,998	3.13	1,086
10	Nutritional deficiencies	44,539	3.10	493
11	Road traffic collisions	39,573	2.75	1,230
12	Chronic obstructive pulmonary disease	38,158	2.65	2,660
13	Congenital abnormalities	36,557	2.54	652
14	Tuberculosis	33,287	2.31	1,669
15	Falls	30,950	2.15	347
16	Maternal conditions	26,101	1.81	497
17	Self-inflicted	25,095	1.74	893
18	Sexually transmitted diseases excluding HIV	19,747	1.37	178
19	Alcohol use	18,743	1.30	60
20	Bipolar disorder	16,368	1.14	6

From World Health Organization: The World Health Report 2000: Health systems. Improving performance. Geneva, Switzerland: World Health Organization, 2000. Reprinted by Michaud CM, Murray CJL, Bloom BR: Burden of disease: Implications for future research. JAMA 285:535–539, 2001.

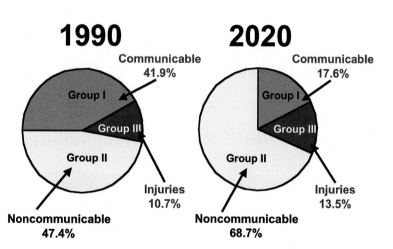

Figure 4-26. The "epidemiologic transition": distribution of deaths from communicable and non-communicable causes in developing countries, 1990 and projected in 2020. (From Murray CJL, Lopez AD: The Global Burden of Disease. Cambridge, MA, Harvard University Press, 1996.)

───────────────── **REFERENCES** ─────────────────

1. De Beauvoir, S: A Very Easy Death. Translated by Patrick O'Brian. New York, Pantheon Books, 1965.

2. Premature mortality in the United States: Public health issues in the use of years of potential life lost, 1986. MMWR 35(Suppl 2S):1s–11s, 1986.

3. National Center for Health Statistics: Instructions for Classifying the Underlying Cause of Death, 1983. Hyattsville, MD, 1983.

4. Chamblee RF, Evans MC: TRANSAX: The NCHS System for Producing Multiple Cause-of-Death Statistics, 1968–1978. Vital and Health Statistics, series 1, No. 20, DHHS publication No. (PHS) 86–1322. Washington, DC, Bureau of Vital and Health Statistics, June 1986.

5. Savage G, Rohde FC, Grant B, Dufour MC: Liver Cirrhosis Mortality in the United States, 1970–90: Surveillance Report

No. 29. Bethesda, MD, Department of Health and Human Services, December 1993.

6. Analysis Group, Pan American Health Organization Special Program for Health Analysis (SHA): Standardization: A classic epidemiological method for the comparison of rates. Epidemiol Bull 23(3):9–12, 2002.

7. Anderson RN, Rosenberg HM: Age Standardization of Death Rates: Implementation of the Year 2000 Standard. National Vital Statistics Reports, Vol. 47, No. 3, pp 1–16. Hyattsville, MD, National Center for Health Statistics, October 7, 1998.

8. Murray CJL, Lopez AD: The Global Burden of Disease. Cambridge, MA, Harvard University Press, 1996.

9. Michaud CM, Murray CJL, Bloom BR: Burden of disease: Implications for future research. JAMA 285:535–539, 2001.

REVIEW QUESTIONS FOR CHAPTER 4

Questions 1 and 2 are based on the information given below:

In an Asian country with a population of 6 million people, 60,000 deaths occurred during the year ending December 31, 1995. These included 30,000 deaths from cholera in 100,000 people who were sick with cholera.

1. What was the cause-specific mortality rate from cholera in 1995?

2. What was the case-fatality rate from cholera in 1995?

3. Age-adjusted death rates are used to:
   a. Correct death rates for errors in the statement of age
   b. Determine the actual number of deaths that occurred in specific age groups in a population
   c. Correct death rates for missing age information
   d. Compare deaths in persons of the same age group
   e. Eliminate the effects of differences in the age distributions of populations in comparing death rates

4. The mortality rate from disease X in city A is 75/100,000 in persons 65 to 69 years old. The mortality rate from the same disease in city B is 150/100,000 in persons 65 to 69 years old. The inference that disease X is two times more prevalent in persons 65 to 69 years old in city B than it is in persons 65 to 69 years old in city A is:
   a. Correct
   b. Incorrect, because of failure to distinguish between prevalence and mortality
   c. Incorrect, because of failure to adjust for differences in age distributions
   d. Incorrect, because of failure to distinguish between period and point prevalence
   e. Incorrect, because a proportion is used when a rate is required to support the inference

5. The incidence rate of a disease is five times greater in women than in men, but the prevalence rates show no sex difference. The best explanation is that:
   a. The crude all-cause mortality rate is greater in women
   b. The case-fatality rate for this disease is greater in women
   c. The case-fatality rate for this disease is lower in women
   d. The duration of this disease is shorter in men
   e. Risk factors for the disease are more common in women

Question 6 is based on the information given below:

Annual Cancer Death in White Male Workers in Two Industries				
	INDUSTRY A		INDUSTRY B	
	No. of Deaths	% of All Cancer Deaths	No. of Deaths	% of All Cancer Deaths
Respiratory system	180	33	248	45
Digestive system	160	29	160	29
Genitourinary	80	15	82	15
All other sites	130	23	60	11
Total	550	100	550	100

Based on the preceding information, it was concluded that workers in industry B are at higher risk of death from respiratory system cancer than workers in industry A. (Assume that the age distributions of the workers in the two industries are nearly identical.)

6. Which of the following statements is true?
   a. The conclusion reached is correct
   b. The conclusion reached may be incorrect because proportionate mortality rates were used when age-specific mortality rates were needed
   c. The conclusion reached may be incorrect because there was no comparison group
   d. The conclusion reached may be incorrect because proportional mortality was used when cause-specific mortality rates were needed
   e. None of the above

7. The following are standardized mortality ratios (SMRs) for lung cancer in England:

	STANDARDIZED MORTALITY RATIO	
Occupation	1949–1960	1968–1979
Carpenters	209	135
Bricklayers	142	118

Based on these SMRs *alone*, it is possible to conclude that:
   a. The number of deaths from lung cancer in carpenters in 1949–1960 was greater than the number of deaths from lung cancer in bricklayers during the same period
   b. The proportionate mortality from lung cancer in bricklayers in 1949–1960 was greater than the proportionate mortality from lung cancer in the same occupational group in 1968–1979
   c. The age-adjusted rate of death from lung cancer in bricklayers was greater in 1949–1960 than it was in 1968–1979
   d. The rate of death from lung cancer in carpenters in 1968–1979 was greater than would have been expected for a group of men of similar ages in all occupations
   e. The proportionate mortality rate from lung cancer in carpenters in 1968–1979 was 1.35 times greater than would have been expected for a group of men of similar ages in all occupations

Questions 8 and 9 are based on the information given below:

	COMMUNITY X		COMMUNITY Y	
Age	No. of People	No. of Deaths from Disease Z	No. of People	No. of Deaths from Disease Z
Young	8,000	69	5,000	48
Old	11,000	115	3,000	60

Calculate the age-adjusted death rate for disease Z in communities X and Y by the direct method, using the total of both communities as the standard population.

8. The age-adjusted death rate from disease Z for community X is: _____

9. The proportionate mortality from disease Z for community Y is: _____
   a. 9.6/1,000
   b. 13.5/1,000
   c. 20.0/1,000
   d. 10.8/1,000
   e. None of the above

10. For a disease such as pancreatic cancer, which is highly fatal and of short duration:
   a. Incidence rates and mortality rates will be similar
   b. Mortality rates will be much higher than incidence rates

c. Incidence rates will be much higher than mortality rates

d. Incidence rates will be unrelated to mortality rates

e. None of the above

11. In 1990, there were 4,500 deaths due to lung diseases in miners aged 20 to 64 years. The expected number of deaths in this occupational group, based on age-specific death rates from lung diseases in all males aged 20 to 64 years, was 1,800 during 1990.

What was the standardized mortality ratio (SMR) for lung diseases in miners? _____

Chapter 5

Assessing the Validity and Reliability of Diagnostic and Screening Tests

A normal individual is a person who has not been sufficiently examined.
—Anonymous

To understand how a disease is transmitted and develops and to provide appropriate and effective health care, it is necessary to distinguish between people in the population who have the disease and those who do not. This is an important challenge, both in the clinical arena, where patient care is the issue, and in the public health arena, where secondary prevention programs that involve early disease detection and intervention are being considered and where etiologic studies are being conducted to provide a basis for primary prevention. Thus, the quality of screening and diagnostic tests is a critical issue. Regardless of whether the test is a physical examination, a chest X-ray, an electrocardiogram, or a blood or urine assay, the same issue arises: How good is the test in separating populations of people with and without the disease in question? This chapter addresses the question of how we assess the quality of newly available screening and diagnostic tests to make reasonable decisions about their use and interpretation.

BIOLOGIC VARIATION OF HUMAN POPULATIONS

In using a test to distinguish between individuals with normal and abnormal results, it is important to understand how characteristics are distributed in human populations.

Figure 5-1 shows the distribution of tuberculin test results in a population. The size of the induration (area of hardness at the site of the injection) in millimeters is shown on the horizontal axis and the number of individuals is indicated on the vertical axis. A large group centers on the value of 0 mm—no induration—and another group centers near 20 mm of induration. This type of distribution, in which there are two peaks, is called a *bimodal curve*. The

bimodal distribution permits the separation of individuals who had no prior experience with tuberculosis (people with no induration, seen on the left) from those who had prior experience with tuberculosis (those with about 20 mm of induration, seen on the right). Although some individuals fall into the "gray zone" in the center, and may belong to either curve, most of the population can be easily distinguished using the two curves. Thus, when a characteristic has a bimodal distribution, it is relatively easy to separate most of the population into two groups (e.g., ill and not ill, having a certain condition or abnormality and not having that condition or abnormality).

In general, however, most human characteristics are not distributed bimodally. Figure 5-2 shows the distribution of systolic blood pressures in a group of men. In this figure there is no bimodal curve; what we see is a *unimodal curve*—a single peak. Therefore, if we want to separate those in the group who are hypertensive from those who are not hypertensive, a cutoff level of blood pressure must be set above which people are designated hypertensive and below which they are designated normotensive. No obvious level of blood pressure distinguishes normotensive from hypertensive individuals. Although we could choose a cutoff for hypertension based on statistical considerations, we would ideally like to choose a cutoff on the basis of biologic information; that is, we would want to know that a pressure above the chosen cutoff level is associated with increased risk of subsequent disease, such as stroke, myocardial infarction, or subsequent mortality. Unfortunately, for many human characteristics, we do not have such information to serve as a guide in setting this level.

In either distribution—unimodal or bimodal—it is relatively easy to distinguish between the extreme values of abnormal and normal. With either type of

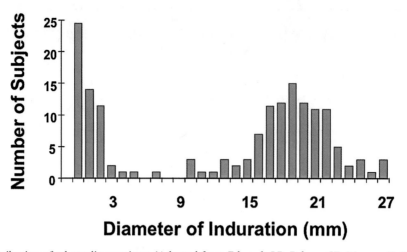

Figure 5-1. Distribution of tuberculin reactions. (Adapted from Edwards LB, Palmer CE, Magnus K: BCG Vaccination: Studies by the WHO Tuberculosis Research Office, Copenhagen. WHO Monograph No. 12. Geneva, WHO, 1953.)

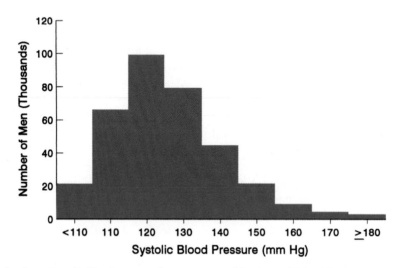

Figure 5-2. Distribution of systolic blood pressure for men screened for the Multiple Risk Factor Intervention Trial. (Data from Stamler J, Stamler R, Neaton JD: Blood pressure, systolic and diastolic, and cardiovascular risks: U.S. population data. Arch Intern Med 153:598–615, 1993.)

curve, however, uncertainty remains about cases that fall into the gray zone.

VALIDITY OF SCREENING TESTS

The *validity* of a test is defined as its ability to distinguish between who has a disease and who does not. Validity has two components: sensitivity and specificity. The *sensitivity* of the test is defined as the ability of the test to identify correctly those who *have* the disease. The *specificity* of the test is defined as the ability of the test to identify correctly those who *do not have* the disease.

Tests with Dichotomous Results (Positive or Negative)

Suppose we have a hypothetical population of 1,000 people, of whom 100 have a certain disease and 900 do not. A test is available that can yield either positive or negative results. We want to use this test to try to distinguish persons who have the disease from those who do not. The results obtained by applying the test to this population of 1,000 people are shown in Table 5-1.

How good was the test? First, how good was the test in correctly identifying those who had the disease?

TABLE 5-1. Concept of the Sensitivity and Specificity of Screening Examinations

Example: Assume a population of 1,000 people, of whom 100 have a disease and 900 do not have the disease. *A Screening Test Is Used to Identify the 100 People with the Disease*

TRUE CHARACTERISTICS IN THE POPULATION

Results of Screening	Disease	No Disease	Total
Positive	80	100	180
Negative	20	800	820
Total	100	900	1,000

$$\text{Sensitivity} = \frac{80}{100} = 80\%$$

$$\text{Specificity} = \frac{800}{900} = 89\%$$

Table 5-1 indicates that of the 100 people with the disease, 80 were correctly identified as "positive" by the test, and a positive identification was missed in 20. Thus, the *sensitivity* of the test, which is defined as the proportion of diseased people who were correctly identified as "positive" by the test, is 80/100, or 80%.

Second, how good was the test in correctly identifying those who did not have the disease? Looking again at Table 5-1, of the 900 people who did not have the disease, the test correctly identified 800 as "negative." The *specificity* of the test, which is defined as the proportion of nondiseased people who are correctly identified as negative by the test, is therefore 800/900, or 89%.

Note that to calculate the sensitivity and specificity of a test, we must know who "really" has the disease and who does not from a source other than the test we are using. We are, in fact, comparing our test results with some "gold standard"—an external source of "truth" regarding the disease status of each individual in the population. Sometimes this truth may be the result of another test that has been in use, and sometimes it is the result of a more definitive, and often more invasive, test (e.g., cardiac catheterization or tissue biopsy). However, in real life, when we use a test to identify diseased and nondiseased persons in a population, we clearly do not know who has the disease and who does not. (If this were already established, testing would be pointless.) But to quantitatively assess the sensitivity and specificity of a test, we must have another source of truth with which to compare the test results.

Table 5-2 compares the results of a dichotomous test (results either positive or negative) with the actual disease status. Ideally, we would like all of the tested subjects to fall into the two cells shown in the upper left and lower right on the table: people

---

TABLE 5-2. Comparison of the Results of a Dichotomous Test with Disease Status

Test Results	TRUE CHARACTERISTICS IN THE POPULATION	
	With Disease	**Without Disease**
Positive	True positive (TP) = Have disease and have positive test	False positive (FP) = No disease, but have positive test
Negative	False negative (FN) = Have disease, but have negative test	True negative (TN) = No disease and have negative test
	$\text{Sensitivity} = \dfrac{TP}{TP + FN}$	$\text{Specificity} = \dfrac{TN}{TN + FP}$

with the disease who are correctly called "positive" by the test (*true positives*) and people without the disease who are correctly called "negative" by the test (*true negatives*). Unfortunately, such is rarely if ever the case. Some people who do not have the disease are erroneously called "positive" by the test (*false positives*), and some people with the disease are erroneously called "negative" (*false negatives*).

Why are these issues important? When we conduct a screening program, we often have a large group of people who screened positive, including both people who really have the disease (true positives) and people who do not have the disease (false positives). The issue of *false positives* is important because all people who screened positive are brought back for more sophisticated and more expensive tests. Of the several problems that result, the first is a burden on the health care system. Another is the anxiety and worry induced in persons who have been told that they have tested positive. Considerable evidence indicates that many people who are labeled "positive" by a screening test never have that label completely erased, even if the results of a subsequent evaluation are negative. For example, children labeled "positive" in a screening program for heart disease were handled as handicapped by parents and school personnel even after being told that subsequent more definitive tests were negative. In addition, such individuals may be limited in regard to employment and insurability by erroneous interpretation of positive screening test results, even if subsequent tests fail to substantiate any positive finding.

Why is the problem of *false negatives* important? If a person has the disease but is erroneously informed that the test result is negative, and if the disease is a serious one for which effective intervention is available, the problem is indeed critical. For example, if the disease is a type of cancer that is curable only in its early stages, a false-negative result could represent a virtual death sentence. Thus, the importance of false-negative results depends on the nature and severity of the disease being screened for, the effectiveness of available intervention measures, and whether the effectiveness is greater if the intervention is administered early in the natural history of the disease.

Tests of Continuous Variables

So far we have discussed a test with only two possible results: positive or negative. But we often test for a continuous variable, such as blood pressure or blood glucose level, for which there is no "positive" or "negative" result. A decision must therefore be made in establishing a cutoff level above which a test result is considered positive and below which a result is considered negative. Let us consider the diagrams shown in Figure 5-3.

Figure 5-3A shows a population of 20 diabetics and 20 nondiabetics who are being screened using a blood sugar test whose scale is shown along the vertical axis from high to low. The diabetics are represented by blue circles and the nondiabetics by red circles. We see that although blood sugar levels tend to be higher in diabetics than in nondiabetics, no level clearly separates the two groups; there is some overlap of diabetics and nondiabetics at every blood sugar level. Nevertheless, we must select a cutoff point so that those whose results fall above the cutoff can be called "positive," and can be called back for further testing, and those whose results fall below that point are called "negative," and are not called back for further testing.

Suppose a relatively high cutoff level is chosen (Fig. 5-3B). Clearly, many of the diabetics will not be identified as positive; on the other hand, most of the nondiabetics will be correctly identified as negative. If these results are distributed on a 2 × 2 table, the sensitivity of the test using this cutoff level will be 25% (5/20) and the specificity will be 90% (18/20).

What if a low cutoff level is chosen (Fig. 5-3C)? Very few diabetics would be misdiagnosed. What then is the problem? A large proportion of the nondiabetics are now identified as positive by the test. As seen in the 2 × 2 table, the sensitivity is now 85% (17/20), but the specificity is only 30% (6/20).

The difficulty is that in the real world, no vertical line separates the diabetics and nondiabetics, and they are, in fact, mixed together (Fig. 5-3D); in fact, they are not even distinguishable by red or blue circles (Fig. 5-3E). So if a high cutoff level is used (Fig. 5-3F), all those with results below the line will be assured they do not have the disease and will not be followed further; if the low cutoff is used (Fig. 5-3G), all those with results above the line will be brought back for further testing.

Figure 5-4A shows actual data regarding the distribution of blood sugar levels in diabetics and nondiabetics. Suppose we were to screen this population. If we decide to set the cutoff level so that we identify all of the diabetics (100% sensitivity), we could set the level at 80 mg/dL (Fig. 5-4B). The problem is, however, that in so doing we will also call many of the nondiabetics positive—that is, the specificity will be very low. On the other hand, if we set the level at

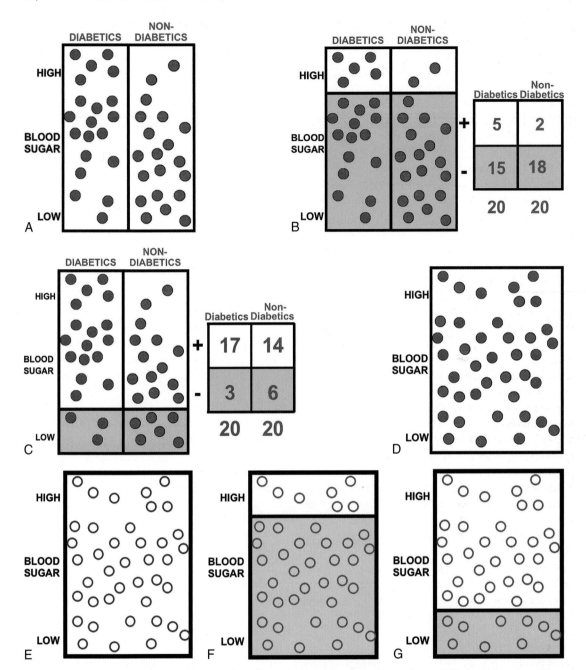

Figure 5-3. Screening for diabetes in a hypothetical population with a prevalence of 50%. Effects of choosing different cutoff levels for a positive test.

200 mg/dL (Fig. 5-4C) so that we call all the nondiabetics negative (100% specificity), we now miss many of the true diabetics because the sensitivity will be very low. Thus, there is a trade-off between sensitivity and specificity: if we increase the sensitivity by lowering the cutoff level, we decrease the specificity; if we increase the specificity by raising the cutoff

level, we decrease the sensitivity. To quote an unknown sage: "There is no such thing as a free lunch."

The dilemma involved in deciding whether to set a high cutoff or a low cutoff rests in the problem of the false positives and the false negatives that result from the testing. It is important to remember that in

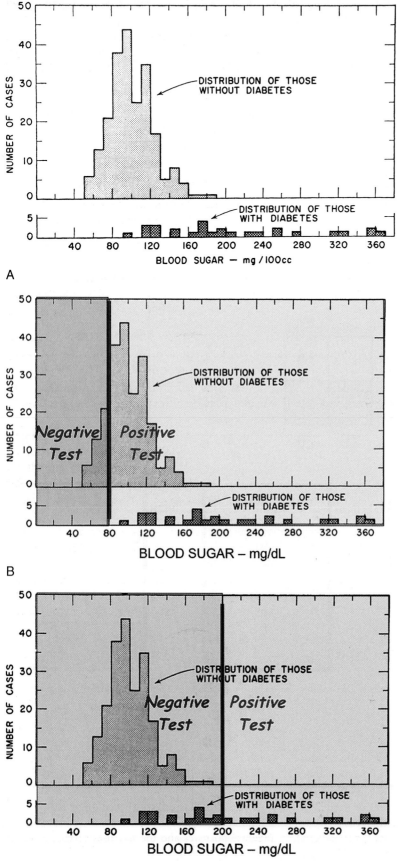

Figure 5-4. A, Distribution of blood sugar levels in diabetics and nondiabetics. **B**, Distribution of blood sugar levels in diabetics and nondiabetics with a low cutoff for positive and negative test results. **C**, Distribution of blood sugar levels in diabetics and nondiabetics with a high cutoff for positive and negative test results. (Adapted from Blumberg M: Evaluating health screening procedures. Operations Res 5:351–360, 1957.)

DISEASE

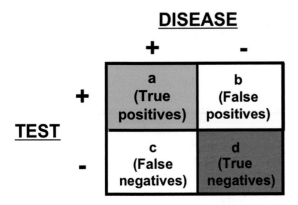

Figure 5-5. Diagram showing four possible groups resulting from screening with a dichotomous test.

screening we end up with groups classified only on the basis of their test results, such as positives and negatives. We have no information regarding their true disease status, which, of course, is the reason for the screening. In effect, the results yield not four groups, as seen in Figure 5-5, but rather two groups: one group of people who tested positive and who will be brought back for additional examinations and one group who tested negative who will not be brought back for further testing (Fig. 5-6).

The choice of a high or a low cutoff level for screening therefore depends on the importance we attach to false positives and false negatives. False positives are associated with costs—emotional and financial—as well as with the difficulty of "delabeling" a person who tests positive and is later found not to have the disease. In addition, false positive results pose a major burden to the health care system in that a large group of people need to be brought back

DISEASE

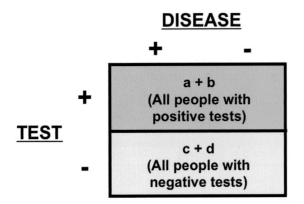

Figure 5-6. Diagram grouping all people with positive test results and all people with negative test results on screening.

for a retest, when only a few of them may have the disease. Those with false negative results, on the other hand, will be told they do not have the disease and will not be followed, so serious disease might possibly be missed at an early treatable stage. Thus, the choice of cutoff level relates to the relative importance of false positivity and false negativity for the disease in question.

USE OF MULTIPLE TESTS

Often several screening tests may be applied in the same individuals—either sequentially or simultaneously. The results of these approaches are described in this section.

Sequential (Two-stage) Testing

In sequential or two-stage screening, a less expensive, less invasive, or less uncomfortable test is generally performed first, and those who screen positive are recalled for further testing with a more expensive, more invasive, or more uncomfortable test, which may have greater sensitivity and specificity. It is hoped that bringing back for further testing only those who screen positive will reduce the problem of false positives.

Consider the hypothetical example in Figure 5-7, in which a population is screened for diabetes using a test with a sensitivity of 70% and a specificity of 80%. How are the data shown in this table obtained? The disease prevalence in this population is given as 5%, so that in the population of 10,000, 500 persons have the disease. With a sensitivity of 70%, the test will correctly identify 350 of the 500 people who have the disease. With a specificity of 80%, the test will correctly identify as nondiabetic 7,600 of the 9,500 people who are free of diabetes; however, 1,900 of these 9,500 will have positive

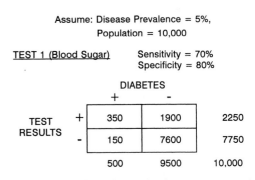

Figure 5-7. Hypothetical example of a two-stage screening program: I.

Assume: Disease Prevalence = 5%, Population = 10,000

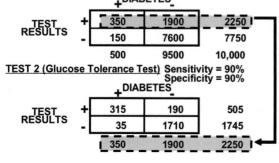

Figure 5-8. Hypothetical example of a two-stage screening program: II.

results. Thus a total of 2,250 people will test positive and will be brought back for a second test. (Remember that in real life we do not have the vertical line separating diabetics and nondiabetics, and we do not know that 350 of the 2,250 have diabetes.)

Now those 2,250 people are brought back and screened using a second test (such as a glucose tolerance test), which for purposes of this example is assumed to have a sensitivity of 90% and a specificity of 90%. Figure 5-8 again shows test 1 together with test 2, which deals only with the 2,250 people who tested positive in the first screening test and have been brought back for second-stage screening.

Since 350 people (of the 2,250) have the disease and the test has a sensitivity of 90%, 315 of those 350 will be correctly identified as positive. Because 1,900 (of the 2,250) do not have diabetes and the test specificity is 90%, 1,710 of the 1,900 will be correctly identified as negative and 190 will be false positives.

We are now able to calculate the *net sensitivity* and the *net specificity* of using both tests in sequence. After finishing both tests, 315 people of the total 500 people with diabetes in this population of 10,000 will have been correctly called positive: 315/500 = 63% *net sensitivity*. Thus, there is a loss in net sensitivity by using both tests. To calculate *net specificity*, note that 7,600 people of the 9,500 in this population who do not have diabetes were correctly called negative in the first-stage screening and were not tested further; an additional 1,710 of those 9,500 nondiabetics were correctly called negative in the second-stage screening. Thus a total of 7,600 + 1,710 of the 9,500 nondiabetics were correctly called negative: 9,310/9,500 = 98% *net specificity*. Thus, use of both tests has resulted in a gain in *net specificity*.

Simultaneous Testing

Let us now turn to the use of simultaneous tests. Let us assume that, in a population of 1,000 people, the prevalence of a disease is 20%. Therefore, 200 people have the disease, but we do not know who they are. In order to identify the 200 people who have this disease, we screen this population of 1,000 using 2 tests for this disease, test A and test B, at the same time. Let us assume that the sensitivity and specificity of the two tests are as follows:

Test A	Test B
Sensitivity = 80%	Sensitivity = 90%
Specificity = 60%	Specificity = 90%

Net Sensitivity Using Two Simultaneous Tests

The first question we ask is, "What is the *net sensitivity* using test A and test B *simultaneously*?" To be considered positive and therefore included in the numerator for net sensitivity for two tests used simultaneously, a person must be identified as positive by test A, test B, or both tests.

To calculate net sensitivity, let us first consider the results of screening with test A whose sensitivity is 80%: of the 200 people who have the disease, 160 test positive (Table 5-3). In Figure 5-9A, the oval represents the 200 people who have the disease. In Figure 5-9B the pink circle within the oval represents the 160 who test positive with test A. These 160 are the true positives using test A.

Consider next the results of screening with test B whose sensitivity is 90% (Table 5-4). Of the 200 people who have the disease, 180 test positive by test B. In Figure 5-9C, the oval again represents the 200 people who have the disease. The blue circle within

TABLE 5-3. **Results of Screening with Test A**		
	POPULATION	
Results of Screening	**Disease**	**No Disease**
Positive	160	320
Negative	40	480
Total	200	800
	Sensitivity = 80%	
	Specificity = 60%	

TABLE 5-4. **Results of Screening with Test B**		
	POPULATION	
Results of Screening	**Disease**	**No Disease**
Positive	180	80
Negative	20	720
Total	200	800
	Sensitivity = 90%	
	Specificity = 90%	

TABLE 5-5. **Results of Screening with Test A**		
	POPULATION	
Results of Screening	**Disease**	**No Disease**
Positive	160	320
Negative	40	480
Total	200	800
	Sensitivity = 80%	
	Specificity = 60%	

the oval represents the 180 who test positive with test B. These 180 are the true positives using test B.

In order to calculate the numerator for net sensitivity, we cannot just add the number of persons who tested positive using test A to those who tested positive using test B because some people tested positive on both tests. These people are shown in lavender by the overlapping area of the two circles, and we do not want to count them twice (Fig. 5-9D). How do we determine how many people tested positive on both tests?

Test A has a sensitivity of 80% and thus identifies as positive 80% of the 200 who have the disease (160 people). Test B has a sensitivity of 90%. Therefore, it identifies as positive 90% of the same 160 people who are identified by test A (144 people). Thus, when tests A and B are used simultaneously, 144 people are identified as positive by both tests (Fig. 5-9E).

Recall that test A correctly identified 160 people with the disease as positive. Because 144 of them were identified by both tests, $160 - 144$, or 16 people, were correctly identified *only* by test A.

Test B correctly identified 180 of the 200 people with the disease as positive. Because 144 of them were identified by both tests, $180 - 144$, or 36 people, were correctly identified *only* by test B. Thus, as seen in Figure 5-9F, the net sensitivity using tests A and B simultaneously

$$= \frac{16 + 144 + 36}{200} = \frac{196}{200} = 98\%$$

Net Specificity Using Two Simultaneous Tests

The next question is, "What is the *net specificity* using test A and test B simultaneously?" To be included in the numerator for net specificity for two tests used

simultaneously, a person must be identified as *negative by both tests*. In order to calculate the numerator for net specificity, we therefore need to determine how many people had negative results on both tests. How do we do this?

Test A has a specificity of 60% and thus correctly identifies 60% of the 800 who do not have the disease (480 people) (Table 5-5). In Figure 5-10A, the oval represents the 800 people who do not have the disease. The green circle within the oval in Figure 5-10B represents the 480 people who test negative on test A. These are the true negatives using test A.

Test B has a specificity of 90% and thus identifies as negative 90% of the 800 people who do not have the disease (720 people) (Table 5-6 and the yellow circle in Fig. 5-10C). However, to be called negative in simultaneous tests, only people who test negative on both tests are considered to have had negative results (Fig. 5-10D). These people are shown in light green

TABLE 5-6. **Results of Screening with Test B**		
	POPULATION	
Results of Screening	**Disease**	**No Disease**
Positive	180	80
Negative	20	720
Total	200	800
	Sensitivity = 90%	
	Specificity = 90%	

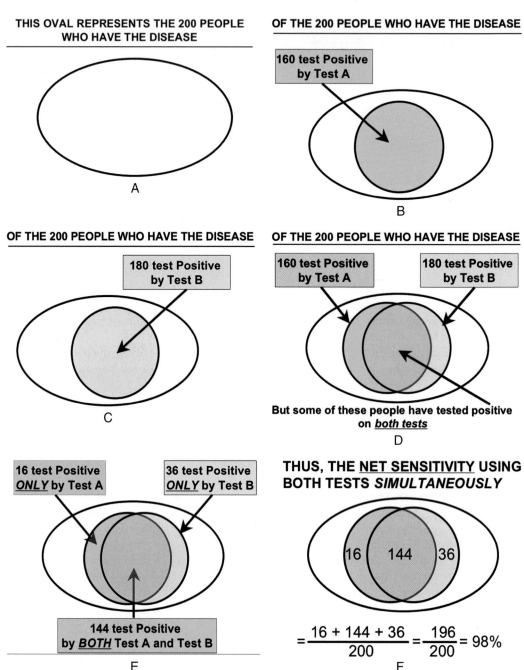

Figure 5-9. Hypothetical example of simultaneous testing: Net sensitivity.

by the overlapping area of the two circles. Test B also identifies as negative 90% of the same 480 people identified as negative by test A (432 people). Thus, as shown by the overlapping circles, when tests A and B are used simultaneously, 432 people are identified as negative by both tests (Fig. 5-10E). Thus, when tests A and B are used simultaneously (Fig. 5-10F), the net specificity = 432/800 = 54%.

Comparison of Simultaneous and Sequential Testing

Thus, when two simultaneous tests are used, there is a net gain in sensitivity (from 80% using test A and 90% using test B to 98% using both tests simultaneously). However, there is a net loss in specificity (net specificity = 54%) compared to using either test alone (specificity of 60% using test A and 90% using test B).

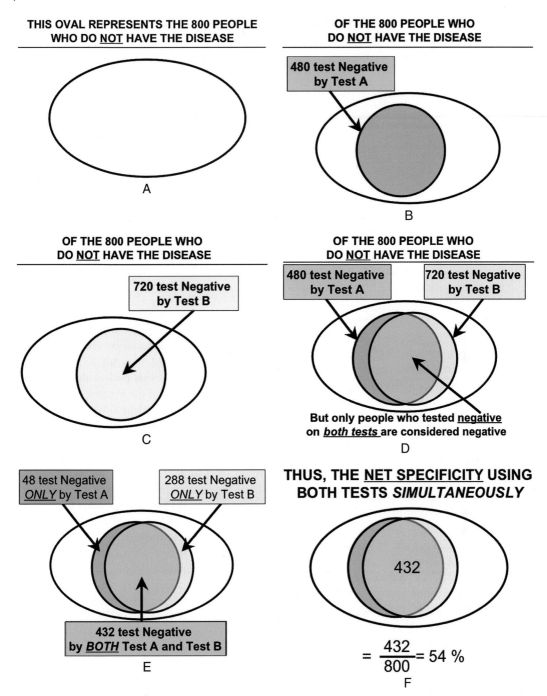

Figure 5-10. Hypothetical example of simultaneous testing: Net specificity.

In a clinical setting, multiple tests are often used simultaneously. For example, a patient admitted to a hospital may have an array of tests performed at the time of admission. When multiple tests are used simultaneously to detect a specific disease, the individual is generally considered to have tested "positive" if he or she has a positive result on any one or more of the tests. The individual is considered to have tested "negative" if he or she tests negative on all of the tests. The effects of such a testing approach on sensitivity and specificity differ from those that result from sequential testing. In sequential testing, when we retest those who tested positive on the first test, there is a loss in net sensitivity and a gain in net

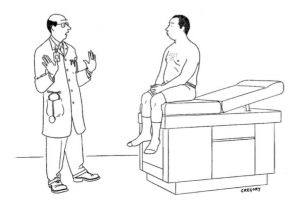

"Whoa—way too much information."

Figure 5-11. "Whoa—*way* too much information." A physician comments on excessive information. (© The New Yorker Collection 2002. Alex Gregory from cartoonbank. com. All rights reserved.)

specificity. In simultaneous testing, because an individual who tests positive on *any* one or multiple tests is considered positive, there is a gain in net sensitivity. However, to be considered negative, a person would have to test negative on *all* the tests performed. As a result, there is a loss in net specificity.

In summary, as we have seen previously, when two sequential tests are used and those who test positive by the first test are brought in for the second test, there is a net loss in sensitivity, but a net gain in specificity, compared with either test alone. However, when two simultaneous tests are used, there is a net gain in sensitivity and a net loss in specificity, compared with either test alone.

Given these results, the decision to use either sequential or simultaneous testing often is based both on the objectives of the testing, including whether testing is being done for screening or diagnostic purposes, and on practical considerations related to the setting in which the testing is being done, including the length of hospital stay, costs, and degree of invasiveness of each of the tests as well as the extent of third-party insurance coverage. Figure 5-11 shows a physician dealing with perceived information overload.

PREDICTIVE VALUE OF A TEST

So far, we have asked, "How good is the test at identifying people with the disease and people without the disease?" This is an important issue, particularly in screening free-living populations. In effect, we are asking, "If we screen a population, what proportion of people who have the disease will be correctly identified?" This is clearly an important public health consideration. In the clinical setting, however, a different question may be important for the physician: If the test results are positive in this patient, what is the probability that this patient has the disease? This is called the *positive predictive value* of the test. In other words, what proportion of patients who test positive actually have the disease in question? To calculate the predictive value, we divide the number of true positives by the total number who tested positive (true positives + false positives).

Let us return to the example shown in Table 5-1, in which a population of 1,000 persons is screened. As seen in Table 5-7, a 2 × 2 table shows the results of a dichotomous screening test in that population. Of the 1,000 subjects, 180 have a positive test result; of these 180 subjects, 80 have the disease. Therefore, the *positive predictive value* is 80/180, or 44%.

A parallel question can be asked about negative test results: "If the test result is negative, what is the probability that this patient does not have the disease?" This is called the *negative predictive value* of the test. It is calculated by dividing the number of true negatives by all those who tested negative (true negatives + false negatives). Looking again at the example in Table 5-7, 820 people have a negative test result, and of these, 800 do not have the disease. Thus, the *negative predictive value* is 800/820, or 98%. In the discussion of predictive value that follows, the term *predictive value* is used to denote the positive predictive value of the test.

Every test that a physician performs—history, physical examination, laboratory tests, X-rays, electrocardiograms, and other procedures—is used to enhance the physician's ability to make a correct diagnosis. What he or she wants to know after administering a test to a patient is: "Given this positive test result, what is the likelihood that the patient has the disease?"

Unlike the sensitivity and specificity of the test, which can be considered characteristic of the test being used, the predictive value is affected by two factors: the prevalence of the disease in the population tested and, when the disease is infrequent, the specificity of the test being used. Both of these relationships are discussed in the following sections.

Relationship between Predictive Value and Disease Prevalence

The relationship between predictive value and *disease prevalence* can be seen in the example given in Table

TABLE 5-7. Predictive Value of a Test

| Results of Screening | POPULATION | | Total |
	Disease	No Disease	
Positive	80	100	180
Negative	20	800	820
Total	100	900	1,000

$$\text{Positive predictive value} = \frac{80}{180} = 44\%$$

$$\text{Negative predictive value} = \frac{800}{820} = 98\%$$

5-8. First, let us direct our attention to the upper part of the table. Assume that we are using a test with a sensitivity of 99% and a specificity of 95% in a population of 10,000 people in which the disease prevalence is 1%. Because the prevalence is 1%, 100 of the 10,000 persons have the disease and 9,900 do not. With a sensitivity of 99%, the test correctly identifies 99 of the 100 people who have the disease. With a specificity of 95%, the test correctly identifies as negative 9,405 of the 9,900 people who do not have the disease. Thus, in this population with a 1% prevalence, 594 people are identified as positive by the test (99 + 495). However, of these 594 people, 495 (83%) are false positives and the positive predictive value is therefore 99/594, or only 17%.

Let us now apply the same test—with the same sensitivity and specificity—to a population with a higher disease prevalence, 5%, as seen in the lower part of Table 5-8. Using calculations similar to those used in the upper part of the table, the positive predictive value is now 51%. Thus, the higher prevalence

in the screened population has led to a marked increase in the positive predictive value using the same test. Figure 5-12 shows the relationship between disease prevalence and predictive value. Clearly, most of the gain in predictive value occurs with increases in prevalence at the lowest rates of disease prevalence.

Why should we be concerned about the relationship between predictive value and disease prevalence? As we have seen, the higher the prevalence, the higher the predictive value. Therefore, a screening program is most productive and efficient if it is directed to a high-risk target population. Screening a total population for a relatively infrequent disease can be very wasteful of resources and may yield few previously undetected cases relative to the amount of effort involved. However, if a high-risk subset can be identified and screening can be directed to this group, the program is likely to be far more productive. In addition, a high-risk population may be more motivated to participate in such a screening program and more

TABLE 5-8. Relationship of Disease Prevalence to Positive Predictive Value

EXAMPLE: SENSITIVITY = 99%, SPECIFICITY = 95%

Disease Prevalence	Test Results	Sick	Not Sick	Totals	Positive Predictive Value
1%	+	99	495	594	$\dfrac{99}{594} = 17\%$
	−	1	9,405	9,406	
	Totals	100	9,900	10,000	
5%	+	495	475	970	$\dfrac{495}{970} = 51\%$
	−	5	9,025	9,030	
	Totals	500	9,500	10,000	

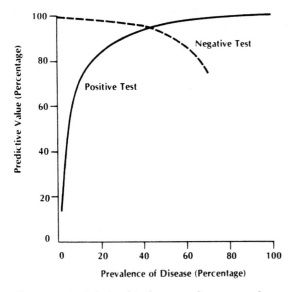

Figure 5-12. Relationship between disease prevalence and predictive value in a test with 95% sensitivity and 95% specificity. (From Mausner JS, Kramer S: Mausner and Bahn Epidemiology: An Introductory Text. Philadelphia, WB Saunders, 1985, p 221.)

likely to take recommended action if their screening results are positive.

The relationship between predictive value and disease prevalence also shows that the results of any test must be interpreted in the context of the prevalence of the disease in the population from which the subject originates. An interesting example is seen with the measurement of the α-fetoprotein (AFP) level in amniotic fluid for prenatal diagnosis of spina bifida. Figure 5-13 shows the distribution of AFP levels in amniotic fluid in normal pregnancies and in pregnancies in which the fetus has spina bifida, which is a neural tube defect. Although the distribution is bimodal, there is a range in which the curves overlap,

and within that range, it may not always be clear to which curve the mother and fetus belong. Sheffield and coworkers[1] reviewed the literature and constructed artificial populations of 10,000 women screened for amniotic fluid AFP to identify fetuses with spina bifida. They created two populations: one at high risk for spina bifida and the other at normal risk.

Table 5-9 shows the calculations for both high-risk and low-risk women. Which women are at high risk for having a child with spina bifida? It is known that women who have previously had a child with a neural tube defect are at increased risk because the defect is known to repeat in siblings. In these calculations, the positive predictive value is found to be 82.9%. Which women are at low risk, but would still have an amniocentesis? These are older women who are undergoing amniocentesis because of concern about possible Down syndrome or some other defect associated with pregnancy at an advanced maternal age. The risk of spina bifida, however, is not related to maternal age, so these women are not at increased risk for having a child with spina bifida. The calculation shows that, using the same test for AFP as was used for the high-risk women, the positive predictive value of the test is only 41.7%, considerably less than it was in a high-risk group.

Thus, we see that the same test can have a very different predictive value when it is administered to a high-risk (high prevalence) population or to a low-risk (low prevalence) population. This has clear clinical implications: A woman may make a decision to terminate a pregnancy and a physician may formulate advice to such a woman on the basis of the test results. However, the same test result may be interpreted differently, depending on whether the woman comes from a pool of high-risk or low-risk women, which will be reflected in the positive predictive value of the test. Consequently, by itself, the test result

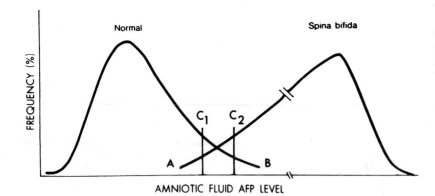

Figure 5-13. Amniotic fluid α-fetoprotein (AFP) levels in normal subjects and subjects with spina bifida. (From Sheffield LI, Sackett DL, Goldsmith CH, et al: A clinical approach to the use of predictive values in the prenatal diagnosis of neural tube defects. Am J Obstet Gynecol 145:319–324, 1983.)

TABLE 5-9. Calculations of Predictive Values for Neural Tube Defects (NTD)* for α-Fetoprotein (AFP) Test in High- and Low-Risk Women

		PREGNANCY OUTCOME			
	AFP Test	NTD	Normal	Totals	Predictive Value (%)
High-risk women	Abnormal	87	18	105	82.9
	Normal	13	9,882	9,895	99.9
	Totals	100	9,900	10,000	
Low-risk women	Abnormal	128	179	307	41.7
	Normal	19	99,674	99,693	99.98
	Totals	147	99,853	100,000	

*Spina bifida or encephalocele.
From Sheffield LI, Sackett DL, Goldsmith CH, et al: A clinical approach to the use of predictive values in the prenatal diagnosis of neural tube defects. Am J Obstet Gynecol 145:319–324, 1983.

may not be sufficient to serve as a guide without taking into account the other considerations just described.

The following true examples highlight the importance of this issue:

The head of a firefighters' union consulted a university cardiologist because the fire department physician had read an article in a leading medical journal reporting that a certain electrocardiographic finding was highly predictive of serious, generally unrecognized, coronary heart disease. On the basis of this article, the fire department physician was disqualifying many young, able-bodied firefighters from active duty. The cardiologist read the paper and found that the study had been carried out in hospitalized patients.

What was the problem? Because hospitalized patients have a much higher prevalence of heart disease than does a group of young firefighters, the fire department physician had erroneously taken the high predictive value obtained in studying a high-prevalence population and inappropriately applied it to a low-prevalence population of healthy firefighters, in whom the same test would actually have a much lower predictive value.

Another example:

A physician visited his general internist for a regular annual medical examination, which included a stool examination for occult blood. One of the three stool specimens examined in the test was positive. The internist told his physician-patient that the result was of no significance because he regularly encountered many false-positive test results in his busy practice. The test was repeated, and all three stool specimens were now negative. Nevertheless, sensing his patient's lingering concerns, the internist referred his physician-patient to a gastroenterologist. The gastroenterologist said, "In my experience, the positive stool finding is serious. Such a finding is almost always associated with pathologic gastrointestinal disorders. The subsequent negative test results mean nothing, because you could have a tumor that only bleeds intermittently."

Who was correct in this episode? The answer is that both the general internist and the gastroenterologist were correct. The internist gave his assessment of predictive value based on his experience in his general medical practice—a population with a low prevalence of serious gastrointestinal disease. On the other hand, the gastroenterologist gave his assessment of the predictive value of the test based on his experience in his referral practice—a practice in which most patients are referred because of a likelihood of serious gastrointestinal illness—a high-prevalence population.

Relationship between Positive Predictive Value and Specificity of the Test

A second factor that affects the positive predictive value of a test is the *specificity* of the test. Examples of this are shown first in graphical form and then in tabular form. Figure 5-14A through D diagrams the results of screening a population; however, the 2 × 2 tables in these figures differ from those shown in earlier figures. Each cell is drawn with its size proportional to the population it represents. In each figure the cells that represent persons who tested positive

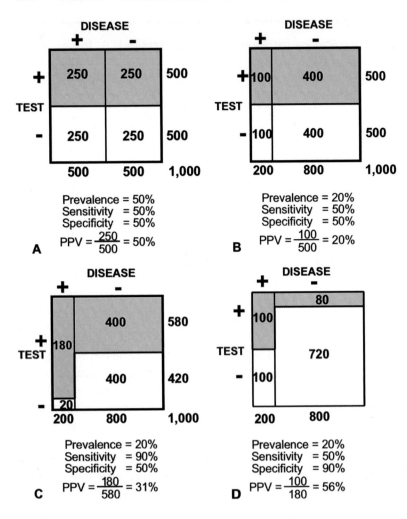

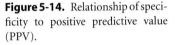

Figure 5-14. Relationship of specificity to positive predictive value (PPV).

are shaded blue; these are the cells that will be used in calculating the positive predictive value.

Figure 5-14A presents the baseline screened population that is used in our discussion: a population of 1,000 people in whom the prevalence is 50%; thus, 500 people have the disease and 500 do not. In analyzing this figure, we also assume that the screening test that was used has a sensitivity of 50% and a specificity of 50%. Because 500 people tested positive, and 250 of these have the disease, the predictive value is 250/500, or 50%.

Fortunately, the prevalence of most diseases is much lower than 50%; we are generally dealing with relatively infrequent diseases. Therefore, Figure 5-14B assumes a lower prevalence of 20% (although even this would be an unusually high prevalence for most diseases). Both the sensitivity and the specificity remain at 50%. Now only 200 of the 1000 people have the disease, and the vertical line separating dis-

eased from nondiseased persons is shifted to the left. The predictive value is now calculated as 100/500, or 20%.

Given that we are screening a population with the lower prevalence rate, can we improve the predictive value? What would be the effect on predictive value if we increased the sensitivity of the test? Figure 5-14C shows the results when we leave the prevalence at 20% and the specificity at 50% but increase the sensitivity to 90%. The predictive value is now 180/580, or 31%, a modest increase.

What if, instead of increasing the sensitivity of the test, we increase its specificity? Figure 5-14D shows the results when prevalence remains 20% and sensitivity remains 50%, but specificity is increased to 90%. The predictive value is now 100/180, or 56%. Thus, an increase in specificity resulted in a much greater increase in predictive value than did the same increase in sensitivity.

TABLE 5-10. Relationship of Specificity to Predictive Value

EXAMPLE: PREVALENCE = 10%, SENSITIVITY = 100%

Specificity	Test Results	Sick	Not Sick	Totals	Predictive Value
70%	+	1,000	2,700	3,700	$\dfrac{1,000}{3,700} = 27\%$
	−	0	6,300	6,300	
	Totals	1,000	9,000	10,000	
95%	+	1,000	450	1,450	$\dfrac{1,000}{1,450} = 69\%$
	−	0	8,550	8,550	
	Totals	1,000	9,000	10,000	

Why does specificity have a greater effect than sensitivity on predictive value? The answer becomes clear by examining these figures. Because we are dealing with infrequent diseases, most of the population falls to the right of the vertical line. Consequently, any change to the right of the vertical line affects a greater number of people than would a comparable change to the left of the line. Thus, a change in specificity has a greater effect on predictive value than does a comparable change in sensitivity. If we were dealing with a high-prevalence disease, the situation would be different.

The effect of changes in specificity on predictive value is also seen in Table 5-10 in a form similar to that used in Table 5-8. As seen in this example, even with 100% sensitivity, a change in specificity from 70% to 95% has a dramatic effect on the positive predictive value (PPV).

RELIABILITY (REPEATABILITY) OF TESTS

Let us consider another aspect of assessing diagnostic and screening tests—the question of whether a test is reliable or repeatable. Can the results obtained be replicated if the test is repeated? Clearly, regardless of the sensitivity and specificity of a test, if the test results cannot be reproduced, the value and usefulness of the test are minimal. The rest of this chapter focuses on the reliability or repeatability of diagnostic and screening tests. The factors that contribute to the variation between test results are discussed first: intrasubject variation (variation within individual subjects), intraobserver variation (variation in the reading of test results by the same reader), and interobserver variation (variation between those reading the test results).

Intrasubject Variation

The values obtained in measuring many human characteristics often vary over time, even during a short period. Table 5-11 shows changes in blood pressure readings over a 24-hour period in three individuals. Variability over time is considerable. This, as well as the conditions under which certain tests are conducted (e.g., postprandially or postexercise, at home or in a physician's office), clearly can lead to different results in the same individual. Therefore, in evaluating any test result, it is important to consider the conditions under which the test was performed, including the time of day.

TABLE 5-11. Examples Showing Variation in Blood Pressure Readings during a 24-Hour Period

Blood Pressure (mm Hg)	Female Aged 27 yrs	Female Aged 62 yrs	Male Aged 33 yrs
Basal	110/70	132/82	152/109
Lowest hour	86/47	102/61	123/78
Highest hour	126/79	172/94	153/107
Casual	108/64	155/93	157/109

From Richardson DW, Honour AJ, Fenton GW, et al: Variation in arterial pressure throughout the day and night. Clin Sci 26:445, 1964.

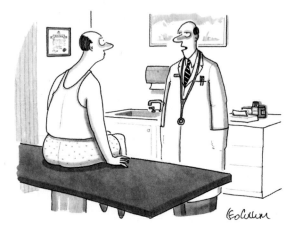

"This is a second opinion. At first, I thought you had something else."

Figure 5-15. "This *is* a second opinion. At first, I thought you had something else." One view of a second opinion. (© The New Yorker Collection 1995. Leo Cullum from cartoonbank.com. All rights reserved.)

Intraobserver Variation

Sometimes variation occurs between two or more readings of the same test results made by the same observer. For example, a radiologist who reads the same group of X-rays at two different times may read one or more of the X-rays differently the second time. Tests and examinations differ in the degree to which subjective factors enter into the observer's conclusions, and the greater the subjective element in the reading, the greater the intraobserver variation in readings is likely to be (Fig. 5-15).

Interobserver Variation

Another important consideration is variation between observers. Two examiners often do not derive the same result. The extent to which observers agree or disagree is an important issue, whether we are considering physical examinations, laboratory tests, or other means of assessing human characteristics. We therefore need to be able to express the extent of agreement in quantitative terms.

Overall Percent Agreement

Table 5-12 shows a schema for examining variation between observers. Two observers were instructed to categorize each test result into one of the following four categories: abnormal, suspect, doubtful, and normal. This diagram might refer, for example, to readings performed by two radiologists. In this diagram, the readings of observer 1 are cross-tabulated against those of observer 2. The number of readings in each cell is denoted by a letter of the alphabet. Thus, A X-rays were read as abnormal by both radiologists. C X-rays were read as abnormal by radiologist 2 and as doubtful by radiologist 1. M X-rays were read as abnormal by radiologist 1 and as normal by radiologist 2.

As seen in Table 5-12, to calculate the overall percent agreement, we add the numbers in all of the cells in which readings by both radiologists agreed (A + F + K + P), divide that sum by the total number of X-rays read, and multiply the result by 100 to yield a percentage. Figure 5-16A shows the use of this approach for a test with possible readings of either "positive" or "negative."

In general, most persons who are tested have negative results. This is shown in Figure 5-16B, in which the size of each cell is drawn in proportion to the number of people in that cell. There is likely to be considerable agreement between the two observers about these negative, or normal, subjects (cell d). Therefore, when percent agreement is calculated for all study subjects, its value may be high only because of the large number of clearly negative findings (cell

	Reading No. 1			
Reading No. 2	*Abnormal*	*Suspect*	*Doubtful*	*Normal*
Abnormal	$\boxed{A}$ +	B	C	D
Suspect	E	$\boxed{F}$ +	G	H
Doubtful	I	J	$\boxed{K}$ +	L
Normal	M	N	O	$\boxed{P}$

$$\text{Percent agreement} = \frac{A + F + K + P}{\text{Total readings}} \times 100$$

TABLE 5-12. **Observer or Instrument Variation: Percent Agreement**

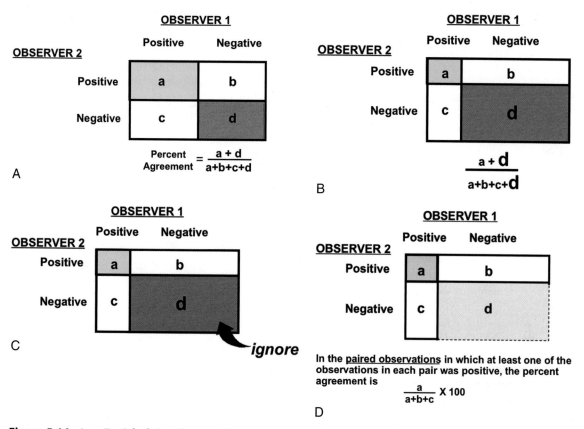

Figure 5-16. A to **D,** Calculating the overall percent agreement between two observers. **A,** Percent agreement when examining paired observations between observer 1 and observer 2. **B,** Percent agreement when examining paired observations between observer 1 and observer 2, considering that cell d (agreement on the negatives) is very high. **C,** Percent agreement when examining paired observations between observer 1 and observer 2, ignoring cell d. **D,** Percent agreement when examining paired observations between observer 1 and observer 2, using only cells a, b, and c for the calculation.

d) on which the observers agree. Thus, the high value may conceal significant disagreement between the observers in identifying subjects who are considered positive by at least one observer.

One approach to this problem, seen in Figure 5-16C, is to disregard the subjects who were labeled negative by both observers (cell d) and to calculate percent agreement using as a denominator only the subjects who were labeled abnormal by at least one observer (cells a, b, and c) (Fig. 5-16D).

Thus, in the paired observations in which at least one of the findings in each pair was positive, the following equation is applicable:

$$\text{Percent agreement} = \frac{a}{a + b + c} \times 100$$

Kappa Statistic
Percent agreement is also significantly affected by the fact that even if two observers use completely different criteria to identify subjects as positive or negative,

we would expect the observers to agree solely as a function of chance.

This can be shown intuitively in the following example: You are the director of a radiology department that is understaffed one day, and a large number of chest X-rays remain to be read. To solve your problem, you go out to the street and ask a few neighborhood residents, who have no background in biology or medicine, to read X-rays as either positive or negative. The first person goes through the pile of X-rays, reading them haphazardly as positive, negative, negative, positive, and so on. The second person does the same, in the same way. Given that both readers have no knowledge, criteria, or standards for reading X-rays, would any of their readings on a specific X-ray agree? The answer is clearly yes; they would agree in some cases, purely by chance.

However, if we want to know how well two observers read X-rays, we might ask, "To what extent do their readings agree *beyond what we would expect by chance alone?*" In other words, to what extent does the agreement between the two observers exceed the level of agreement that would result just from chance? One approach to answering this question is to calculate the kappa statistic, proposed by Cohen in 1960.[2]

In order to understand kappa, we ask two questions. First, how much better is the agreement between the observers' readings than would be expected by chance alone? This can be calculated as the percent agreement observed minus the percent agreement we would expect by chance alone. This is the numerator of kappa:

(Percent agreement observed)

  − (Percent agreement expected by chance alone)

Our second question is, "What is the most that the two observers could have improved their agreement over the agreement that would be expected by chance alone?" Clearly, the maximum that they could agree would be 100% (full agreement—the two observers agree completely). Therefore, the most that we could expect them to be able to improve would be:

100% − (Percent agreement expected by chance alone)

This is the denominator of kappa.

Kappa expresses the extent to which the observed agreement exceeds that which would be expected by chance alone (numerator) relative to the most that the observers could hope to improve their agreement (i.e., 100% − agreement expected by chance alone) [denominator].

Thus kappa quantifies the extent to which the observed agreement that the observers achieved exceeds that which would be expected by chance alone, and expresses it as the proportion of the maximum improvement that could occur beyond the agreement expected by chance alone. The kappa statistic can be defined by the equation:

Kappa =

$$\frac{\left(\begin{array}{c}\text{Percent agreement}\\\text{observed}\end{array}\right)-\left(\begin{array}{c}\text{Percent agreement}\\\text{expected by chance alone}\end{array}\right)}{100\%-\left(\begin{array}{c}\text{Percent agreement}\\\text{expected by chance alone}\end{array}\right)}$$

To calculate the numerator for kappa, we must first calculate the amount of agreement that might be expected on the basis of chance alone. Let us consider data reported on the histologic classification of lung cancer that focused on the reproducibility of the decisions of pathologists in subtyping cases of non–small cell lung carcinoma.[3] Figure 5-17A shows data comparing the findings of two pathologists in subtyping 75 such cases.

The first question is, "What is the observed agreement between the two pathologists?" Figure 5-17B shows the readings by pathologist A along the bottom of the table and those of pathologist B along the right margin. Thus, pathologist A identified 45 (or 60%) of all of the 75 slides as grade II and 30 (or 40%) of the slides as grade III. Pathologist B identified 44 (or 58.7%) of all of the slides as grade II and 31 (or 41.3%) of the slides as grade III. As discussed earlier, the percent agreement is calculated by the following equation:

$$\text{Percent agreement} = \frac{41+27}{75} \times 100 = 90.7\%$$

That is, the two pathologists agreed on 90.7% of the readings.

The next question is, "If the two pathologists had used entirely different sets of criteria, how much agreement would have been expected solely on the basis of chance?" Pathologist A read 60% of all 75 slides (45 slides) as being grade II and 40% (30 slides) as grade III. If his or her readings had used criteria independent of those used by pathologist B (e.g., if pathologist A were to read 60% of any group of slides as grade II), we would expect that pathologist A would read as grade II both 60% of the slides that pathologist B had called grade II and 60% of the slides that pathologist B had called grade III. Therefore, we would expect that 60% (26.4) of the 44 slides called grade II by pathologist B would be called grade II by pathologist A and that 60% (18.6) of the 31 slides called grade III by pathologist B would also be called grade II by pathologist A (Fig. 5-17C). Of the 31 slides called grade III by pathologist B, 40% (12.4) would also be classified as grade III by pathologist A.

Thus, the agreement expected by chance alone would

$$= \frac{26.4}{75} + \frac{12.4}{75} = \frac{38.8}{75} = 51.7\%$$

of all slides read.

Having calculated the figures needed for the numerator and denominator, kappa can now be calculated as follows:

$$\text{Kappa} = \frac{\left(\begin{array}{c}\text{Percent}\\\text{observed}\\\text{agreement}\end{array}\right)-\left(\begin{array}{c}\text{Percent agreement}\\\text{expected by}\\\text{chance alone}\end{array}\right)}{100\%-\left(\begin{array}{c}\text{Percent agreement}\\\text{expected by}\\\text{chance alone}\end{array}\right)}$$

$$= \frac{90.7\% - 51.7\%}{100\% - 51.7\%} = \frac{39\%}{48.3\%} = 0.81$$

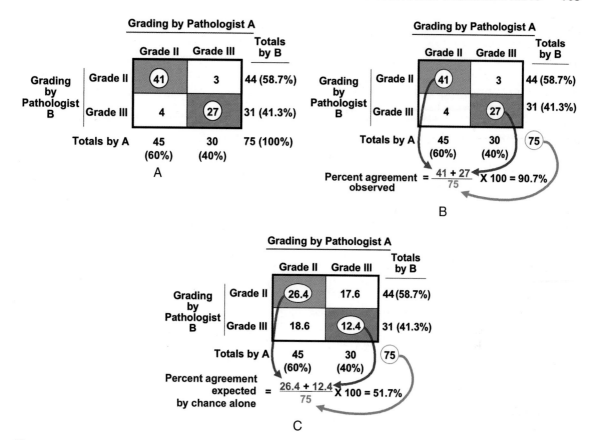

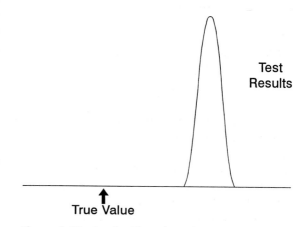

Figure 5-17. A, Histologic classification by subtype of 75 slides of non–small cell carcinoma, by two pathologists (A and B). **B,** Percent agreement by pathologist A and pathologist B. **C,** Percent agreement by pathologist A and pathologist B *expected by chance alone.* (Adapted from Ghandur-Mnaymneh L, Raub WA, Sridhar KS, et al: The accuracy of the histological classification of lung carcinoma and its reproducibility: A study of 75 archival cases of adenosquamous carcinoma. Cancer Invest 11:641, 1993.)

Landis and Koch[4] suggested that a kappa greater than 0.75 represents excellent agreement beyond chance, a kappa below 0.40 represents poor agreement, and a kappa of 0.40 to 0.75 represents intermediate to good agreement. Testing for the statistical significance of kappa is described by Fleiss.[5] Considerable discussion has arisen about the appropriate use of kappa, a subject addressed by MacLure and Willett.[6]

RELATIONSHIP BETWEEN VALIDITY AND RELIABILITY

To conclude this chapter, let us compare validity and reliability using a graphical presentation.

The horizontal line in Figure 5-18 is a scale of values for a given variable, such as blood glucose level, with the true value indicated. The test results obtained are shown by the curve. The curve is narrow, indicating that the results are quite reliable (repeatable); unfortunately, however, they cluster

far from the true value, so they are not valid. Figure 5-19 shows a curve that is broad and therefore has low reliability. However, the values obtained cluster around the true value and, thus,

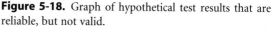

Figure 5-18. Graph of hypothetical test results that are reliable, but not valid.

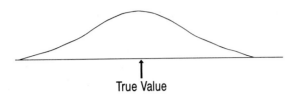

Figure 5-19. Graph of hypothetical test results that are valid, but not reliable.

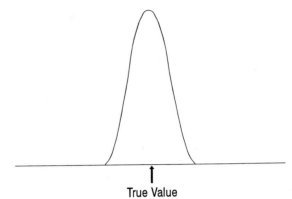

Figure 5-20. Graph of hypothetical test results that are both valid and reliable.

are valid. Clearly, what we would like to achieve are results that are both valid and reliable (Fig. 5-20).

It is important to point out that in Figure 5-19, in which the distribution of the test results is a broad curve centered on the true value, we describe the results as valid. However, the results are valid only for a group (i.e., they tend to cluster around the true value). It is important to remember that what may be valid for a group or a population may not be so for an individual in a clinical setting. When the reliability or repeatability of a test is poor, the validity of the test for a given individual also may be poor. The distinction between group validity and individual validity is therefore important to keep in mind when assessing the quality of diagnostic and screening tests.

CONCLUSION

This chapter has discussed the validity of diagnostic and screening tests as measured by their sensitivity and specificity, their predictive value, and the reliability or repeatability of these tests. Clearly, regardless of how sensitive and specific a test may be, if its results cannot be replicated, the test is of little use. All these characteristics must, therefore, be borne in mind when evaluating such tests, together with the purpose for which the test will be used.

REFERENCES

1. Sheffield LJ, Sackett DL, Goldsmith CH, et al: A clinical approach to the use of predictive values in the prenatal diagnosis of neural tube defects. Am J Obstet Gynecol 1465:319, 1983.
2. Cohen J: A coefficient of agreement for nominal scales. Educ Psychol Meas 20:37, 1960.
3. Ghandur-Mnaymneh L, Raub WA, Sridhar KS, et al: The accuracy of the histological classification of lung carcinoma and its reproducibility: A study of 75 archival cases of adenosquamous carcinoma. Cancer Invest 11:641, 1993.
4. Landis JR, Koch GG: The measurement of observer agreement for categorical data. Biometrics 33:159, 1977.
5. Fleiss JL: Statistical Methods for Rates and Proportions, 2nd ed. New York, John Wiley & Sons, 1981.
6. MacLure M, Willett WC: Misinterpretation and misuse of the kappa statistic. Am J Epidemiol 126:161, 1987.

REVIEW QUESTIONS FOR CHAPTER 5

Questions 1, 2, and 3 are based on the information given below:

A physical examination was used to screen for breast cancer in 2,500 women with biopsy-proven adenocarcinoma of the breast and in 5,000 age- and race-matched control women. The results of the physical examination were positive (i.e., a mass was palpated) in 1,800 cases and in 800 control women, all of whom showed no evidence of cancer at biopsy.

1. The sensitivity of the physical examination was:

_____

2. The specificity of the physical examination was:

_____

3. The positive predictive value of the physical examination was: _____

Question 4 is based on the following information:

A screening test is used in the same way in two similar populations, but the proportion of false-positive results among those who test positive in population A is lower than that among those who test positive in population B.

4. What is the likely explanation for this finding?
   a. It is impossible to determine what caused the difference
   b. The specificity of the test is lower in population A
   c. The prevalence of disease is lower in population A
   d. The prevalence of disease is higher in population A
   e. The specificity of the test is higher in population A

Question 5 is based on the following information:

A physical examination and an audiometric test were given to 500 persons with suspected hearing problems, of whom 300 were actually found to have them. The results of the examinations were as follows:

PHYSICAL EXAMINATION

Result	HEARING PROBLEMS	
	Present	Absent
Positive	240	40
Negative	60	160

AUDIOMETRIC TEST

Result	HEARING PROBLEMS	
	Present	Absent
Positive	270	60
Negative	30	140

5. Compared with the physical examination, the audiometric test is:
   a. Equally sensitive and specific
   b. Less sensitive and less specific
   c. Less sensitive and more specific
   d. More sensitive and less specific
   e. More sensitive and more specific

Question 6 is based on the following information:

Two pediatricians want to investigate a new laboratory test that identifies streptococcal infections. Dr. Kidd uses the standard culture test, which has a sensitivity of 90% and a specificity of 96%. Dr. Childs uses the new test, which is 96% sensitive and 96% specific.

6. If 200 patients undergo culture with both tests, which of the following is correct?
   a. Dr. Kidd will correctly identify more people with streptococcal infection than Dr. Childs
   b. Dr. Kidd will correctly identify fewer people with streptococcal infection than Dr. Childs
   c. Dr. Kidd will correctly identify more people without streptococcal infection than Dr. Childs
   d. The prevalence of streptococcal infection is needed to determine which pediatrician will correctly identify the larger number of people with the disease

Questions 7 and 8 are based on the following information:

A colon cancer screening study is being conducted in Nottingham, England. Individuals 50 to 75 years old will be screened with the Hemoccult test. In this test, a stool sample is tested for the presence of blood.

7. The Hemoccult test has a sensitivity of 70% and a specificity of 75%. If Nottingham has a prevalence of 12/1,000 for colon cancer, what is the positive predictive value of the test?

8. If the Hemoccult test result is negative, no further testing is done. If the Hemoccult test result is positive, the individual will have a second stool sample tested with the Hemoccult II test. If this second sample also tests positive for blood, the individual will be referred for more extensive evaluation. What is the effect on net sensitivity and net specificity of this method of screening?
   a. Net sensitivity and net specificity are both increased
   b. Net sensitivity is decreased and net specificity is increased
   c. Net sensitivity remains the same and net specificity is increased
   d. Net sensitivity is increased and net specificity is decreased
   e. The effect on net sensitivity and net specificity cannot be determined from the data

Questions 9 through 12 are based on the information given below:

Two physicians were asked to classify 100 chest X-rays as abnormal or normal independently. The comparison of their classification is shown in the following table:

Classification of Chest X-Rays by Physician 1 Compared with Physician 2			
	Physician 2		
Physician 1	*Abnormal*	*Normal*	**Total**
Abnormal	40	20	60
Normal	10	30	40
Total	50	50	100

9. The simple, overall percent agreement between the two physicians out of the total is: _____
10. The overall percent agreement between the two physicians, excluding the X-rays that both physicians classified as normal, is: _____
11. The value of kappa is: _____
12. This kappa represents what level of agreement? _____

   a. Excellent
   b. Intermediate to good
   c. Poor

Chapter 6

The Natural History of Disease: Ways of Expressing Prognosis

At this point, we have learned how diagnostic and screening tests permit the categorization of sick and healthy individuals. Once a person is identified as having a disease, the question arises, "How can we characterize the natural history of the disease in quantitative terms?" Such quantification is important for several reasons. First, it is necessary to describe the severity of a disease to establish priorities for clinical services and public health programs. Second, patients often ask questions about prognosis (Fig. 6-1). Third, such quantification is important to establish a baseline for natural history, so that as new treatments become available, the effects of these treatments can be compared with the expected outcome without them. Furthermore, if different types of therapy are available for a given disease, such as surgical or medical treatments or two different types of surgical procedures, we want to be able to compare the effectiveness of the various types of therapy. Therefore, to allow such a comparison, we need a quantitative means of expressing the prognosis in groups receiving different treatments.

This chapter describes some of the ways in which prognosis can be described in quantitative terms for a group of patients. Thus, the natural history of disease (prognosis) is discussed in this chapter; later chapters discuss the issue of how to intervene in the natural history of disease to improve prognosis: Chapters 7 and 8 discuss how randomized trials are used to select the most appropriate drug or other treatment, and Chapter 18 discusses how disease can be detected at an earlier point than usual in its natural history to maximize the effectiveness of treatment.

To discuss prognosis, let us begin with a schematic representation of the natural history of disease in a patient, as shown in Figure 6-2.

Point A marks the biologic onset of disease. Often, this point cannot be identified because it occurs subclinically, perhaps as a subcellular change, such as an alteration in DNA. At some point in the progression of the disease process (point P), pathologic evidence of disease could be obtained if it were sought. Subsequently, signs and symptoms of the disease develop in the patient (point S), and at some time after that, the patient may seek medical care (point M). The patient may then receive a diagnosis (point D), after which treatment may be given (point T). The subsequent course of the disease might result in cure, control of the disease (with or without disability), or even death.

At what point do we begin to quantify survival time? Ideally, we might prefer to do so from the onset of disease. Generally, this is not possible, because the time of biologic onset in an individual is not known. If we were to count from the time at which symptoms begin, we would introduce considerable subjective variability in measuring length of survival. In general, in order to standardize the calculations, duration of survival is counted from the time of diagnosis. However, even with the use of this starting point, variability occurs, because patients differ in the point at which they seek medical care. In addition, some diseases, such as certain types of arthritis, are indolent and develop slowly, so that patients may not be able to pinpoint the onset of symptoms or the point in time at which they sought medical care. Furthermore, when survival is counted from the time of diagnosis, any patients who may have died before a diagnosis was made are excluded from the count. What effect would this problem have on our estimates of prognosis?

An important related question is, "How is the diagnosis made?" Is there a clear pathognomonic test for the disease in question? Such a test is often not available. Sometimes a disease may be diagnosed by the isolation of an infectious agent, but because people can be carriers of organisms without actually being infected, we do not always know that the isolated organism is the cause of disease. For some diseases, we might prefer to make a diagnosis by tissue confirmation, but there is often variability in the interpretation of tissue slides by different

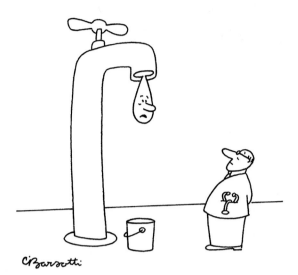

"How much time do I have, Doc?"

Figure 6-1. "How much time do I have, Doc?" Concern about prognosis. (© The New Yorker Collection 2001. Charles Barsotti from cartoonbank.com. All rights reserved.)

pathologists. An additional issue is that in certain health problems, such as headaches, lower back pain, and dysmenorrhea, there may not be a specific tissue diagnosis. Consequently, when we say that survivorship is measured from the time of diagnosis, the time frame is not always clear. These issues should be kept in mind as we proceed to discuss different approaches to estimating prognosis.

Prognosis can be expressed either in terms of deaths from the disease or in terms of survivors with the disease. Both approaches are used in the following discussion. Finally, the endpoint used for the purposes of our discussion is death. Because death is inevitable, we are not talking about dying versus not dying, but rather about extending the interval until death occurs. Other endpoints might be used, including the interval from diagnosis to recurrence of disease or from diagnosis to the time of functional impairment, disability, or changes in the patient's quality of life, all of which may be affected by the invasiveness of the available treatment or the extent to which some of the symptoms can be relieved, even if the patient's life span cannot be extended. These are all important measures, but they are not discussed in this chapter.

CASE-FATALITY RATE

The first way to express prognosis is the *case-fatality rate*, which was discussed in Chapter 4. The case-fatality rate is defined as the number of people who die of a disease divided by the number of people who have the disease. Given that a person has the disease, what is the likelihood that he or she will die of the disease? Note that the denominator for the case-fatality rate is the number of people who have the disease. This differs from a *mortality rate*, in which the denominator includes anyone at risk of dying of the disease—both persons who have the disease and persons who do not (yet) have the disease, but in whom it could develop.

The case-fatality rate does not include any explicit statement of time. However, time is expressed implicitly, because case-fatality is generally used for acute diseases in which death, if it occurs, occurs relatively soon after diagnosis. Thus, if the usual natural history of the disease is known, the term *case-fatality* refers to the period after diagnosis during which death might be expected to occur.

The case-fatality rate is ideally suited to diseases that are short-term, acute conditions. In chronic diseases, in which death may occur many years after diagnosis and the possibility of death from other causes becomes more likely, the case-fatality rate becomes a less useful measure. We therefore use different approaches for expressing prognosis in such diseases.

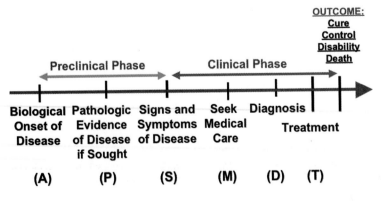

Figure 6-2. The natural history of disease in a patient.

PERSON-YEARS

A useful way of expressing mortality is in terms of the number of deaths divided by the person-years over which a group is observed. Because individuals are often observed for different periods of time, the unit used for counting observation time is the person-year. (Person-years were previously discussed in Chapter 3.) The number of person-years for two people, each of whom is observed for 5 years, is equal to that of 10 people, each of whom is observed for 1 year, that is, 10 person-years. The numbers of person-years can then be added together and the number of events (e.g., deaths) calculated per number of person-years observed.

One problem in using person-years is that each person-year is assumed to be equivalent to every other person-year (i.e., the risk in any person-year observed is the same). However, this may not be true. Consider the example in Figure 6-3 showing two examples of 10 person-years: two people each observed for 5 years and five people each observed for 2 years. Are they equivalent?

Suppose the situation is that shown in Figure 6-4, in which the period of greatest risk of dying is from shortly after diagnosis until about 20 months after diagnosis. Clearly, most of the person-years in the first example, that is, two persons observed for 5 years, will be outside the period of greatest risk (Fig. 6-5). In contrast, most of the 2-year intervals of the five persons shown in the second example will occur during the period of highest risk (Fig. 6-6). Consequently, when we compare the two examples (Fig. 6-7), more deaths would be expected in the example of five persons observed for 2 years than in the example of two persons observed for 5 years. Despite

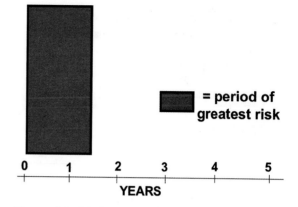

Figure 6-4. Timing of period of greatest risk is from shortly after diagnosis until about 20 months after diagnosis.

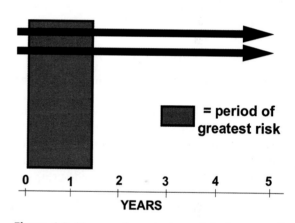

Figure 6-5. Two people, each observed for 5 years, and the relation to the period of greatest risk.

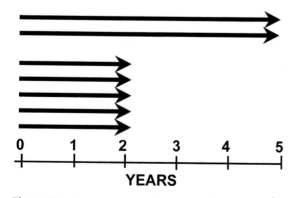

Figure 6-3. Two examples of 10 person-years: five people, each observed for 2 years, and two people, each observed for 5 years.

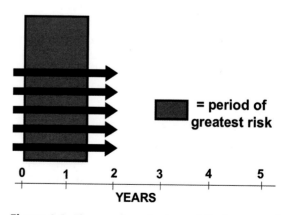

Figure 6-6. Five people, each observed for 2 years, and the relation to the period of greatest risk.

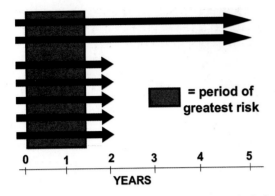

Figure 6-7. Two examples of 10 person-years in which the period of greatest risk is from shortly after diagnosis until about 20 months after diagnosis.

this issue, person-years are useful as denominators of rates of events in many situations, such as randomized trials (see Chapters 7 and 8) and cohort studies (see Chapter 9).

FIVE-YEAR SURVIVAL RATE

Another measure used to express prognosis is the *5-year survival rate*. This term is frequently used in clinical medicine, particularly in evaluating treatments for cancer.

The 5-year survival rate is the percentage of patients who are alive 5 years after treatment begins or 5 years after diagnosis. Despite the widespread use of the 5-year interval, it should be pointed out that there is nothing magical about 5 years. Certainly, no significant biologic change occurs abruptly at 5 years in the natural history of a disease that would justify its use as an endpoint. However, most deaths from cancer occur during this period after diagnosis, so 5-year survival has been used as an index of success in cancer treatment.

One problem with the use of the 5-year survival rate has become more prominent in recent years with the advent of screening programs. Let us examine a hypothetical example: Figure 6-8 shows a timeline for a woman who had biologic onset of breast cancer

in 2000. Because the disease was subclinical at that time, she had no symptoms. In 2008, she felt a lump in her breast which precipitated a visit to her physician, who made the diagnosis. The patient then underwent a mastectomy. In 2010, she died of metastatic cancer. As measured by the 5-year survival rate, which is often used in oncology as a measure of whether therapy has been successful, this patient is not a "success," because she survived for only 2 years after diagnosis.

Let us now imagine that this woman lived in a community in which there was an aggressive breast cancer screening campaign (lower timeline in Fig. 6-9). As before, biologic onset of disease occurred in 2000, but in 2005, she was identified through screening as having a very small mass in her breast. She had surgery in 2005 and died in 2010. Because she survived for 5 years after diagnosis and therapy, she would now be identified as a therapeutic success in terms of 5-year survival. However, this apparently longer survival is an artifact. Death still occurred in 2010; the patient's life was not lengthened by early detection and therapy. What has happened is that the interval between her diagnosis (and treatment) and her death was increased through earlier diagnosis, but there was no delay in the time of death. (The interval between the earlier diagnosis in 2005, made possible by screening, and the later usual time of diagnosis in 2008 is called the *lead time*. This concept is discussed in detail in Chapter 18 in the context of evaluating screening.) It is misleading to conclude that, given the patient's 5-year survival, the outcome of the second scenario is any better than that of the first, because no change in the natural history of the disease has occurred, as reflected by the year of death. Indeed, the only change that has taken place is that when the diagnosis was made 3 years earlier (2005 vs. 2008), the patient received medical care for breast

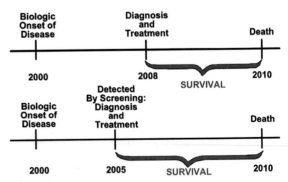

Figure 6-9. The problem of 5-year survival in a screened population: II. Earlier disease detection by screening.

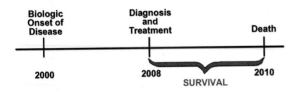

Figure 6-8. The problem of 5-year survival in a screened population: I. Situation without screening.

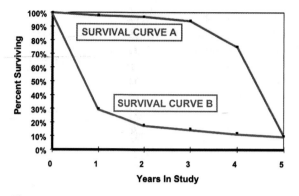

Figure 6-10. Five-year survival curves in two hypothetical populations.

cancer, with all its attendant difficulties, for an additional 3 years. Thus, when screening is performed, a higher 5-year survival rate may be observed, not because people live longer, but only because an earlier diagnosis has been made. This type of potential bias must be taken into account in evaluating any screening program before it can be concluded that the screening is beneficial.

Another problem with 5-year survival is that if we want to look at the survival experience of a group of patients who were diagnosed less than 5 years ago, we clearly cannot use this criterion, because 5 years of observation are necessary in these patients to calculate 5-year survival. Therefore, if we want to assess a therapy that was introduced less than 5 years ago, 5-year survival is not an appropriate measure.

A final issue relating to 5-year survival is shown in Figure 6-10. Here we see survival curves for two populations, A and B. Five-year survival is about 10%. However, the curves leading to the same 5-year survival are quite different. For although survival at 5 years is the same in both groups, most of the deaths

in group A did not occur until the fifth year, whereas most of the deaths in group B occurred in the first year. Thus, despite the identical 5-year survivals, survival during the 5 years is clearly better for those in group A.

OBSERVED SURVIVAL

Rationale for the Life Table

Another approach is to use the actual observed survival over time. For this purpose, we use a *life table*. Let us examine the conceptual framework underlying the calculation of survival rates using a life table.

Table 6-1 shows a hypothetical study of treatment results in patients who were treated from 2000 to 2004 and followed to 2005. (By just glancing at this table, you can tell that the example is hypothetical, because the title indicates that none were lost to follow-up.)

For each calendar year of treatment, the table shows the number of patients enrolled in treatment and the number of patients alive at each calendar year after the initiation of that treatment. For example, of 84 patients enrolled in treatment in 2000, 44 were alive in 2001, a year after beginning treatment; 21 were alive in 2002; and so on.

The results in Table 6-1 are of all the data available for assessing the treatment. If we want to describe the prognosis in these treated patients using all of the data in the table, obviously we cannot use the 5-year survival rate, because the entire group of 375 patients has not been observed for 5 years. We could calculate the 5-year survival rate using only the 84 patients who were enrolled in 2000 and observed until 2005, because they were the only ones observed for 5 years. However, this would require us to discard the rest of the data, which would be unfortunate, given the

---

TABLE 6-1. **Hypothetical Study of Treatment Results in Patients Treated from 2000 to 2004 and Followed to 2005 (None Lost to Follow-up)**

Year of Treatment	Number of Patients Treated	NUMBER ALIVE ON ANNIVERSARY OF TREATMENT				
		2001	2002	2003	2004	2005
2000	84	44	21	13	10	8
2001	62		31	14	10	6
2002	93			50	20	13
2003	60				29	16
2004	76					43

TABLE 6-2. Rearrangement of Data in Table 6-1, Showing Survival Tabulated by Years since Enrollment in Treatment (None Lost to Follow-up)

Year of Treatment	No. of Patients Treated	NUMBER ALIVE AT END OF YEAR				
		1st Year	2nd Year	3rd Year	4th Year	5th Year
2000	84	44	21	13	10	8
2001	62	31	14	10	6	
2002	93	50	20	13		
2003	60	29	16			
2004	76	43				

effort and expense involved in obtaining the data, and also given the additional light that the survival experience of those patients would cast on the effectiveness of the treatment. The question is: how can we use *all* of the information in Table 6-1 to describe the survival experience of the patients in this study?

To use all of the data, we rearrange the data from Table 6-1 as shown in Table 6-2. In this table, the data are shown as the number of patients who started treatment each calendar year and the number of those who are alive on each anniversary of the initiation of treatment. The patients who started treatment in 2004 were observed for only 1 year, because the study ended in 2005.

With the data in this format, how do we use the table? First we ask, "What is the probability of surviving for 1 year after the beginning of treatment?" To answer this, we divide the total number of patients who were alive 1 year after the initiation of treatment (197) by the total number of patients who started

treatment (375) (Table 6-3). The probability of surviving the first year (P_1) is:

$$P_1 = \frac{197}{375} = .525$$

Next, we ask, "What is the probability that, having survived the first year after beginning treatment, the patient will survive the second year?" We see in Table 6-4 that 197 people survived the first year, but for 43 of them (the ones who were enrolled in 2004), we have no further information because they were observed for only 1 year. Because 71 survived the second year, we calculate the probability of surviving the second year, if the patient survived the first year (P_2), as:

$$P_2 = \frac{71}{197 - 43} = .461$$

In the denominator we subtract the 43 patients for whom we have no data for the second year.

TABLE 6-3. Analysis of Survival in Patients Treated from 2000 to 2004 and Followed to 2005 (None Lost to Follow-up): I

Year of Treatment	No. of Patients Treated	NUMBER ALIVE AT END OF YEAR				
		1st Year	2nd Year	3rd Year	4th Year	5th Year
2000	84	44	21	13	10	8
2001	62	31	14	10	6	
2002	93	50	20	13		
2003	60	29	16			
2004	76	43				
Totals	375	197				

$$P_1 = \text{Probability of surviving the 1st year} = \frac{197}{375} = .525$$

TABLE 6-4. Analysis of Survival in Patients Treated from 2000 to 2004 and Followed to 2005 (None Lost to Follow-up): II

		NUMBER ALIVE AT END OF YEAR				
Year of Treatment	No. of Patients Treated	1st Year	2nd Year	3rd Year	4th Year	5th Year
2000	84	44	21	13	10	8
2001	62	31	14	10	6	
2002	93	50	20	13		
2003	60	29	16			
2004	76	[43]				
Totals		197	71			

$$P_2 = \text{Probability of surviving the 2nd year} = \frac{71}{197-43} = .461$$

Following this pattern, we ask, "Given that a person has survived to the end of the second year, what is the probability that he or she will survive to the end of the third year?"

In Table 6-5, we see that 36 survived the third year. Although 71 had survived the second year, we have no further information on survival for 16 of them because they were enrolled late in the study. Therefore, we subtract 16 from 71 and calculate the probability of surviving the third year, given survival to the end of the second year (P_3), as:

$$P_3 = \frac{36}{71-16} = .655$$

We then ask, "If a person survives to the end of the third year, what is the probability that he or she will survive to the end of the fourth year?"

As seen in Table 6-6, a total of 36 people survived the third year, but we have no further information for 13 of them. Because 16 survived the fourth year, the probability of surviving the fourth year, if the person has survived the third year (P_4), is:

$$P_4 = \frac{16}{36-13} = .696$$

Finally, we do the same calculation for the fifth year (Table 6-7). We see that 16 people survived the fourth year, but that no further information is available for 6 of them.

Because 8 people were alive at the end of the fifth year, the probability of surviving the fifth year, if the person has survived the fourth year (P_5), is:

$$P_5 = \frac{8}{16-6} = .800$$

TABLE 6-5. Analysis of Survival in Patients Treated from 2000 to 2004 and Followed to 2005 (None Lost to Follow-up): III

		NUMBER ALIVE AT END OF YEAR				
Year of Treatment	No. of Patients Treated	1st Year	2nd Year	3rd Year	4th Year	5th Year
2000	84	44	21	13	10	8
2001	62	31	14	10	6	
2002	93	50	20	13		
2003	60	29	[16]			
2004	76	43				
Totals			71	36		

$$P_3 = \text{Probability of surviving the 3rd year} = \frac{36}{71-16} = .655$$

TABLE 6-6. Analysis of Survival in Patients Treated from 2000 to 2004 and Followed to 2005 (None Lost to Follow-up): IV

Year of Treatment	No. of Patients Treated	NUMBER ALIVE AT END OF YEAR				
		1st Year	2nd Year	3rd Year	4th Year	5th Year
2000	84	44	21	13	10	8
2001	62	31	14	10	6	
2002	93	50	20	[13]		
2003	60	29	16			
2004	76	43				
Totals					36	16

$$P_4 = \text{Probability of surviving the 4th year} = \frac{16}{36 - 13} = .696$$

TABLE 6-7. Analysis of Survival in Patients Treated from 2000 to 2004 and Followed to 2005 (None Lost to Follow-up): V

Year of Treatment	No. of Patients Treated	NUMBER ALIVE AT END OF YEAR				
		1st Year	2nd Year	3rd Year	4th Year	5th Year
2000	84	44	21	13	10	8
2001	62	31	14	10	[6]	
2002	93	50	20	13		
2003	60	29	16			
2004	76	43				
Totals					16	8

$$P_5 = \text{Probability of surviving the 5th year} = \frac{8}{16 - 6} = .800$$

Using all of the data that we have calculated, we ask, "What is the probability of surviving for all 5 years?" Table 6-8 shows all of the probabilities of surviving for each individual year that we have calculated.

Now we can answer the question, "If a person is enrolled in the study, what is the probability that he or she will survive 5 years after beginning treatment?" The probability of surviving for 5 years is the product of each of the probabilities of surviving each year, shown in Table 6-8. So the probability of surviving for 5 years is:

$$= P_1 \times P_2 \times P_3 \times P_4 \times P_5$$
$$= .525 \times .461 \times .655 \times .696 \times .800$$
$$= .088, \text{ or } 8.8\%$$

The probabilities for surviving different lengths of time are shown in Table 6-9. These calculations can

be presented graphically in a survival curve, as seen in Figure 6-11. Note that these calculations use all of the data we have obtained, including the data for patients who were not observed for the full 5 years of the study. As a result, the use of data is economical and efficient.

Calculating a Life Table

Let us now view the data from this example in the standard tabular form in which they are usually presented for calculating a life table. In the example just discussed, the persons for whom data were not available for the full 5 years of the study were those who were enrolled sometime after the study had started, so they were not observed for the full 5-year period. In virtually every survival study, however, subjects are also lost to follow-up. Either they cannot be found or they decline to continue participating in the

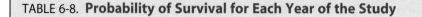

TABLE 6-8. **Probability of Survival for Each Year of the Study**

P_1 = Probability of surviving the 1st year = $\dfrac{197}{375}$ = .525 = 52.5%

P_2 = Probability of surviving the 2nd year given survival to the end of the 1st year = $\dfrac{71}{197-43}$ = .461 = 46.1%

P_3 = Probability of surviving the 3rd year given survival to the end of the 2nd year = $\dfrac{36}{71-16}$ = .655 = 65.5%

P_4 = Probability of surviving the 4th year given survival to the end of the 3rd year = $\dfrac{16}{36-13}$ = .696 = 69.6%

P_5 = Probability of surviving the 5th year given survival to the end of the 4th year = $\dfrac{8}{16-6}$ = .800 = 80.0%

TABLE 6-9. **Cumulative Probabilities of Surviving Different Lengths of Time**

Probability of surviving 1 year = P_1 = .525 = 52.5%
Probability of surviving 2 years = $P_1 \times P_2$ = .525 × .461 = .242 = 24.2%
Probability of surviving 3 years = $P_1 \times P_2 \times P_3$ = .525 × .461 × .655 = .159 = 15.9%
Probability of surviving 4 years = $P_1 \times P_2 \times P_3 \times P_4$ = .525 × .461 × .655 × .696 = .110 = 11.0%
Probability of surviving 5 years = $P_1 \times P_2 \times P_3 \times P_4 \times P_5$ = .525 × .461 × .655 × .696 × .800 = .088 = 8.8%

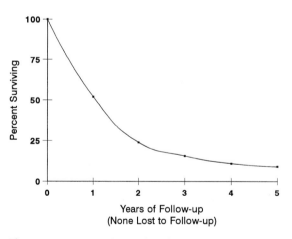

Figure 6-11. Survival curve for a hypothetical example of patients treated from 2000 to 2004 and followed until 2005.

study. In calculating the life table, persons for whom data are not available for the full period of follow-up—either because follow-up was not possible or because they were enrolled after the study was started—are called "withdrawals" (or losses to follow-up).

Table 6-10 shows the data from this example with information provided about the number of deaths and the number of withdrawals in each interval. The

columns are numbered merely for reference. The row directly under the column labels gives the terms that are often used in life table calculations. The next five rows of the table give data for the 5 years of the study.

The columns are as follows:

Column (1): The interval since beginning treatment.

Column (2): The number of subjects who were alive at the beginning of each interval.

Column (3): The number of study subjects who died during that interval.

Column (4): The number who "withdrew" during the interval, that is, the number who could not be followed for the full study period, either because they were lost to follow-up or because they were enrolled after the study had started.

Table 6-11 adds four additional columns to Table 6-10. These columns show the calculations. The new columns are as follows:

Column (5): The number of people who are effectively at risk of dying during the interval. Losses to follow-up (withdrawals) during each time interval are assumed to have occurred uniformly during the entire interval. (This assumption is most likely

TABLE 6-10. **Rearrangement of Data in Standard Format for Life Table Calculations**

(1) Interval Since Beginning Treatment	(2) Alive at Beginning of Interval	(3) Died during Interval	(4) Withdrew during Interval
x	l_x	d_x	w_x
1st year	375	178	0
2nd year	197	83	43
3rd year	71	19	16
4th year	36	7	13
5th year	16	2	6

to hold when the interval is short.) We therefore assume that on average they were at risk for half the interval. Consequently, to calculate the number of people at risk during each interval, we subtract half the withdrawals during that interval as indicated in the heading for column 5.

Column (6): The proportion who died during the interval is calculated by dividing:

$$\frac{\text{The number who died during the interval (column 3)}}{\text{The number who were effectively at risk of dying during the interval (column 5)}}$$

Column (7): The proportion who did not die during the interval, that is, the proportion of those who were alive at the beginning of the interval and who survived that entire interval = 1 − proportion who died during the interval (column 6).

Column (8): The proportion who survived from the point at which they were enrolled in the study to the end of this interval (cumulative survival). This is obtained by multiplying the proportion who were alive at the beginning of this interval and who survived this interval by the proportion who had survived from enrollment through the end of the previous interval. Thus, each of the figures in column 8 gives the proportion of people enrolled in the study who survived to the end of this interval. This will be demonstrated by calculating the first two rows of Table 6-11.

Let us look at the data for the first year. (In these calculations, we will round the results at each step and use the rounded figures in the next calculation. In reality, however, when life tables are calculated, the unrounded figures are used for calculating each subsequent interval, and at the end of all the calculations, all the figures are rounded for purposes of presenting the results.) There were 375 subjects

TABLE 6-11. **Calculating a Life Table**

(1) Interval Since Beginning Treatment	(2) Alive at Beginning of Interval	(3) Died during Interval	(4) Withdrew during Interval	(5) Effective Number Exposed to Risk of Dying during Interval: Col (2) − $\frac{1}{2}$[Col (4)]	(6) Proportion Who Died during Interval: Col (3) Col (5)	(7) Proportion Who Did Not Die during Interval: 1 − Col (6)	(8) Cumulative Proportion Who Survived from Enrollment to End of Interval: Cumulative Survival
x	l_x	d_x	w_x	l'_x	q_x	p_x	P_x
1st year	375	178	0	375.0	.475	.525	.525
2nd year	197	83	43	175.5	.473	.527	.277
3rd year	71	19	16	63.0	.302	.698	.193
4th year	36	7	13	29.5	.237	.763	.147
5th year	16	2	6	13.0	.154	.846	.124

enrolled in the study who were alive at the beginning of the first year after enrollment (column 2). Of these, 178 died during the first year (column 3). All subjects were followed for the first year, so there were no withdrawals (column 4). Consequently, 375 people were effectively at risk for dying during this interval (column 5). The proportion who died during this interval was 0.475: 178 (the number who died [column 3]) divided by 375 (the number who were at risk for dying [column 5]). The proportion who did not die during the interval is 1 − [the proportion who died (1 − 0.475)] = 0.525 (column 7). For the first year after enrollment, this is also the proportion who survived from enrollment to the end of the interval (column 8).

Now let us look at the data for the second year. At the start of the second year, 197 subjects were alive at the beginning of the interval (375 − 178 [column 2]). Of these, 83 died during the second year (column 3). There were 43 withdrawals who had been observed for only 1 year (column 4). As discussed earlier, we subtract half of the withdrawals, 21.5 (43/2), from the 197 who were alive at the start of the interval, yielding 175.5 people who were effectively at risk for dying during this interval (column 5). The proportion who died during this interval (column 6) was 0.473, that is, 83 (the number who died [column 3]) divided by 175.5 (the number who were at risk for dying [column 5]). The proportion who did not die during the interval is 1 − the proportion who died (1 − 0.473) = 0.527 (column 7). The proportion of subjects who survived from the start of treatment to the end of the second year is the product of 0.525 (the proportion who had survived from the start of treatment to the end of the first year, that is, the beginning of the second year) multiplied by 0.527 (the proportion of people who were alive at the beginning of the second year and survived to the end of the second year) = 0.277 (column 8). Thus, 27.7% of the subjects survived from the beginning of treatment to the end of the second year. Looking at the last entry in column 8, we see that 12.4% of all individuals enrolled in the study survived to the end of the fifth year.

Work through the remaining years in Table 6-11 to be sure you understand the concepts and calculations involved.

THE KAPLAN-MEIER METHOD

In contrast to the approach just demonstrated, in the Kaplan-Meier method,[1] predetermined intervals, such as 1 month or 1 year, are not used. Rather, we

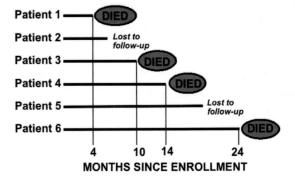

Figure 6-12. Hypothetical example of a study of six patients analyzed by the Kaplan-Meier method.

identify the exact point in time when each death occurred so that each death terminates the previous interval and a new interval (and a new row in the life table) is started. The number of persons who died at that point is used as the numerator, and the number alive up to that point (including those who died at that time point) is used as the denominator, after any withdrawals that occurred before that point are subtracted.

Let us look at the small study shown in Figure 6-12. Six patients were studied, of whom four died and two were lost to follow-up. The deaths occurred at 4, 10, 14, and 24 months after enrollment in the study. The data are set up as shown in Table 6-12:

Column (1): The times for each death from the time of enrollment (time that treatment was initiated).
Column (2): The number of patients who were alive and followed at the time of that death, including those who died at that time.
Column (3): The number who died at that time.
Column (4): The proportion of those who were alive and followed (column 2) who died at that time (column 3) [column 3/column 2].
Column (5): The proportion of those who were alive and survived (1 − column 4).
Column (6): Cumulative survival (the proportion of those who were initially enrolled and survived to that point).

Let us consider the first row of the table. The first death occurred at 4 months, at which time six patients were alive and followed (see Fig. 6-12). One death occurred at this point (column 3), for a proportion of 1/6 = 0.167 (column 4). The proportion who survived at that time is 1 − column 4, or 1 − 0.167 = .833 (column 5), which is also the cumulative survival at this point (column 6).

TABLE 6-12. **Calculating Survival Using the Kaplan-Meier Method***

(1) Times to Deaths from Starting Treatment (months)	(2) Number Alive at Each Time	(3) Number Who Died at Each Time	(4) Proportion Who Died at That Time: $\frac{Col (3)}{Col (2)}$	(5) Proportion Who Survived at That Time: 1 − Col (4)	(6) Cumulative Proportion Who Survived to That Time: Cumulative Survival
4	6	1	.167	.833	.833
10	4	1	.250	.750	.625
14	3	1	.333	.667	.417
24	1	1	1.000	.000	.000

*See text and Figure 6-12 regarding withdrawals.

The next death occurred 10 months after the initial enrollment of the six patients in the study, and data for this time are seen in the next row of the table. Although only one death had occurred before this one, the number alive and followed is only four because there had also been a withdrawal before this point (not shown in the table, but seen in Fig. 6-12). Thus, there was one death (column 3), and, as seen in Table 6-12, the proportion who died is 1/4 or 0.250 (column 4). The proportion who survived is 1 − column 4, or 1 − 0.250 = 0.750 (column 5). Finally, the cumulative proportion surviving (column 6) is the product of the proportion who survived to the end of the previous interval (until just before the previous death) seen in column 6 of the first row (0.833) and the proportion who survived from that time until just before the second death (second row in column 5, 0.750). The product = 0.625, that is, 62.5% of the original enrollees survived to this point. Review the next two rows of the table to be sure that you understand the concepts and calculations involved.

The values calculated in column 6 are plotted as seen in Figure 6-13. Note that the data are plotted in a stepwise fashion rather than in a smoothed slope because, after each death, survival remains unchanged until the next death occurs.

When information on the exact time of death is available, the Kaplan-Meier method clearly makes fullest use of this information because the data are used to define the intervals. Although the method is well suited to studies with small numbers of patients, today, computer programs are readily available that make this method applicable to large data sets as well. Many of the studies in the published literature now

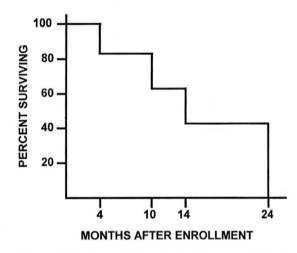

Figure 6-13. Kaplan-Meier plot of the survival study shown in Figure 6-12.

report data on survival using the Kaplan-Meier method. For example, in 2000, Rosenhek and colleagues reported a study of patients with asymptomatic, but severe, aortic stenosis.[2] An unresolved issue is whether patients with asymptomatic disease should have their aortic valves replaced. The investigators examined the natural history of this condition to assess the overall survival of these patients and to identify predictors of outcome. Figure 6-14A shows their Kaplan-Meier analysis of survival among 126 patients with aortic stenosis compared with age- and sex-matched people in the general population. Although survival was slightly worse in patients with aortic stenosis, the difference was not significant. When they examined several risk factors, they found that moderate and severe calcification of the aortic

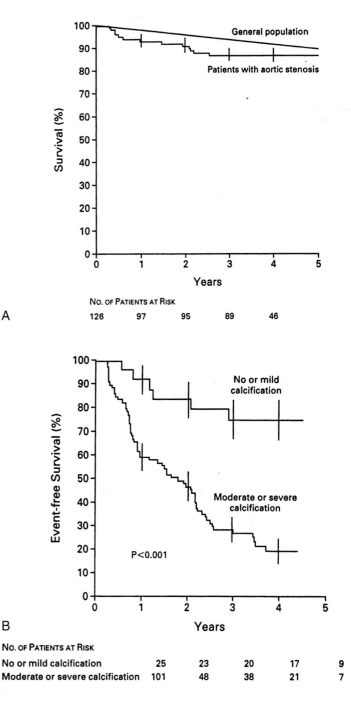

Figure 6-14. A, Kaplan-Meier analysis of overall survival among 126 patients with asymptomatic, but severe, aortic stenosis, compared with age- and sex-matched persons in the general population. This analysis included perioperative and postoperative deaths among patients who required valve replacement during follow-up. **B,** Kaplan-Meier analysis of event-free survival among 25 patients with no or mild aortic valve calcification, compared with 101 patients with moderate or severe calcification. The vertical bars indicate standard errors.

valve was a significant predictor of subsequent cardiac events and very poor prognosis (see Fig. 6-14B). Event-free survival was much worse in patients with moderate or severe valve calcification than in patients with no or mild calcification. The authors concluded that such patients should be considered for early valve replacement rather than have surgery delayed until symptoms develop.

ASSUMPTIONS MADE IN USING LIFE TABLES

Two important assumptions are made in using life tables. The first is that there has been no secular (temporal) change in the effectiveness of treatment or in survivorship over calendar time. That is, we assume that over the period of the study, there has been no improvement in treatment and that survivorship in one calendar year of the study is the same as in another calendar year of the study. Clearly, if a study is conducted over many years, this assumption may not be valid because, fortunately, therapies improve over time. If we are concerned that the effectiveness of therapy may have changed over the course of the study, we could examine the early data separately from the later data. If they seem to differ, the early and later periods could be analyzed separately.

The second assumption relates to follow-up of persons enrolled in the study. In virtually every real-life study, participants are lost to follow-up. People can be lost to follow-up for many reasons. Some may die and may not be traced. Some may move or seek care elsewhere. Some may be lost because their disease disappears and they feel well. In most studies, we do not know the actual reasons for loss to follow-up. How can we deal with the problem of people lost to follow-up for whom we therefore have no further information on survival? Because we have baseline data on these people, we could compare their characteristics with those of persons who remained in the study, but the problem nevertheless remains. If a large proportion of the study population is lost to follow-up, the findings will be less valid. The challenge is to minimize loss to follow-up. In any case, the second assumption made in life tables is that the survival experience of people who are lost to follow-up is the same as the experience of those who are followed up. Although this assumption is made for purposes of calculation, in actual fact its validity may often be questionable.

Although the term *life table* might suggest that these methods are useful only for calculating survival, this is not so. Death need not be the endpoint in these calculations. For example, *survival* can be calculated as time to the development of hypertension, time to the development of a recurrence of cancer, or survival time free of treatment side effects. Furthermore, although we can look at a single survival curve, often, the greatest interest lies in comparing two or more survival curves, such as for those who are treated and those who are not treated in a randomized trial. In conducting such comparisons, statistical methods are available to determine whether one curve is significantly different from another.

Example of Use of a Life Table

Life tables are used in virtually every clinical area. They are the standard means by which survival is expressed and compared. Let us examine a few examples. One of the great triumphs of pediatrics in recent decades has been the treatment of leukemia in children. However, the improvement has been much greater for whites than for blacks, and the reasons for this difference are not clear. At a time when survival rates from childhood acute leukemia were increasing rapidly, a study was conducted to explore the racial differences in survivorship. Figures 6-15 through 6-17 show data from this study.[3] The curves are based on life tables that were constructed using the approach discussed earlier.

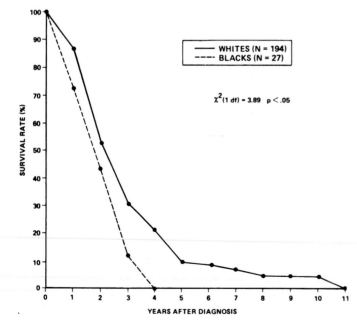

Figure 6-15. Survival of children aged 0 to 19 years with acute lymphocytic leukemia by race, metropolitan Baltimore, 1960–1975. (From Szklo M, Gordis L, Tonascia J, Kaplan E: The changing survivorship of white and black children with leukemia. Cancer 42:59–66, 1978. Copyright © 1978 American Cancer Society. Reprinted by permission of Wiley-Liss, Inc., a subsidiary of John Wiley & Sons, Inc.)

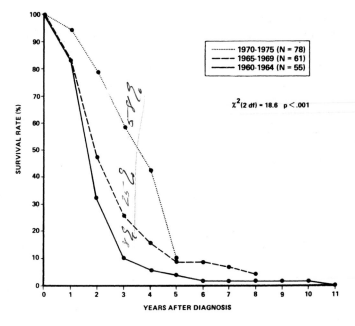

Figure 6-16. Temporal changes in survival of white children aged 0 to 19 years with acute lymphocytic leukemia, metropolitan Baltimore, 1960–1975. (From Szklo M, Gordis L, Tonascia J, Kaplan E: The changing survivorship of white and black children with leukemia. Cancer 42:59–66, 1978. Copyright © 1978 American Cancer Society. Reprinted by permission of Wiley-Liss, Inc., a subsidiary of John Wiley & Sons, Inc.)

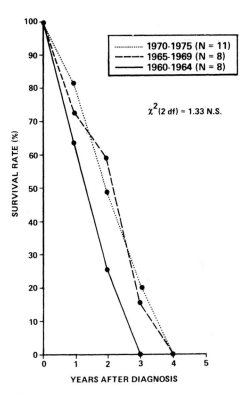

Figure 6-17. Temporal changes in survival of black children aged 0 to 19 years with acute lymphocytic leukemia, metropolitan Baltimore, 1960–1975. (From Szklo M, Gordis L, Tonascia J, Kaplan E: The changing survivorship of white and black children with leukemia. Cancer 42:59–66, 1978. Copyright © 1978 American Cancer Society. Reprinted by permission of Wiley-Liss, Inc., a subsidiary of John Wiley & Sons, Inc.)

Figure 6-15 shows survival for white and black children with leukemia in Baltimore over a 16-year period. No black children survived longer than 4 years, but some white children survived as long as 11 years in this 16-year period of observation.

What changes took place in survivorship during the 16 years of the study? Figure 6-16 and Figure 6-17 show changes in leukemia mortality over time in whites and blacks, respectively. The 16-year period was divided into three periods: 1960 to 1964 *(solid line)*, 1965 to 1969 *(dashed line)*, and 1970 to 1975 *(dotted line)*.

In whites (see Fig. 6-16), survivorship increased in each successive period. For example, if we examine 3-year survival by looking at the 3-year point on each successive curve, we see that survival improved from 8% to 25% to 58%. In contrast, in blacks (see Fig. 6-17) there was much less improvement in survival over time; the curves for the two later 5-year periods almost overlap.

What accounts for this racial difference? First, we must take account of the small numbers involved and the possibility that the differences could have been due to chance. Let us assume, however, that the differences are real. During the past several decades, tremendous strides have occurred in the treatment of leukemia through combined therapy, including central nervous system radiation added to chemotherapy. Why, then, does a racial difference exist in survivorship? Why is it that the improvement in therapy that has been so effective in white children has not had a comparable benefit in black children? Further analyses of the interval from the time the mother noticed symptoms to the time of diagnosis and treatment indicated that the differences in survival did not appear to be due to a delay in black parents seeking or obtaining medical care. Because acute leukemia is more severe in blacks and more advanced at the time of diagnosis, the racial difference could reflect biologic differences in the disease, such as a more aggressive and rapidly progressive form of the illness. The definitive explanation is not yet clear.

APPARENT EFFECTS ON PROGNOSIS OF IMPROVEMENTS IN DIAGNOSIS

We have discussed the assumption made in using a life table that *no improvement in the effectiveness of treatment* has occurred over calendar time during the period of the study. Another issue in calculating and interpreting survival rates is the possible effect of *improvements in diagnostic methods* over calendar time.

An interesting example was reported by Feinstein, Sosin, and Wells.[4] They compared survival in a cohort

of patients with lung cancer first treated in 1977 with survival in a cohort of patients with lung cancer treated from 1953 to 1964. Six-month survival was higher in the later group for both the total group and for subgroups formed on the basis of stage of disease. The authors found that the apparent improvement in survival was due in part to *stage migration*, a phenomenon shown in Figures 6-18A–C.

In Figure 6-18A, patients with cancer are divided into "good" and "bad" stages on the basis of whether they had detectable metastases in 1980. Some patients who would have been assigned to a "good" stage in 1980 may have had micro-metastases at that time which would have been unrecognized (Fig. 6-18B). However, by 2000, as diagnostic technology improved, many of these patients would have been assigned to a "bad" stage, because their micro-metastases would now have been recognized using improved diagnostic technology that had become available (Fig. 6-18C). If this had occurred, survival by stage would appear to have improved even if treatment had not become any more effective during this time.

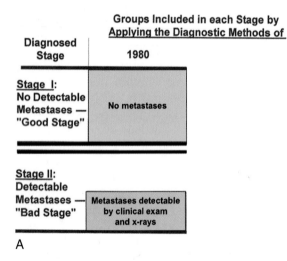

A

B

C

Figure 6-18. Stage migration. **A,** Classification of cases by presence or absence of detectable metastases in 1980. **B,** Presence of undetectable micro-metastases in 1980. **C,** Impact of improved diagnosis of micro-metastases in 2000, on the stage-specific case-fatality rate.

Let us consider a hypothetical example that illustrates this effect of such stage migration. Figures 6-19A–C show a hypothetical study of cancer case-fatality rates for 300 patients in two time periods, 1980 and 2000, *assuming no improvement in the effectiveness of available therapy between the two periods.* We will assume that as shown in Figure 6-19A, in both time periods, the case-fatality rate is 10% for patients who have no metastases, 30% for those with micro-metastases, and 80% for those with metastases. Looking at Figure 6-19B, we see that in 1980, 200 patients were classified as stage I. One hundred of these patients had no metastases and 100 had unrecognized micro-metastases. Their case-fatality rates were thus 10% and 30%, respectively. In 1980, 100 patients had clearly evident metastases and were classified as stage II; their case-fatality rate was 80%.

As a result of improved diagnostic technology in 2000, micro-metastases were detected in the 100 affected patients, and these patients were classified as stage II (Fig. 6-19C). Because the prognosis of the patients with micro-metastases is worse than that of the other patients in stage I, and because, in the later study period, patients with micro-metastases are no longer included in the stage I group (because they have migrated to stage II), the case-fatality rate for stage I patients appears to decline from 20% in the early period to 10% in the later period. However, although the prognosis of the patients who migrated from stage I to stage II was worse than that of the others in stage I, the prognosis for these patients was still better than that of the other patients in stage II, who had larger, more easily diagnosed metastases and a case-fatality rate of 80%. Consequently, the case-fatality rate for patients in stage II also appears to have improved, having declined from 80% in the early period to 55% in the later period, *even in the absence of any improvement in treatment effectiveness.*

The apparent improvements in survival in both stage I and stage II patients result only from the changed classification of patients with micro-metastases in the later period. Looking at the bottom line of the figure, we see that the case-fatality rate of 40% for all 300 patients has not changed from the early period to the later period. Only the apparent stage-specific case-fatality rates have changed. It is therefore important to exclude the possibility of stage migration before attributing any apparent improvement in prognosis to improved effectiveness of medical care.

The authors call this the "Will Rogers phenomenon." The reference is to Will Rogers, an American humorist during the time of the economic depression of the 1930s. At that time, because of economic

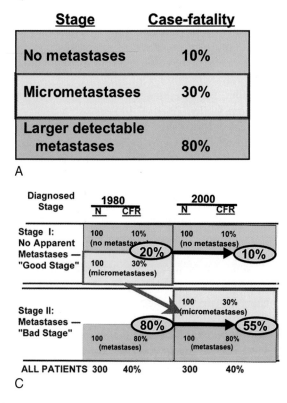

A

C

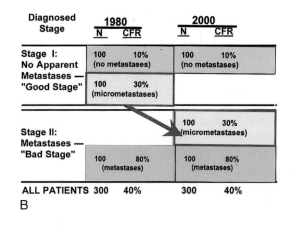

B

Figure 6-19 Hypothetical example of stage migration. **A,** Assumed case-fatality by stage. **B,** Impact of improved diagnosis of micro-metastases on stage-specific case-fatality (CFR). **C,** Apparent improvements in stage-specific survival as a result of stage migration even without any improvement in effectiveness of treatment.

TABLE 6-13. **Five-Year Observed and Relative Survival Rates (%) by Age for Colon and Rectum Cancer: SEER Program (Surveillance, Epidemiology, and End Results Study), 1990–1998**

Age (yr)	Observed Rate (%)	Relative Rate (%)
<50	60.4	61.5
50–64	59.4	63.7
65–74	53.7	63.8
>75	35.8	58.7

From Edwards BK, Howe HL, Ries LAG, et al: Annual report to the nation on the status of cancer, 1973–1999, featuring implications of age and aging on U.S. cancer burden. Cancer 94:2766–2792, 2002.

hardship, many residents of Oklahoma left the state and migrated to California. Rogers commented, "When the Okies left Oklahoma and moved to California, they raised the average intelligence level in both states."

MEDIAN SURVIVAL TIME

Another approach to expressing prognosis is the *median survival time*, which is defined as the length of time that half of the study population survives. Why should we use median survival time rather than mean survival time, which is an average of the survival times? Median survival offers two advantages over mean survival. First, it is less affected by extremes, whereas the mean is significantly affected by even a single outlier. One or two persons with a very long survival time could significantly affect the mean, even if all of the other survival times were much shorter. Second, if we used mean survival, we would have to observe all of the deaths in the study population before the mean could be calculated. However, to calculate median survival, we would only have to observe the deaths of half of the group.

RELATIVE SURVIVAL RATE

Let us consider the 5-year survival rate for a group of 30-year-old men with colorectal cancer. What would we expect their 5-year survival to be if they did not have

colorectal cancer? Clearly, it would be nearly 100%. Thus, we are comparing the survival rate observed in young men with colorectal cancer to a survival rate of almost 100% that is expected in those without colorectal cancer. What if we consider a group of 80-year-old men with colorectal cancer? We would not expect anything near 100% 5-year survival in a population of this age, even if they do not have colorectal cancer. We would want to compare the observed survival in 80-year-old men with colorectal cancer to the expected survival of 80-year-old men without colorectal cancer. So for any group of people with a disease, we want to compare their survival to the survival we would expect in this age group even if they did *not* have the disease. This is known as the *relative survival rate*.

The relative survival rate is thus defined as the ratio of the observed survival to the expected survival rate:

$$\text{Relative survival rate} = \frac{\text{Observed survival in people with the disease}}{\text{Expected survival if disease were absent}}$$

Does relative survival really make any difference?

Table 6-13 shows data for patients with cancer of the colon and rectum, both relative survival and observed survival from 1990 to 1998. When we look at the older age groups, which have high rates of mortality from other causes, there is a large difference between the observed and the relative survival rates. However, in young persons, who generally do not die of other causes, observed and relative survival rates for cancer of the colon and rectum do not differ significantly.

Another way to view relative survival is by examining the hypothetical 10-year survival curves of 80-year-old men shown in Figures 6-20 through 6-23. For reference, Figure 6-20 shows a perfect survival curve of 100% (the horizontal curve at the top) over the 10 years of the study period. Figure 6-21 adds a curve of observed survival, that is, the actual survival observed in this group of patients with the disease over the 10-year period. As seen in Figure 6-22, the expected survival for this group of 80-year-old men is clearly less than 100% because deaths from other causes are significant in this age group. The relative survival is the ratio of observed survival to expected survival. Since expected survival is less than perfect (100%) survival, and expected survival is the denominator for these calculations, the relative survival will be higher than the observed survival (Fig. 6-23).

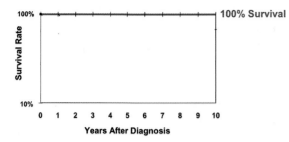

Figure 6-20. Relative survival rate I: 100% survival over 10 years.

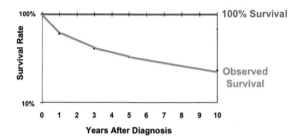

Figure 6-21. Relative survival rate II: Observed survival.

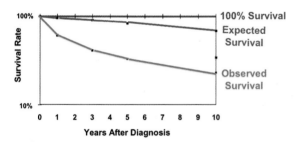

Figure 6-22. Relative survival rate III: Observed and expected survival.

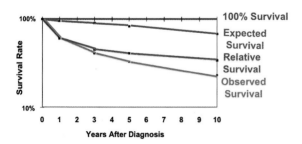

Figure 6-23. Relative survival rate IV: Observed, expected, and relative survival.

GENERALIZABILITY OF SURVIVAL DATA

A final point in connection with the natural history and prognosis of disease is the question of which patients are selected for study. Let us look at one example.

Febrile seizures are common in infants. Children who are otherwise healthy often experience a seizure in association with high fever. The question arises as to whether these children should be treated with a regimen of phenobarbital or another long-term anticonvulsant medication. That is, is a febrile seizure a warning of subsequent epilepsy, or is it simply a phenomenon associated with fever in infants, in which case children are unlikely to have subsequent nonfebrile seizures?

To make a rational decision about treatment, the question we must ask is, "What is the risk that a child who has had a febrile seizure will have a subsequent nonfebrile seizure?" Figure 6-24 shows the results of an analysis by Ellenberg and Nelson of published studies.[5]

Each dot shows the percentage of children with febrile seizures who later developed nonfebrile seizures in a different study. The authors divided the studies into two groups: population-based studies and studies based in individual clinics, such as epilepsy or pediatric clinics. The results from different clinic-based studies show a considerable range in the

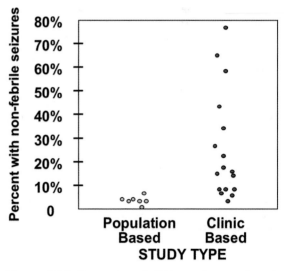

Figure 6-24. Percentage of children who experienced nonfebrile seizures after one or more febrile seizures, by study design. (Adapted from Ellenberg JH, Nelson KB: Sample selection and the natural history of disease: Studies on febrile seizures. JAMA 243:1337–1340, 1980.)

risk of later development of nonfebrile seizures. However, the results of population-based studies show little variation in risk, and the results of all of these studies tend to cluster at a low level of risk.

Why should the two types of studies differ? Which results would you believe? Each of the clinics probably had different selection criteria and different referral patterns. Consequently, the different risks observed in the different clinic-based studies are probably the result of the selection of different populations in each of the clinics. In contrast, in the population-based studies, this type of variation due to selection is reduced or eliminated, which accounts for the clustering of the data, and for the resultant finding that the risk of nonfebrile seizures is very low. The important point is that it may be very tempting to look at patient records in one hospital and generalize the findings to all patients in the general population. However, this is not a legitimate approach because patients who come to a certain clinic or hospital often are not representative of all patients in the community. This does not mean that studies conducted at a single hospital or clinic cannot be of value. Indeed, there is much to be learned from conducting studies at single hospitals. However, these studies are particularly prone to selection bias, and this possibility must always be kept in mind when the findings from such studies and their potential generalizability are being interpreted.

TABLE 6-14. **Five Approaches to Expressing Prognosis**
1. Case-fatality rate
2. 5-year survival
3. Observed survival rate
4. Median survival time
5. Relative survival rate

CONCLUSION

This chapter has discussed five ways of expressing prognosis (Table 6-14). Which approach is best depends on the type of data that are available and on the purpose of data analysis. Chapters 7 and 8 address the use of randomized trials for selecting the optimal means of intervention.

REFERENCES

1. Kaplan EL, Meier P: Nonparametric estimation from incomplete observations. J Am Stat Assoc 53:457–481, 1958.
2. Rosenhek R, Binder T, Porenta G, et al: Predictors of outcome in severe, asymptomatic aortic stenosis. N Engl J Med 343: 611–617, 2000.
3. Szklo M, Gordis L, Tonascia J, Kaplan E: The changing survivorship of white and black children with leukemia. Cancer 42:59–66, 1978.
4. Feinstein AR, Sosin DM, Wells CK: The Will Rogers phenomenon: Stage migration and new diagnostic techniques as a source of misleading statistics for survival in cancer. N Engl J Med 312:1604–1608, 1985.
5. Ellenberg JH, Nelson KB: Sample selection and the natural history of disease: Studies on febrile seizures. JAMA 243: 1337–1340, 1980.

REVIEW QUESTIONS FOR CHAPTER 6

1. Which of the following is a good index of the severity of a short-term, acute disease?
   a. Cause-specific death rate
   b. 5-year survival
   c. Case-fatality rate
   d. Standardized mortality ratio
   e. None of the above

Question 2 is based on the information given in the table at right:

Year of Treatment	No. of Patients Treated	NO. OF PATIENTS ALIVE ON EACH ANNIVERSARY		
		1st	2nd	3rd
1991	75	60	56	48
1992	63	55	31	
1993	42	37		
Total	180	152	87	48

One hundred eighty patients were treated for disease X from 1991 to 1993, and their progress was followed to 1994. The treatment results are given in the table. No patients were lost to follow-up.

2. What is the probability of surviving for 3 years?

_____

3. An important assumption in this type of analysis is that:
   a. Treatment has improved during the period of the study
   b. The quality of record-keeping has improved during the period of the study
   c. No change has occurred in the effectiveness of the treatment during the period of the study
   d. An equal number of men and women were enrolled each year
   e. None of the above

4. A diagnostic test has been introduced that will detect a certain disease 1 year earlier than it is usually detected. Which of the following is *most likely* to happen to the disease within the 10 years after the test is introduced? (Assume that early detection has no effect on the natural history of the disease. Also assume that no changes in death certification practices occur during the 10 years.)
   a. The period prevalence rate will decrease
   b. The apparent 5-year survival rate will increase

   c. The age-adjusted mortality rate will decrease
   d. The age-adjusted mortality rate will increase
   e. The incidence rate will decrease

5. Which of the following statements about relative survival is true?
   a. It refers to survival of first-degree relatives
   b. It is generally closer to observed survival in elderly populations
   c. It is generally closer to observed survival in young populations
   d. It generally differs from observed survival by a constant amount, regardless of age
   e. None of the above

Questions 6 to 8 are based on the data in the table at the bottom of this page. The data were obtained from a study of 248 patients with AIDS who were given a new treatment and followed to determine survival. The study population was followed for 36 months.

Note: Carry your calculations in the table to four decimal places (i.e., 0.1234), but give the final answer to three decimal places (e.g., 0.123 or 12.3%).

6. For those people who survived the second year, what is the probability of dying in the third year?

_____

7. What is the probability that a person enrolled in the study will survive to the end of the third year?

_____

Survival of Patients with AIDS after Diagnosis

(1) Interval since Beginning Treatment (months)	(2) Alive at Beginning of Interval	(3) Died during Interval	(4) Withdrew during Interval	(5) Effective Number Exposed to Risk of Dying during Interval: Col (2) − $\frac{1}{2}$[Col (4)]	(6) Proportion Who Died during Interval: $\frac{Col (3)}{Col (5)}$	(7) Proportion Who Did Not Die during Interval: 1 − Col (6)	(8) Cumulative Proportion Who Survived from Enrollment to End of Interval: Cumulative Survival
x	l_x	d_x	w_x	l'_x	q_x	p_x	P_x
1–12	248	96	27				
13–24	125	55	13				
25–36	57	55	2				

8. Before reporting the results of this survival analysis, the investigators compared the baseline characteristics of the 42 persons who withdrew from the study before its end with those of the participants who had complete follow-up. This was done for which of the following reasons:

a. To test whether randomization was successful

b. To check for changes in prognosis over time

✓c. To check whether those who remained in the study represent the total study population

d. To determine whether the outcome of those who remained in the study is the same as the outcome of the underlying population

e. To check for confounders in the exposed and nonexposed groups

Assessing the Efficacy of Preventive and Therapeutic Measures: Randomized Trials

All who drink of this treatment recover in a short time,
Except those whom it does not help, who all die,
It is obvious, therefore, that it fails only in incurable cases.
—Galen[1] (129–c. 199 CE)

Some ways of quantifying the natural history of disease and of expressing disease prognosis were discussed in Chapter 6. Our objective, both in public health and in clinical practice, is to modify the natural history of a disease so as to prevent or delay death or disability and to improve the health of the patient or the population. The challenge is to select the best available preventive or therapeutic measures to achieve this goal. To do so, we need to carry out studies that determine the value of these measures. The randomized trial is considered the ideal design for evaluating both the effectiveness and the side effects of new forms of intervention.

The notion of using a rigorous methodology to assess the efficacy of new drugs, or of any new modalities of care, is not recent. In 1883, Sir Francis Galton, the British anthropologist, explorer, and eugenicist, who had a strong interest in human intelligence, wrote as follows:

It was asserted by some that men possess the faculty of obtaining results over which they have little or no direct personal control, by means of devout and earnest prayer, while others doubt the truth of this assertion. The question regards a matter of fact, that has to be determined by observation and not by authority; and it is one that appears to be a very suitable topic for statistical inquiry. . . . Are prayers answered or are they not? . . . Do sick persons, who pray or are prayed for, recover on the average more rapidly than others?[2]

As with many pioneering ideas in science and medicine, many years were to pass before this suggestion was actually implemented. In 1965, Joyce and Welldon reported the results of a double-blind clinical trial of the efficacy of prayer.[3] The findings of this study did not indicate that patients who were prayed for derived any benefits from that prayer. A more recent study by Byrd,[4] however, evaluated the effectiveness of intercessory prayer in a coronary care unit population using a randomized double-blind protocol. The findings from this study suggested that prayer had a beneficial therapeutic effect.

In this chapter and the one following, we discuss possible study designs that can be used for evaluating new approaches to treatment and prevention, and focus on the randomized trial. Although the term *randomized clinical trial* is often used together with its acronym, RCT, the randomized trial design also has major applicability to studies outside the clinical setting, such as community-based trials. For this reason, we use the term *randomized trial*. To facilitate our discussion, reference is generally made to treatments and drugs; the reader should bear in mind that the principles described apply equally to evaluations of preventive and other measures.

Suggestions of many of the elements that are important to randomized trials can be seen in many anecdotal descriptions of early trials. In a review of the history of clinical trials, Bull described an unintentional trial conducted by Ambroise Paré (1510–1590), a leading figure in surgery during the Renaissance.[5] Paré lived at a time when the standard treatment for war wounds was the application of boiling oil. In 1537, Paré was responsible for the treatment of the wounded after the capture of the castle of Villaine. The wounded were so numerous that, he says:

> At length my oil lacked and I was constrained to apply in its place a digestive made of yolks of eggs, oil of roses and turpentine. That night I could not sleep at my ease, fearing that by lack of cauterization I would find the wounded upon which I had not used the said oil, dead from the poison. I raised myself early to visit them, when beyond my hope I found those to whom I had applied the digestive medicament feeling but little pain, their wounds neither swollen nor inflamed, and having slept through the night. The others to whom I had applied the boiling oil were feverish with much pain and swelling about their wounds. Then I determined never again to burn thus so cruelly the poor wounded.

Although this was not a randomized trial, it was a form of unplanned trial, which has been carried out many times when a therapy thought to be the best available has been in short supply and has not been available for all of the patients who needed it.

A planned trial was described by the Scottish surgeon James Lind in 1747.[6] Lind became interested in scurvy, which killed thousands of British seamen each year. He was intrigued by the story of a sailor who had developed scurvy and had been put ashore on an isolated island where he subsisted on a diet of grasses and then recovered from the scurvy. Lind conducted an experiment which he described as follows:

> I took 12 patients in the scurvy on board the Salisbury at sea. The cases were as similar as I could have them . . . they lay together in one place and had one diet common to them all. Two of these were ordered a quart of cider per day. . . . Two others took 25 gutts of elixir vitriol. . . . Two others took two spoonfuls of vinegar. . . . Two were put under a course of sea water. . . . Two others had two oranges and one lemon given them each day. . . . Two others took the bigness of nutmeg. The most sudden and visible good effects were perceived from the use of oranges and lemons, one of those who had taken them being at the end of 6 days fit for duty. . . . The other . . . was appointed nurse to the rest of the sick.

Interestingly, the idea of a dietary cause of scurvy proved unacceptable in Lind's day. Only 47 years later did the British Admiralty permit him to repeat his experiment—this time on an entire fleet of ships. The results were so dramatic that, in 1795, the Admiralty made lemon juice a required part of the standard diet of British seamen and later changed this to lime juice. Scurvy essentially disappeared from British sailors, who, even today, are referred to as "limeys."

Randomized trials can be used for many purposes. They can be used for evaluating new drugs and other treatments of disease, including tests of new health and medical care technology. Such trials can be used to assess new programs for screening and early detection, or new ways of organizing and delivering health services.

The basic design of a randomized trial is shown in Figure 7-1.

We begin with a defined population that is randomized to receive either new treatment or current treatment, and we follow the subjects in each group to see how many are improved in the new treatment group compared with the current treatment group. If the new treatment is associated with a better outcome, we would expect to find better outcome in more of the new treatment group than the current treatment group.

We may choose to compare two groups receiving different therapies, or we may compare more than two groups. Although, at times, a new treatment may be compared with no treatment, often a decision is made not to use an untreated group. For example, if we wanted to evaluate a newly developed therapy for acquired immunodeficiency syndrome (AIDS), would we be willing to have a group of AIDS patients in our study who were untreated? The answer is clearly no; we would compare the newly developed therapy with a currently recommended regimen, which would clearly be better than no therapy at all.

Let us now turn to some of the issues that must be considered in the design of randomized trials.

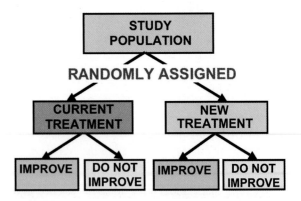

Figure 7-1. Design of a randomized trial.

SELECTION OF SUBJECTS

The criteria for determining who will or will not be included in the study must be spelled out with great precision, and *in writing*. An excellent test of the adequacy of these written criteria is to ask: If we have spelled out our criteria in writing, and someone walks in off the street and applies our criteria to the same population, will they select the same subjects whom we would have selected? There should be no element of subjective decision-making on the part of the investigator in deciding who is included or not included in the study. Any study must in principle be replicable by others, just as is the case with laboratory experiments. Clearly, this is easier said than done, because in randomized trials we are often dealing with relatively large populations. The principle is nevertheless important, and the selection criteria must therefore be precisely stated.

ALLOCATION OF SUBJECTS TO TREATMENT GROUPS

Before discussing the process of randomization, let us ask whether there might not be some alternatives to randomization that could be used.

Studies without Comparison

The first possible alternative is the *case study* or *case series*. In this type of study, no comparison is made with an untreated group or with a group that is receiving some other treatment. The following story was told by Dr. Earl Peacock when he was chairman of the Department of Surgery at the University of Arizona:

> One day when I was a junior medical student, a very important Boston surgeon visited the school and delivered a great treatise on a large number of patients who had undergone successful operations for vascular reconstruction. At the end of the lecture, a young student at the back of the room timidly asked, "Do you have any controls?" Well, the great surgeon drew himself up to his full height, hit the desk, and said, "Do you mean did I not operate on half of the patients?" The hall grew very quiet then. The voice at the back of the room very hesitantly replied, "Yes, that's what I had in mind." Then the visitor's fist really came down as he thundered, "Of course not. That would have doomed half of them to their death." God, it was quiet then, and one could scarcely hear the small voice ask, "Which half?"[7]

The issue of comparison is important because we want to be able to derive a causal inference regarding the relationship of a treatment and subsequent outcome. The problem of inferring a causal relationship from a sequence of events without any comparison is demonstrated in a story cited by Ederer.[8]

> During World War II, rescue workers, digging in the ruins of an apartment house blown up in the London blitz, found an old man lying naked in a bathtub, fully conscious. He said to his rescuers, "You know, that was the most amazing experience I ever had. When I pulled the plug and the water started down the drain, the whole house blew up."

The problem exemplified by this story is: If we administer a drug and the patient improves, can we attribute the improvement to the administration of that drug? Professor Hugo Muensch of Harvard University articulated his Second Law: "Results can always be improved by omitting controls."[9]

Studies with Comparison

If we therefore recognize the need for our study to include some type of comparison, what are the possible designs?

Historical Controls

We could use a comparison group from the past, called *historical controls*. We have a therapy today that we believe will be quite effective, and we would like to test it in a group of patients; we realize that we need a comparison group. So, for comparison, we will go back to the records of patients with the same disease who were treated before the new therapy became available. This type of design seems inherently simple and attractive.

What are the problems in using historical controls? First, if today we decide to carry out the study just described, we may set up a very meticulous system for data collection from the patients currently being treated. But, of course, we cannot do that for the patients who were treated in the past, for whom we must abstract data from medical records. Those records were generated for clinical purposes at the time and not for research purposes. Consequently, if at the end of the study we find a difference in outcome between patients treated in the early period (historical controls) and patients treated in the later (current) period, we will not know whether there was a true difference in outcome or whether the observed difference was due only to a difference in the quality of the data collection. The data obtained from the study groups must be comparable in kind and quality; in studies using historical controls, this is often not the case.

The second problem is that if we observe a difference in outcome between the early group and the later group, we will not be sure that the difference is due to the therapy, because many things other than the therapy change over calendar time (e.g., ancillary supportive therapy, living conditions, nutrition, and lifestyles). Hence, if we observe a difference and if we have ruled out differences in data quality as the reason for the observed difference, we will not know whether the difference is a result of the drug we are studying or of changes that take place in many other factors over calendar time.

At times, however, this type of design may be useful. For example, when a disease is uniformly fatal and a new drug becomes available, a decline in case-fatality that parallels use of the drug would strongly support the conclusion that the new drug is having an effect. Nevertheless, the possibility that the decline could have resulted from other changes in the environment would still have to be ruled out.

Simultaneous Nonrandomized Controls

Because of the importance of the problems posed by historical controls and the difficulties of dealing with changes over calendar time, an alternative approach is to use simultaneous controls that are not selected in a randomized manner. The problem with selecting simultaneous controls in a nonrandomized manner is illustrated by the following story:

> A sea captain was given samples of anti-nausea pills to test during a voyage. The need for controls was carefully explained to him. Upon return of the ship, the captain reported the results enthusiastically. "Practically every one of the controls was ill, and not one of the subjects had any trouble. Really wonderful stuff." A skeptic asked how he had chosen the controls and the subjects. "Oh, I gave the stuff to my seamen and used the passengers as controls."[10]

There are a number of possible approaches for selecting controls in such a nonrandomized fashion. One is to assign patients by the day of the month on which the patient is admitted to the hospital: for example, if admission is on an odd-numbered day of the month the patient is in group A, and if admission is on an even-numbered day of the month the patient is in group B. In a trial of anticoagulant therapy after World War II, in which this day-of-the-month method was used, it was discovered that more patients

than expected were admitted on odd-numbered days. The investigators reported that "as physicians observed the benefits of anticoagulant therapy, they speeded up, where feasible, the hospitalization of those patients . . . who would routinely have been hospitalized on an even day in order to bring as many as possible under the odd-day deadline."[11]

The problem here is that the assignment system was predictable: it was possible for the physicians to know what the assignment of the next patient would be. The goal of randomization is to eliminate the possibility that the investigator will know what the assignment of the next patient will be, because such knowledge introduces the possibility of selection bias.

Many years ago a study was carried out of the effects of bacillus Calmette-Guérin (BCG) vaccination against tuberculosis in children from tuberculous families in New York City.[12] The physicians were told to divide the group of eligible children into a group to be immunized and a control group.

As seen in Table 7-1, tuberculosis mortality was almost five times higher in the controls than in the vaccinated children. However, as the investigators wrote:

> Subsequent experience has shown that by this method of selection, the tendency was to inoculate the children of the more intelligent and cooperative parents and to keep the children of the noncooperative parents as controls. This was probably of considerable error since the cooperative parent will not only keep more careful precautions, but will usually bring the child more regularly to the clinic for instruction as to child care and feeding.[12]

Recognizing that the vaccinations were selectively performed in children from families that were more

---

TABLE 7-1. Results of a Trial of Bacillus Calmette-Guérin (BCG) Vaccination: I

	Number of Children	TUBERCULOSIS DEATHS	
		Number	%
Vaccinated	445	3	0.67
Controls	545	18	3.30

Data from Levine MI, Sackett MF: Results of BCG immunization in New York City. Am Rev Tuberculosis 53:517–532, 1946.

TABLE 7-2. Results of a Trial of Bacillus Calmette-Guérin (BCG) Vaccination: II

| | Number of Children | TUBERCULOSIS DEATHS | |
		Number	%
Vaccinated	556	8	1.44
Controls	528	8	1.52

Data from Levine MI, Sackett MF: Results of BCG immunization in New York City. Am Rev Tuberculosis 53:517–532, 1946.

TABLE 7-3. A Table of Random Numbers

	00–04	05–09	10–14	15–19
00	56348	01458	36236	07253
01	09372	27651	30103	37004
02	44782	54023	61355	71692
03	04383	90952	57204	57810
04	98190	89997	98839	76129
05	16263	35632	88105	59090
06	62032	90741	13468	02647
07	48457	78538	22759	12188
08	36782	06157	73084	48094
09	63302	55103	19703	74741

likely to be conscious of health and related issues, the investigators realized that it was possible that the mortality rate from tuberculosis was lower in the vaccinated group not because of the vaccination itself, but because these children were selected from more health-conscious families that had a lower risk of mortality from tuberculosis, with or without vaccination. To address this problem, a change was made in the study design: alternate children were vaccinated and the remainder served as controls. This does not constitute randomization, but it was a marked improvement over the initial design. As seen in Table 7-2, there was now no difference between the groups.

Randomization

In view of the problems discussed, randomization is the best approach in the design of a trial. Randomization means, in effect, tossing a coin to decide the assignment of a patient to a study group. The critical element of randomization is the unpredictability of the next assignment. Figure 7-2 shows a comic strip cited by Ederer to demonstrate the problem of predictability of the next assignment.[13] How is randomization accomplished? In this hypothetical example we use a selection from a table of random numbers

(Table 7-3). (Such random number tables are available in most statistics textbooks or can be generated on computers.) Today, particularly for large trials, randomization is carried out using a computer.

First, how do we look at this table? Note that the table is divided into two groups of five rows each and five columns. This division is only made to enhance readability. The columns are numbered along the top, 00–04, 05–09, and so on. Similarly, the rows are numbered along the left, 00, 01, 02, and so on. Thus, it is possible to refer to any digit in the table by giving its column and row numbers. This is important if the quality of the randomization process is to be checked by an outsider.

How do we use this table? Let us say that we are conducting a study in which there will be two groups: therapy A and therapy B. In this example, we will consider every odd number an assignment to A and every even number an assignment to B. We close our eyes and put a finger anywhere on the table, and write down the column and row number that was our starting point. We also write down the direction we will move in the table from that starting point (horizontally to the right, horizontally to the left, up, or

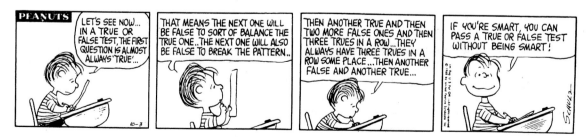

Figure 7-2. How to predict the next patient's treatment assignment in a randomized study. (PEANUTS © UFS. Reprinted by permission.)

down). Let us assume that we point to the "5" at the intersection of column 07 and row 07, and move horizontally to the right. The first patient, then, is designated by an odd number, 5, and will receive therapy A. The second patient is also designated by an odd number, 3, and will receive therapy A. The third is designated by an even number, 8, and will receive therapy B, and so on. Note that the next patient assignment is not predictable; it is *not* a strict alternation, which would be predictable.

There are other ways of using a table of random numbers. For example, we could say that digits 0 to 4 would be treatment A, and digits 5 to 9 treatment B. If we are studying three groups, we could say that digits 1 to 3 are treatment A, digits 4 to 6 treatment B, digits 7 to 9 treatment C, and digit 0 would be ignored. Any of these approaches is valid; the important point is to spell out in writing whatever approach is selected, before the randomization is actually started.

Another way to use the table is to prepare a series of opaque envelopes that are numbered sequentially on the outside: 1, 2, 3, 4, 5, and so on. Inside each envelope a card is placed: a card for therapy A in the first one, for therapy B in the second one, and so on, as determined by the random numbers. The envelopes are then sealed. When the first patient is enrolled, envelope 1 is opened and the assignment is read; this process is repeated for each of the remaining patients in the study.

In a randomized study comparing radical and simple mastectomy for breast cancer, one of the surgeons participating was convinced that radical mastectomy was the treatment of choice and could not reconcile himself to performing simple mastectomy on any of his patients who were included in the study. When randomization was carried out for his patients and an envelope was opened that indicated simple mastectomy for the next assignment, he would set the envelope aside and keep opening envelopes until he reached one with an assignment to radical mastectomy.

What is reflected here is the conflict experienced by many clinicians who enroll their patients in randomized trials. On one hand, the clinician has the obligation to do the best he or she can for the patient; on the other hand, when a clinician participates in a clinical trial, he or she is, in effect, asked to step aside from the usual decision-making role and, essentially, to "flip a coin" to decide which therapy the patient will receive. Thus, there is often an underlying con-

flict between the clinician's role and the role of the physician participating in a clinical trial, and as a result, unintentional biases may occur.

This is such a common problem, particularly in large, multicentered trials, that randomization is not carried out in each clinical center, but is done in a separate coordinating and statistical center. When a new patient is registered at a clinical center, the coordinating center is called and the patient's name is given. A randomized assignment is then made for that patient by the center, and the assignment is noted in both locations.

What do we hope to accomplish by randomization? If we randomize properly, we achieve nonpredictability of the next assignment; we do not have to worry that any subjective biases of the investigators, either overt or covert, may be introduced into the process of selecting patients for one treatment group or the other. Also, in the long run, we hope that randomization will increase the likelihood that the groups will be comparable in regard to characteristics about which we may be concerned, such as sex, age, race, and severity of disease, and that may affect prognosis. However, randomization is not a guarantee of comparability, because chance may play a role in the process, but over the long term, the groups will tend to be similar.

Figure 7-3 presents a hypothetical example of the effect of lack of comparability on a comparison of mortality rates of the groups being studied. Let us assume a study population of 2,000 subjects with myocardial infarctions, of whom half receive an intervention and the other half do not. Let us further assume that of the 2,000 patients, 700 have an arrhythmia and 1,300 do not. Case-fatality in patients with the arrhythmia is 50% and in patients without the arrhythmia it is 10%.

Let us look at the observational study on the left side of Figure 7-3, which shows a study with no randomization. The groups are, therefore, not likely to be comparable in the proportion of patients who have the arrhythmia. By chance, perhaps 200 in the intervention group may have the arrhythmia (with a case-fatality of 50%) and 500 in the no-intervention group may have the arrhythmia (with its 50% case fatality). The resulting case-fatality will be 18% in the intervention group and 30% in the no-intervention group. We might be tempted to conclude that the intervention is effective.

But let us now look at the experimental study on the right side of the figure, in which the groups are randomized. As seen here, the groups are compara-

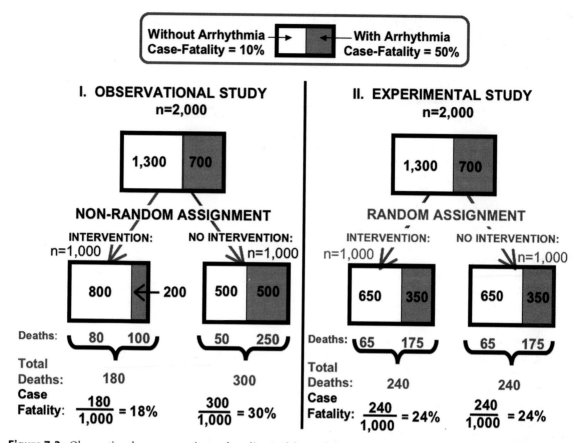

Figure 7-3. Observational versus experimental studies. *I,* If the study is not randomized, the proportions of patients with arrhythmia in the two groups may differ. *II,* If the study is randomized, the proportions of patients with arrhythmia in the two groups are more likely to be similar.

ble, as is likely to occur when we randomize, so that 350 of the 1,000 patients in the intervention group and 350 of the 1,000 patients in the no-intervention group have the arrhythmia. When the case-fatality rate is calculated for this example, it is 24% in both groups. Thus, the difference observed between intervention and no-intervention when the groups were not comparable in terms of the arrhythmia was entirely due to the noncomparability and not to any effects of the intervention itself.

One might ask, if we are so concerned about the comparability of the groups, why not just match the groups on the specific variables about which we are concerned, rather than randomizing? The answer is that we can only match on variables that we know about and that we can measure. Thus, we cannot match on many variables that may affect prognosis, such as an individual's genetic constitution, elements of an individual's immune status, or other variables of which we may not even be aware. Randomization

increases the likelihood that the groups will be comparable not only in terms of variables that we recognize and can measure, but also in terms of variables that we may not recognize and may not be able to measure but that nevertheless may affect prognosis.

Stratified Randomization

Let us say that we are particularly concerned about age as a prognostic variable: prognosis is much worse in older patients. Therefore, we are concerned that the two treatment groups be comparable in terms of age. Although randomization may increase the likelihood of such comparability, it does not guarantee it. It is still possible that after we randomize, we may, by chance, find that most of the older patients are in one group and most of the younger patients are in the other. Our results would then be impossible to interpret because the high-risk patients would be clustered in one group and the low-risk patients in the other. The difference in outcome may then be

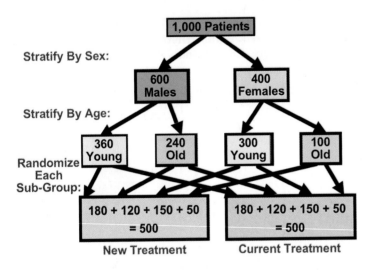

Figure 7-4. Stratified randomization.

attributable to this difference in age distribution rather than to the effects of the intervention.

One approach for dealing with this problem is called *stratified randomization*. In this approach, we first stratify (stratum = layer) our study population by each variable that we consider important, and then randomize participants to treatment groups within each stratum.

Let us consider the example shown in Figure 7-4. We are studying 1,000 patients and are concerned that age and sex are important determinants of prognosis. If we randomize, we do not know what the composition of the groups may be in terms of age and sex; therefore, we decide to use stratified randomization.

We first stratify the 1,000 patients by sex into 600 males and 400 females. We then stratify the males by age and the females by age. We now have four groups (strata): young males, old males, young females, and old females. We now randomize *within each group*, and the result is a new treatment group and a current treatment group for each of the four groups. We end up with two randomized groups, but having initially stratified the groups, we increase the likelihood that the two groups will be comparable in terms of age and sex.

DATA COLLECTION ON SUBJECTS

As mentioned earlier, it is essential that the data collected for each of the study groups be of the same quality. Let us consider some of the variables about which data need to be obtained on the subjects.

Treatment (Assigned and Received)

What data are needed? First, we must know to which treatment group the patient was assigned. In addition, we must know which therapy the patient actually received. It is important to know, for example, if the patient was assigned to receive treatment A, but did not comply. A patient may agree to be randomized, but may later change his or her mind and refuse to comply. Conversely, it is also clearly important to know whether a patient who was not assigned to receive treatment A may have taken treatment A on his or her own, often without realizing it.

Outcome

The need for comparable measurements in all study groups is particularly true for measurements of outcome. Such measurements include both improvement (the desired effect) and any side effects that may appear. There is, therefore, a need for explicitly stated criteria for all outcomes to be measured in a study. Once the criteria are explicitly stated, we must be certain that they are measured comparably in all study groups. In particular, the potential pitfall of outcomes being measured more carefully in those receiving a new drug than in those receiving currently available therapy must be avoided. Blinding (masking), discussed on the next page, can prevent much of this problem, but because blinding is not always possible, attention must be given to ensuring comparability of measurements and of data quality in all of the study groups.

Prognostic Profile at Entry

If we know the risk factors for a bad outcome, we want to verify that randomization has provided reasonable similarity between the two groups in terms of these risk factors. For example, if age is a significant risk factor, we would want to know that randomization has resulted in groups that are comparable for age. Data for prognostic factors should be obtained at the time of subject entry into the study.

Masking (Blinding)

Masking involves several components: First, we would like the subjects not to know which group they are assigned to. This is of particular importance when the outcome is a subjective measure, such as headache or low back pain. If the patient knows that he or she is receiving a new therapy, enthusiasm and certain psychological factors may operate to elicit an improved response.

How can subjects be masked? One way is by using a *placebo*, an inert substance that looks, tastes, and smells like the active agent. However, use of a placebo does not automatically guarantee that the patients are masked (blinded). Some participants may try to determine whether they are taking the placebo or active drug. For example, in a randomized trial of vitamin C for the common cold, patients were blinded by use of a placebo and were then asked whether they knew or suspected which drug they were taking.

As seen in Table 7-4, of the 52 people who were receiving vitamin C and were willing to make a guess, 40 stated they had been receiving vitamin C. Of the 50 who were receiving placebo, 39 said they were receiving placebo. How did they know? They had bitten into the capsule and could tell by the bitter taste. Does it make any difference that they knew? The data suggest that the rate of colds was higher in subjects who received vitamin C but thought they were receiving placebo than in subjects who received placebo but thought they were receiving vitamin C. Thus we must be very concerned about lack of masking or blinding of the subjects and its potential effects on the results of the study, particularly when we are dealing with subjective endpoints.

Use of a placebo is also important for studying the rates of side effects and reactions. The Physicians' Health Study was a randomized trial of the use of aspirin to prevent myocardial infarctions. Table 7-5 shows the side effects that were reported in groups receiving aspirin and those receiving placebo in this study.

Note the high rates of reported reactions in people receiving placebo. Thus, it is not sufficient to say that 34% of the people receiving aspirin had gastrointestinal symptoms; what we really want to know is the extent to which the risk of side effects is increased in people taking aspirin compared to those not taking aspirin (i.e., those taking placebo). Thus, the placebo plays a major role in identifying both the real benefits of an agent and its side effects.

In addition to blinding the subjects, we also want to mask (or blind) the observers or data collectors in regard to which group a patient is in. This is called "double blinding." Some years ago, a study was being conducted to evaluate coronary care units in the treatment of myocardial infarction. It was planned in the following manner:

> *Patients who met strict criteria for categories of myocardial infarction [were to] be randomly assigned either to the group that was admitted immediately to the coronary care unit or to the group that was returned to their homes for domiciliary care. When the preliminary data were presented, it was apparent in the early phases of the experiment that the group of patients labeled as having been admitted to the coronary care unit did somewhat better than the patients sent home. An enthusiast for coronary care units was uncompromising in his insistence that the experiment was unethical and should be terminated and that the data showed that all such patients should be admitted to the coronary care unit. The*

TABLE 7-4. A Randomized Trial of Vitamin C and Placebo for the Common Cold: Results of a Questionnaire Study to Determine Whether Subjects Suspected Which Agent They Had Been Given

Actual Drug	Suspected Drug		
	Vitamin C	*Placebo*	**Total**
Vitamin C	40	12	52
Placebo	11	39	50
Total	51	51	102

$P < .001$.
From Karlowski TR, Chalmers TC, Frenkel LD, et al: Ascorbic acid for the common cold. JAMA 231(10):1038, 1975. Copyright 1975, American Medical Association.

TABLE 7-5. **Physicians' Health Study: Side Effects According to Treatment Group**

Side Effect	Aspirin Group (%)	Placebo Group (%)	P
Gastrointestinal symptoms (except ulcer)	34.8	34.2	.48
Upper gastrointestinal tract ulcers	1.5	1.3	.08
Bleeding problems	27.0	20.4	<.00001

Data from Steering Committee of the Physicians' Health Study Research Group: Final report on the aspirin component of the Ongoing Physicians' Health Study. N Engl J Med 321:129–135, 1989. Copyright 1989, Massachusetts Medical Society. All rights reserved.

statistician then revealed the headings of the data columns had been interchanged and that really the home care group seemed to have a slight advantage. The enthusiast then changed his mind and could not be persuaded to declare coronary care units unethical.[14]

The message of this example is that each of us comes to whatever study we are conducting with a certain number of subconscious or conscious biases and preconceptions. The methods discussed in this chapter and the next are designed to shield the study from the biases of the investigators.

We will now turn to two other aspects of the design of randomized trials: crossover and factorial design.

CROSSOVER

Another important issue in clinical trials is *crossover*. Crossover may be of two types: planned or unplanned.

A *planned crossover* is shown in Figure 7-5. In this example a new treatment is being compared with current treatment. Subjects are randomized to new treatment or current treatment (Fig. 7-5A). After being observed for a certain period of time on one therapy and after any changes are measured (Fig. 7-5B), the patients are switched to the other therapy (Fig. 7-5C). Both groups are then again observed for a certain period of time (Fig. 7-5D). Changes in Group 1 patients while they are on the new treatment can be compared to changes in these patients while they are on current treatment (Fig. 7-5E). Changes in Group 2 patients while they are on the new treatment can also be compared to changes in these patients while they are on current treatment (Fig. 7-5F). Thus, each patient can serve as his or her own control, holding constant the variation between individuals in many characteristics that could potentially affect a comparison of the effectiveness of two agents.

This type of design is very attractive and useful provided that certain cautions are taken into account. First is that of *carryover*: For example, if a subject is changed from therapy A to therapy B and observed under each therapy, the observations under therapy B will be valid only if there is no residual carryover from therapy A. There must be enough of a washout period to be sure none of therapy A, or its effects, remains. Second, the order in which the therapies are given may elicit psychological responses. Patients may react differently to the first therapy given in a study as a result of the enthusiasm that is often accorded a new study; this enthusiasm may diminish over time. We therefore want to be sure that any differences observed are indeed due to the agents being evaluated, and not to any effect of order. Finally, the planned crossover design is clearly not possible if the new therapy is surgical or if the new therapy cures the disease.

A more important consideration is that of an *unplanned crossover*. Figure 7-6 shows the design of a randomized trial of coronary bypass surgery, comparing it with medical care for coronary heart disease. Randomization is carried out after informed consent has been obtained. Although the initial design is straightforward, in reality, unplanned crossovers may occur. Some subjects assigned by the randomization to bypass surgery may begin to have second thoughts and decide not to have the surgery (Fig. 7-7A). They are therefore crossovers into the medical care group. In addition, the condition of some subjects assigned to medical care may begin to deteriorate and urgent bypass surgery may be required (Fig. 7-7B)—these subjects are crossovers from the medical to the

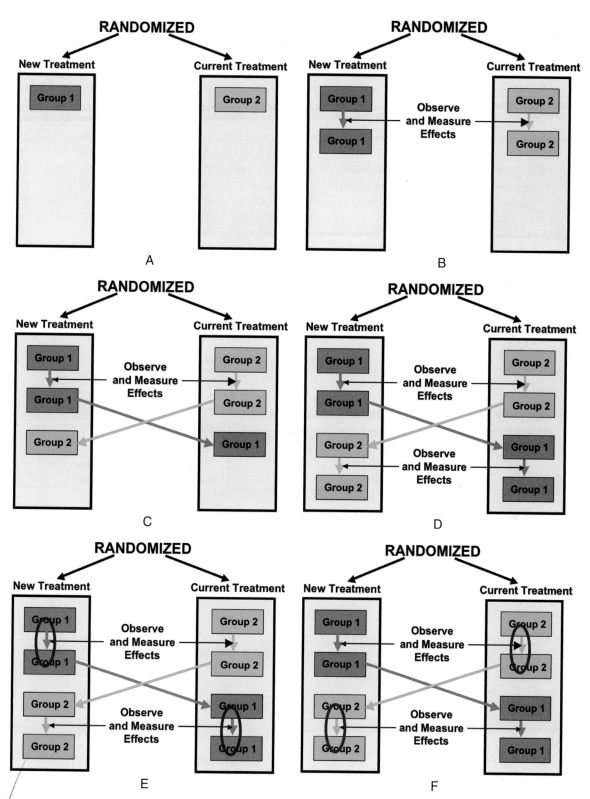

Figure 7-5. **A–F,** Design of a planned crossover trial.

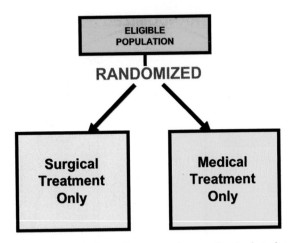

Figure 7-6. Unplanned crossover in a randomized study of cardiac bypass surgery: I. Original study design.

surgical care group. The patients seen on the left in Figure 7-7C are now treated surgically and those on the right in this figure are treated medically. Those treated surgically include some who were randomized to surgery and some who crossed over to surgery. Those treated medically include some who were randomized to medical treatment and some who crossed over to medical treatment. However, if we want to carry out an intention to treat analysis, we would compare the groups shown in Figure 7-7D who are shown in blue with those who are shown in yellow. That is, we would compare the patients according to their original assignments following randomization.

This problem poses a serious challenge in analyzing the data. If we analyze according to the original assignment (intention to treat), we will include in the

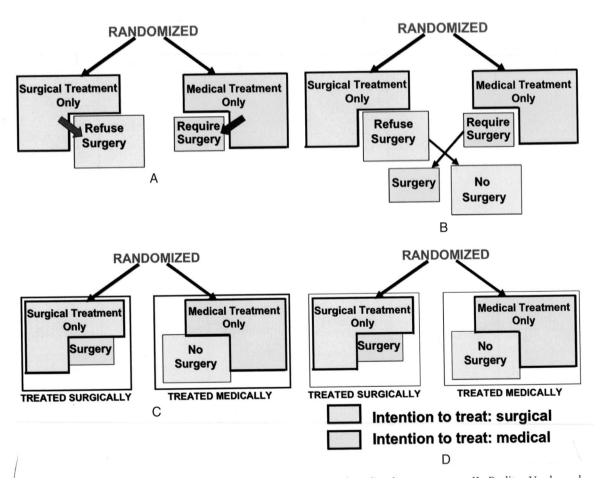

Figure 7-7. A–D, Unplanned crossover in a randomized study of cardiac bypass surgery: II. Reality: Unplanned crossovers.

surgical group some patients who received only medical care, and we will include in the medical group some patients who had surgery. If, however, we analyze according to the treatment that the patients actually receive, we will have broken the randomization and will not have analyzed by intention to treat.

No perfect solution is available for this dilemma. Current practice is to perform the primary analysis by intention to treat—according to the original randomized assignment. We would hope that the results of other comparisons would be consistent with this primary approach. The bottom line is that because there are no perfect solutions, the number of unplanned crossovers must be kept to a minimum. Obviously, if we analyze according to original randomization and there have been many crossovers, the meaning of the study results will be questionable. If the number of crossovers becomes large, the problem may be insurmountable.

FACTORIAL DESIGN

An attractive variant on the study designs discussed in these chapters is *factorial design.* Assuming that two drugs are to be tested, the anticipated outcomes for the two drugs are different, and their modes of action are independent, one can economically use the same study population for testing both drugs. This factorial type of design is shown in Figure 7-8.

If the effects of the two treatments are indeed completely independent, we could evaluate the effects of treatment A by comparing the results in cells

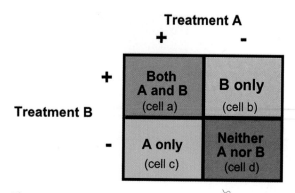

Figure 7-8. Factorial design for studying the effects of two treatments.

$a + c$ to the results in cells $b + d$ (Fig. 7-9A). Similarly, the results for treatment B could be evaluated by comparing the effects in $a + b$ to those in $c + d$ (Fig. 7-9B). In the event that it is decided to terminate the study of treatment A, this design permits continuing the study to determine the effects of treatment B.

An example of a factorial design is seen in the Physicians' Health Study.[15] More than 22,000 physicians were randomized using a 2×2 factorial design that tested aspirin for primary prevention of cardiovascular disease and beta-carotene for primary prevention of cancer. Each physician received one of four possible interventions: both aspirin and beta-carotene, neither aspirin nor beta-carotene, aspirin and beta-carotene placebo, or beta-carotene and aspirin placebo. The resulting four groups are shown

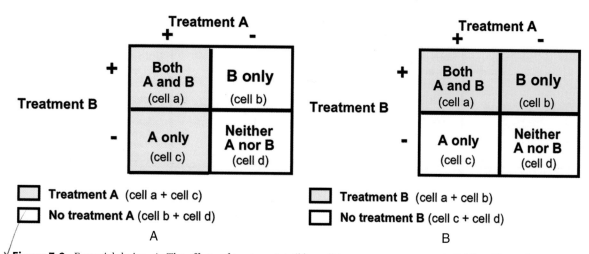

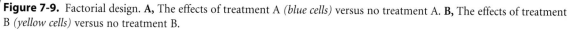

Figure 7-9. Factorial design. **A,** The effects of treatment A *(blue cells)* versus no treatment A. **B,** The effects of treatment B *(yellow cells)* versus no treatment B.

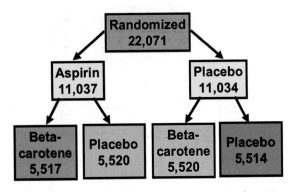

Figure 7-10. Factorial design used in a study of aspirin and beta-carotene.

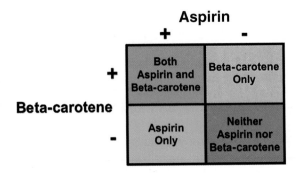

Figure 7-11. Factorial design of the study of aspirin and beta-carotene in 2 × 2 table format.

in Figures 7-10 and 7-11. The aspirin part of the study (Fig. 7-12A) was terminated early, on the advice of the external data monitoring board, because a statistically significant 44% decrease in the risk of first myocardial infarction was observed in the group taking aspirin. The randomized beta-carotene component (Fig. 7-12B) continued until the originally scheduled date of completion. After 12 years of beta-carotene supplementation, no benefit or harm was observed in terms of the incidence of cancer or heart disease or death from all causes. Subsequent reports have reported greater risk of cancer with beta-carotene in smokers.

NONCOMPLIANCE

Patients may agree to be randomized, but following randomization they may not comply with the assigned treatment. Noncompliance may be overt or covert: On the one hand, people may overtly articulate their refusal to comply or may stop participating in the study. These non-compliers are also called *dropouts* from the study. On the other hand, people may just stop taking the agent assigned without admitting this to the investigator or the study staff. Whenever possible, checks on potential noncompliance are built into the study. These may include, for example, urine tests for the agent being tested or for one of its metabolites.

Another problem in randomized trials has been called *drop-ins*. Patients in one group may inadvertently take the agent assigned to the other group. For example, in a trial of the effect of aspirin for prevention of myocardial infarction, patients were randomized to aspirin or to no aspirin. However, a problem arose in that, because of the large number of over-the-counter preparations that contain aspirin, many of the control patients might well be taking aspirin without knowing it. Two steps were taken to address

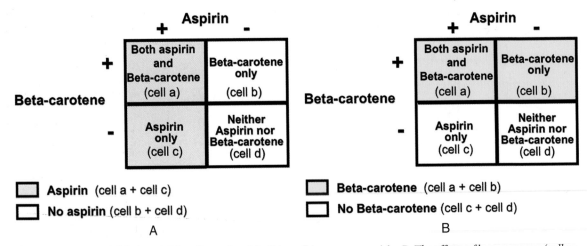

Figure 7-12. Factorial design. **A,** The effects of aspirin (*blue cells*) versus no aspirin. **B,** The effects of beta-carotene (*yellow cells*) versus no beta-carotene.

this problem: (1) controls were provided with lists of aspirin-containing over-the-counter preparations that they should avoid, and (2) urine tests for salicylates were carried out both in the aspirin group and in the controls.

The net effect of noncompliance on the study results will be to reduce any observed differences, because the treatment group will include some who did not receive the therapy, and the no-treatment group may include some who received the treatment. Thus, the groups will be less different in terms of therapy than they would have been had there been no noncompliance, so that even if there is a difference in the effects of the treatments, it will appear much smaller.

One approach that was used in the Veterans Administration Study of the Treatment of Hypertension was to carry out a pilot study in which compliers and noncompliers were identified. When the actual full study was later carried out, the study population was limited to those who had been compliers during the pilot study. The problem with this approach is that when we want to generalize from the results of such a study, we can only do so to other populations of compliers, which may be different from the population in any free-living community, which would consist of both compliers and noncompliers.

Table 7-6 shows data from the Coronary Drug Project reported by Canner and coworkers.[16] This study was a comparison of clofibrate and placebo for lowering cholesterol. The table presents the mortality in the two groups.

No large difference in 5-year mortality was seen between the two groups. The investigators speculated that perhaps this was the result of the patients not having taken their medication. Table 7-7 shows the

---

TABLE 7-7. Coronary Drug Project: Five-Year Mortality in Patients Given Clofibrate or Placebo According to Level of Compliance

	Number of Patients	Mortality (%)
Clofibrate		
Poor complier (<80%)	357	24.6
Good complier (≥80%)	708	15.0
Placebo	2,695	19.4

Adapted from Canner PL, Forman SA, Prud'homme GJ, for the Coronary Drug Project Research Group: Influence of adherence to treatment and response to cholesterol on mortality in the coronary drug project. N Engl J Med 303:1038–1041, 1980.

---

results of separating the clofibrate subjects into good compliers and poor compliers. Here we see the 5-year mortality was 24.6% in the poor-complier group compared to 15% in the good-complier group. We might thus be tempted to conclude that compliance was indeed the factor that produced the results seen in Table 7-7: no significant difference between the clofibrate and placebo groups.

Table 7-8 separates both groups, clofibrate and placebo, into compliers and noncompliers. Even in the placebo group, 5-year mortality in the poor compliers was higher than in the good compliers: 28% compared to 15%.

What can we learn from these tables? People who do not comply or who do not participate in studies differ from those who do comply and who do participate. Therefore, in conducting a study to evaluate a therapy or other intervention, we cannot offer the agent to a population and compare the effects in those who take the agent to the effects in those who refuse or do not, because the two groups are basically different in terms of many demographic, social, psychological, and cultural variables that may have important roles in determining outcome. That is why randomization, or some other approach that reduces selection bias, is essential.

CONCLUSION

The randomized clinical trial is generally considered the "gold standard" of study designs. When hierarchies of study design are created to assess the strength of the available evidence supporting clinical and

---

TABLE 7-6. Coronary Drug Project: Five-Year Mortality in Patients Given Clofibrate or Placebo

	Number of Patients	Mortality (%)
Clofibrate	1,065	18.2
Placebo	2,695	19.4

Adapted from Canner PL, Forman SA, Prud'homme GJ, for the Coronary Drug Project Research Group: Influence of adherence to treatment and response to cholesterol on mortality in the coronary drug project. N Engl J Med 303:1038–1041, 1980.

TABLE 7-8. Coronary Drug Project: Five-Year Mortality in Patients Given Clofibrate or Placebo According to Level of Compliance

Compliance	CLOFIBRATE		PLACEBO	
	Number of Patients	**Mortality (%)**	**Number of Patients**	**Mortality (%)**
Poor (<80%)	357	24.6	882	28.2
Good (≥80%)	708	15.0	1,813	15.1
Total Group	1,065	18.2	2,695	19.4

Adapted from Canner PL, Forman SA, Prud'homme GJ, for the Coronary Drug Project Research Group: Influence of adherence to treatment and response of cholesterol on mortality in the coronary drug project. N Engl J Med 303:1038–1041, 1980.

public health policy, randomized trials are virtually always at the top of the list when study designs are ranked in order of descending quality.

This chapter has discussed many of the components of the randomized trial that are designed to shield the study from any preconceptions and biases of the investigator and of others involved in conducting the study, as well as from other biases that might inadvertently be introduced. In the next chapter we will address some other issues relating to the design of randomized trials and will consider several interesting examples and applications of the randomized trial design. In Chapters 17 and 18 we will discuss the use of randomized trials and other study designs for evaluating health services and for studying the effectiveness of screening.

REFERENCES

1. Cited in Silverman WA: Where's the Evidence? Debates in Modern Medicine. New York, Oxford University Press, 1998.
2. Galton F: Inquiries into Human Faculty and Its Development. London, Macmillan, 1883.
3. Joyce CRB, Welldon RMC: The efficacy of prayer: A double blind clinical trial. J Chronic Dis 18:367, 1965.
4. Byrd RC: Positive therapeutic effects of intercessory prayer in a coronary care unit population. South Med J 81:826, 1988.
5. Bull JP: The historical development of clinical therapeutic trials. J Chronic Dis 10:218, 1959.
6. Lind J: A Treatise of the Scurvy. Edinburgh, Sands, Murray & Cochran, 1753.
7. Peacock E: Cited in Tufte ER: Data Analyses for Politics and Policy. Englewood Cliffs, NJ, Prentice-Hall, 1974.
8. Ederer F: Why do we need controls? Why do we need to randomize? Am J Ophthalmol 79:758, 1975.
9. Bearman JE, Loewenson RB, Gullen WH: Muensch's Postulates, Laws and Corollaries. Biometrics note No. 4. Bethesda, MD, Office of Biometry and Epidemiology, National Eye Institute, April 1974.
10. Wilson EB: Cited in Ederer F: Why do we need controls? Why do we need to randomize? Am J Ophthalmol 79:761, 1975.
11. Wright IS, Marple CD, Beck DF: Cited in Ederer F: Why do we need controls? Why do we need to randomize? Am J Ophthalmol 79:761, 1975.
12. Levine MI, Sackett MF: Results of BCG immunization in New York City. Am Rev Tuberculosis 53:517–532, 1946.
13. Ederer F: Practical problems in collaborative clinical trials. Am J Epidemiol 102:111–118, 1975.
14. Cochrane AL: Cited in Ballintine EJ: Objective measurements and the double masked procedure. Am J Ophthalmol 79:764, 1975.
15. Hennekens CH, Buring JE, Manson JE: Lack of effect of long-term supplementation with beta carotene on the incidence of malignant neoplasms and cardiovascular disease. N Engl J Med 334:1145–1149, 1996.
16. Canner PL, Forman SA, Prud'homme GJ: Influence of adherence to treatment and response of cholesterol on mortality in the coronary drug project. N Engl J Med 303:1038–1041, 1980.

Review Questions for Chapters 7 and 8 are at the end of Chapter 8.

Randomized Trials: Some Further Issues

SAMPLE SIZE

At a scientific meeting some years ago, an investigator presented the results of a study he had conducted to evaluate a new drug in sheep. "After taking the drug," he reported, "one third of the sheep were markedly improved, one third of the sheep showed no change, and the other one ran away."

This story introduces one of the most frequent questions asked by physicians conducting trials of new agents, or for that matter by anyone conducting evaluative studies: "How many subjects do we have to study?" The time to answer this question is *before* the study is done. All too often studies are conducted, large amounts of money and other resources are invested, and only after the study has been completed do the investigators find that from the beginning they had too few subjects to obtain meaningful results.

The question of how many subjects are needed for study is not based on mystique. This section presents the logic of how to approach the question of sample size. Let us begin this discussion of sample size with Figure 8-1.

We have two jars of beads, each containing 100 beads, some white and some blue. The jars are opaque, so (despite their appearance in the figure) we cannot see the colors of the beads in the jars just by looking at the jars. We want to know whether the distribution of the beads by color differs in jars A and B: that is, is there a larger (or smaller) proportion of blue beads in jar A than in jar B?

To answer this question, let us take a sample of 10 beads from jar A in one hand and a sample of 10 beads from jar B in the other. On the basis of the color distribution of the 10 beads in each hand, we will try to reach a conclusion about the color distribution of all the 100 beads in each of the jars.

Let us assume that (as shown in Fig. 8-2) in one hand we have 9 blue beads and 1 white bead from jar A, and in the other hand we have 2 blue beads and 8 white beads from jar B. Can we conclude that 90% of the beads in jar A are blue and that 10% are white? Clearly, we cannot. It is possible, for example, that of the 100 beads in jar A, 90 are white and 10 are blue, but *by chance* our 10-bead sample includes 9 blue and 1 white. This is possible, but highly unlikely. Similarly, in regard to jar B we cannot conclude that 20% of the beads are blue and 80% are white. It is conceivable that 90 of the 100 beads are blue and 10 are white, but that *by chance* the 10-bead sample includes 2 blue beads and 8 white beads. This is conceivable but, again, highly unlikely.

On the basis of the distributions of the 10-bead samples in each hand, could we say that the distributions of the 100 beads in the two jars are different? Given the samples in each hand, could it be, for example, that the distribution of beads in each jar is 50 blue and 50 white? Again, it is possible, but it is not likely. We cannot exclude this possibility on the basis of our samples. We are looking at samples and trying to draw a conclusion regarding a whole universe—the jars from which we have drawn the samples.

Let us consider a second example, shown in Figure 8-3. Again, we draw two samples. This time, the 10-bead sample from jar A consists of 7 blue beads and 3 white beads, and the 10-bead sample from jar B also consists of 7 blue beads and 3 white beads. Could the color distribution of the beads in the two jars be the same? Clearly, it could. Could we have drawn these two samples of 7 blue beads and 3 white beads from both jars if the distribution is actually 90 white beads and 10 blue beads in jar A and 90 blue beads and 10 white beads in jar B? Yes, possibly, but highly unlikely.

When we carry out a study we are only looking at the sample of subjects in our study, such as a sample of patients with a certain illness who are being treated with treatment A or with treatment B. From the study results, we want to draw a conclusion that goes

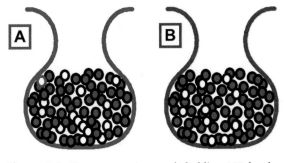

Figure 8-1. Two opaque jars, each holding 100 beads, some blue and some white.

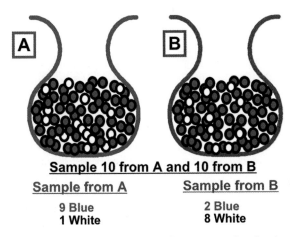

Sample 10 from A and 10 from B

Sample from A	Sample from B
9 Blue	2 Blue
1 White	8 White

Figure 8-2. Samples of 10 beads from jar A and 10 beads from jar B.

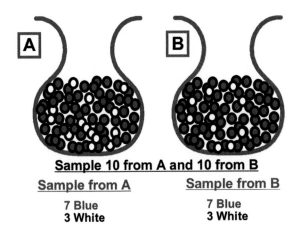

Sample 10 from A and 10 from B

Sample from A	Sample from B
7 Blue	7 Blue
3 White	3 White

Figure 8-3. Samples of 10 beads from jar A and 10 beads from jar B.

beyond the study population—is treatment A more effective than treatment B in the total universe of all patients with this disease who might be treated with treatment A or treatment B? The same issue that arose with the 10-bead samples arises when we want

TABLE 8-1.	**Four Possibilities in Testing Whether the Treatments Differ**

1. The treatments do not differ, and we correctly conclude that they do not differ.
2. The treatments do not differ, but we conclude that they do differ.
3. The treatments differ, but we conclude that they do not differ.
4. The treatments do differ, and we correctly conclude that they do differ.

to derive a conclusion regarding all patients from the sample of patients included in our study. Rarely, if ever, is a study conducted in all patients with a disease or in all patients who might be treated with the drugs in question.

Given this background, let us now consider a trial in which groups receiving one of two therapies, therapy A and therapy B, are being compared. (Keep in mind the sampling of beads just discussed.) Before beginning our study, we can list the four possible study outcomes (Table 8-1):

1. It is possible that in reality there is no difference in efficacy between therapy A and therapy B (i.e., therapy A is no better and no worse than therapy B), and when we do our study we correctly conclude on the basis of our samples that the two groups do not differ.
2. It is possible that in reality there is no difference in efficacy between therapy A and therapy B (i.e., therapy A is no better and no worse than therapy B), but in our study we found a difference between the groups and therefore concluded, on the basis of our samples, that there is a difference between the therapies. This conclusion, based on our samples, is in error.
3. It is possible that in reality there is a difference between therapy A and therapy B, but when we examine the groups in our study we find no difference between them. We therefore conclude, on the basis of our samples, that there is no difference between therapy A and therapy B. This conclusion is in error.
4. It is possible that in reality there is a difference between therapy A and therapy B, and when we examine the groups in our study we find that they differ. On the basis of these samples, we correctly conclude that therapy A differs from therapy B.

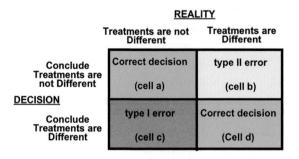

Figure 8-4. Possible outcomes of a randomized trial.

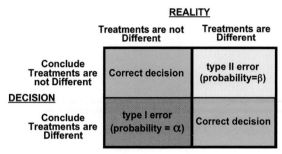

Figure 8-5. Possible outcomes of a randomized trial: type I and type II errors.

These four possibilities constitute the universe of outcomes after we complete our study. Let us look at these four possibilities as presented in a 2 × 2 table (Fig. 8-4): Two columns represent reality—either therapy A differs from therapy B or therapy A does not differ from therapy B. The two rows represent our decision: We conclude either that they differ or that they do not differ. In this figure, the four possibilities that were just listed are represented as four cells in the 2 × 2 table. If there is no difference, and on the basis of the samples included in our study we conclude there is no difference, this is a correct decision *(cell a)*. If there is a difference, and on the basis of our study we conclude that there is a difference *(cell d)*, this too is a correct decision. In the best of all worlds, all of the possibilities would fall into one of these two cells. Unfortunately, this is rarely, if ever, the case. There are times when there is no difference between the therapies, but on the basis of the samples of subjects included in our study, we erroneously conclude that they differ *(cell c)*. This is called a *type I error*. It is also possible that there really is a difference between the therapies, but on the basis of the samples included in our study we erroneously conclude that there is no difference *(cell b);* this is called a *type II error*. (In this situation, the therapies differ, but we fail to detect the difference in our study samples.)

The *probability* that we will make a type I error is designated α, and the *probability* that we will make a type II error is designated β (as shown in Fig. 8-5).

α is the so-called *P* value, which is seen in many published papers and has been sanctified by many years of use. When you see "*P* < .05," the reference is to α. What does *P* < .05 mean? It tells us that we have concluded that therapy A differs from therapy B on the basis of the sample of subjects included in our study, which we found to differ. The probability that such a difference could have arisen by chance alone,

and that this difference between our groups does not reflect any true difference between therapies A and B, is only .05 (or 1 in 20).

Let us now direct our attention to the right half of this 2 × 2 table, which shows the two possibilities when there is a true difference between therapies A and B, as shown in Figure 8-6. If, as seen here, the reality is that there is a difference between the therapies, there are only two possibilities: We might conclude, in error, that the therapies do not differ (type II error). The probability of making a type II error is designated β. Or we might conclude, correctly, that the therapies differ. Because the total of all probabilities must equal 1 and the probability of a type II error = β, the probability that we shall correctly decide on the basis of our study that the therapies differ if there is a difference will equal 1 − β. This probability, 1 − β, is called the *power* of the study. It tells us how good our study is at correctly identifying a difference between the therapies if in reality they are different. How likely is our study not to miss a difference if one exists?

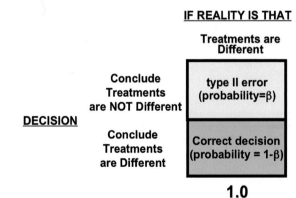

Figure 8-6. Possible outcomes of a randomized trial when the treatments differ.

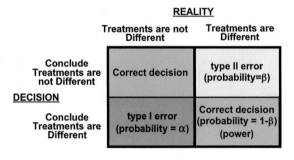

Figure 8-7. Possible outcomes of a randomized trial: summary.

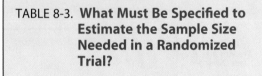

TABLE 8-3. **What Must Be Specified to Estimate the Sample Size Needed in a Randomized Trial?**

1. The difference in response rates to be detected
2. An estimate of the response rate in one of the groups
3. Level of statistical significance (α)
4. The value of the power desired ($1 - \beta$)
5. Whether the test should be one-sided or two-sided

The full 2×2 table in Figure 8-7 includes all of the terms that have been discussed. Table 8-2 provides multiple definitions of these terms.

How do these concepts help us to arrive at an estimate of the sample size that we need? If we ask the question, "How many people do we have to study in a clinical trial?" we must be able to specify a number of items as listed in Table 8-3.

First, we must specify the expected difference in response rate. Let us say that the existing therapy cures 40% of patients, and we are going to test a new therapy. We must be able to say whether we expect the new therapy to cure 50%, 60%, or some other proportion of treated patients. That is, will the new therapy be 10% better than the current therapy and cure 50% of people, 20% better than current therapy and cure 60%, or some other difference? What is the size of the difference between current therapy and new therapy that we want to be able to detect with our study?

How do we generally arrive at such a figure? What if we do not have information on which to base an estimate of the improvement in effectiveness that might be anticipated? Perhaps we are studying a new therapy for which we have no prior experience. One approach is to search for data in human populations for similar diseases and therapies. We can also search for relevant data from animal studies. At times, we simply have no way of producing such an estimate. In this situation, we can make a guess—say, 30% improvement—but *bracket* the estimate: that is, calculate the sample size needed based on a 40% improvement in response rate and also calculate the sample size needed based on a 20% improvement in response rate.

Second, we must have an estimate of the response rate (rate of cure, rate of improvement) in one of the groups. In the example just used, we said the current cure rate (or response rate) is 40%. This is the estimate of the response rate for the current treatment group based on current clinical experience.

Third, we must specify the level of α with which we will be satisfied. The choice is up to the investigator; there is nothing sacred about any specific value, but values of .05 or .01 are commonly used. Fourth, we must specify the power of the study. Again, no specific value is sacred, but powers of 80% or 90% are commonly used.

TABLE 8-2. **Summary of Terms**

Term	Definitions
α	= Probability of making a type I error
	= Probability of concluding the treatments differ when in reality they do not differ
β	= Probability of making a type II error
	= Probability of concluding that the treatments do not differ when in reality they do differ
Power	= 1 − Probability of making a type II error
	= $1 - \beta$
	= Probability of correctly concluding that the treatments differ
	= Probability of detecting a difference between the treatments if the treatments do in fact differ

Finally, we must specify whether the test should be one-sided or two-sided. What does this mean? Our present cure rate is 40% and we are trying a new therapy that we believe will have a higher cure rate—perhaps 50% or 60%. We want to detect a difference that is in the direction of improvement with the new therapy—an increase in cure rate. So we might say we will only test for a difference in that direction because that is the direction in which we are interested—that is, a one-sided test.

The problem is that in the history of medicine and of public health we have at times been surprised, and have found that new therapies that we thought would be beneficial have actually been harmful. If such a possibility exists, we would want to find a difference in cure rate *in either direction* from the current rate in our study—that is, we would use a two-sided test, testing not only for a difference that is better than the current cure rate, but also for one that is worse than the current rate. Clinicians and other investigators often prefer to use a one-sided test in their studies because such tests require smaller sample sizes than do two-sided tests. Because the number of patients available for study is often limited, a one-sided test is attractive. At times investigators may make a practical decision to use a one-sided test, even if there is no conceptual justification for this decision.

Opinions differ on this subject. Some believe that if the investigator is only interested in one direction—improvement—a one-sided test is justified.

Others believe that as long as the difference could go in either direction, a two-sided test is required. In a situation in which a particular disease is currently 100% fatal, any difference with a new therapy could only be in the direction of improvement, and a one-sided test would be appropriate.

Let us now turn to the application of these five factors to estimating the needed sample size from a sample size table. Tables 8-4 and 8-5 are selections from sample size tables published by Gehan in 1979.[1] (Similar tables are available in many standard statistics texts.) Both tables give the number of patients needed *in each group* to detect various differences in cure rates with an α of .05 and a power $(1 - \beta)$ of .80. Table 8-4 is intended to be used for a two-sided test and Table 8-5 for a one-sided test.

Let us say that we are conducting a clinical trial of two therapies: one that is currently in use and one that is new. The current therapy has a cure rate of 40%, and we believe that the new therapy may have a cure rate of 60%—that is, we wish to detect an improvement in cure rate of 20%. How many subjects do we have to study? Let us say we will use an α of .05, a power of 80%, and a two-sided test. We therefore will use Table 8-4. The first column of this table is designated the lower of the two cure rates. As the current cure rate is 40%, and we expect a cure rate of 60% with our new therapy, the lower of the two cure rates is 40%, and we move to that row of the table. We expect the new therapy to have a cure rate of 60%, so the difference in cure rates will be

TABLE 8-4. **Number of Patients Needed in Each Group to Detect Various Differences in Cure Rates; $\alpha = .05$; Power $(1 - \beta) = .80$ (Two-sided Test)**

Lower of the Two Cure Rates	DIFFERENCES IN CURE RATES BETWEEN THE TWO TREATMENT GROUPS													
	.05	.10	.15	.20	.25	.30	.35	.40	.45	.50	.55	.60	.65	.70
.05	420	130	69	44	36	31	23	20	17	14	13	11	10	8
.10	680	195	96	59	41	35	29	23	19	17	13	12	11	8
.15	910	250	120	71	48	39	31	25	20	17	15	12	11	9
.20	1,090	290	135	80	53	42	33	26	22	18	16	12	11	9·
.25	1,250	330	150	88	57	44	35	28	22	18	16	12	11	—
.30	1,380	360	160	93	60	44	36	29	22	18	15	12	—	—
.35	1,470	370	170	96	61	44	36	28	22	17	13	—	—	—
.40	1,530	390	175	97	61	44	35	26	20	17	—	—	—	—
.45	1,560	390	175	96	60	42	33	25	19	—	—	—	—	—
.50	1,560	390	170	93	57	40	31	23	—	—	—	—	—	—

Adapted from Gehan E: Clinical trials in cancer research. Environ Health Perspect 32:31, 1979.

TABLE 8-5. Number of Patients Needed in Each Group to Detect Various Differences in Cure Rates; α = .05; Power (1 − β) = .80 (One-sided Test)

Lower of the Two Cure Rates	DIFFERENCES IN CURE RATES BETWEEN THE TWO TREATMENT GROUPS													
	.05	.10	.15	.20	.25	.30	.35	.40	.45	.50	.55	.60	.65	.70
.05	330	105	55	40	33	24	20	17	13	12	10	9	9	8
.10	540	155	76	47	37	30	23	19	16	13	11	11	9	8
.15	710	200	94	56	43	32	26	22	17	15	11	10	9	8
.20	860	230	110	63	42	36	27	23	17	15	12	10	9	8
.25	980	260	120	69	45	37	31	23	17	15	12	10	9	—
.30	1,080	280	130	73	47	37	31	23	17	15	11	10	—	—
.35	1,160	300	135	75	48	37	31	23	17	15	11	—	—	—
.40	1,210	310	135	76	48	37	30	23	17	13	—	—	—	—
.45	1,230	310	135	75	47	36	26	22	16	—	—	—	—	—
.50	1,230	310	135	73	45	36	26	19	—	—	—	—	—	—

Adapted from Gehan E: Clinical trials in cancer research. Environ Health Perspect 32:31, 1979.

20%. We therefore move down the 20% column (the difference in cure rates) to the point at which it intersects the row of 40% (the lower of the cure rates), where we find the value 97. We need 97 subjects *in each of our study groups.*

Another approach is to use the table in a reverse direction. For example, let us consider a clinic for people who have a certain rare disease. Each year the clinic treats 30 patients with the disease and wishes to test a new therapy. Given this maximum number of 30 patients, we could ask, "What size difference in cure rates could we hope to detect?" We may find a difference of a certain size that may be acceptable, or we may find that the number of subjects available for study is simply too small. If the number of patients is too small, we have several options: We can decide not to do the study, and such a decision should be made early on, before most of the effort has been invested. Or we could decide to extend the study in time to accumulate more subjects. Finally, we could decide to collaborate with investigators at other institutions to increase the total number of subjects available for the study. An advantage of the last approach is that in such a multicenter study, a major selection bias at one of the centers would be manifest in the results in subjects recruited at that center and would differ from the results in the other subjects in the study. The presence of such a bias would be more readily recognizable.

This section has demonstrated the use of a sample size table. Formulas and computer programs are also available for calculating sample size. Sample sizes can be calculated not only for randomized trials but also for cohort and case-control studies.

WAYS OF EXPRESSING THE RESULTS OF RANDOMIZED TRIALS

The results of randomized trials can be expressed in a number of ways. The risks of death or of developing a disease or complication in each group can be calculated, and the *reduction in risk* (efficacy) can then be calculated. *Efficacy* of an agent being tested, such as a vaccine, can be expressed in terms of the rates of developing disease in the vaccine and placebo groups:

$$\text{Efficacy} = \frac{\left(\begin{array}{c}\text{Rate in those who} \\ \text{received placebo}\end{array}\right) - \left(\begin{array}{c}\text{Rate in those who} \\ \text{received the vaccine}\end{array}\right)}{\text{Rate in those who received the placebo}}$$

This formula tells us the extent of the reduction in disease by use of the vaccine. Risks are often calculated per *person-years* of observation.

Another approach is to calculate the *ratio of the risks* in the two treatment groups (the relative risk), which will be discussed in Chapter 11. In addition, often we compare the *survival curves* for each of the groups (Chapter 6) and determine whether they differ.

A major objective of randomized trials is to have an impact on the way clinical medicine and public health are practiced. But at times practitioners may find it difficult to place the findings of such trials in a perspective that seems relevant to their practices. Another approach, therefore, for expressing the results of randomized trials is to estimate the *number of patients who would need to be treated* (NNT) to prevent one adverse outcome such as one death. This can be calculated by

$$NNT = \frac{1}{\left(\begin{array}{c}\text{Rate in}\\\text{untreated group}\end{array}\right) - \left(\begin{array}{c}\text{Rate in}\\\text{treated group}\end{array}\right)}$$

Thus, if, for example, the mortality rate in the untreated group is 17% and mortality in the treated group is 12%, we would need to treat

$$\frac{1}{17\% - 12\%} = \frac{1}{0.05} = 20$$

people to prevent one death. Estimates of NNT are usually rounded up to the next highest whole number. This approach can be used in studies of various interventions including both treatment and prevention. The same approach can also be used to look at the risk of side effects by calculating the *number needed to harm* (NNH) to cause one additional person to be harmed. These estimates are subject to considerable error and are generally presented with 95% confidence intervals so that they can be properly interpreted. In addition, they have other limitations: they do not take into account quality of life and are of limited value to patients. They can nevertheless be helpful in assisting practitioners in estimating the effect they might expect to observe by using the new treatment or preventive measure in their practices.

GENERALIZABILITY OF RESULTS

Whenever we carry out a trial, the ultimate objective is to generalize the results beyond the study population itself. In this context, it is useful to introduce two concepts: internal validity and external validity, as shown in Figure 8-8.

This diagram represents a randomized trial in which the study population is our sample, identified as a subset of some reference population. For example, the reference population might be all patients with lupus erythematosus, and the study population will be patients with the disease attending several clinics in our city. We then randomize the study population to new treatment or current treatment. If the study is properly done without major methodologic problems, and takes into account all the issues discussed thus far, the study is said to have *internal validity.*

Another issue relates to the *generalizability* or *external validity* of the study. If, for example, we carry out a study in one city and find a new therapy to be better than a current therapy, we would like to be able to say that the new therapy is better for the disease

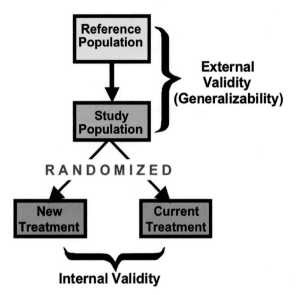

Figure 8-8. Internal and external validity in a randomized trial.

regardless of where the patients are treated, and not just for patients in that city. We want to be able to generalize from the study findings to all patients with the disease. To do so, we must know to what extent the patients we have studied are representative of all patients with the disease in question; to do so, we must characterize those who did not participate in the study and identify characteristics of study patients that might preclude our generalizing the results to other patients who were not in the study. Thus, the issues of internal validity—whether the study was well done and whether the findings are valid—and of external validity or generalizability are basic concerns in the conduct of any randomized trial.

THREE MAJOR U.S. RANDOMIZED TRIALS

The Hypertension Detection and Follow-up Program

Many years ago a Veterans Administration study demonstrated that treating people who have large increases in blood pressure can significantly reduce their mortality.[2] The question of whether antihypertensive therapy benefits people with only a slight increase in blood pressure (diastolic blood pressure of 90 to 104 mm Hg) was left unanswered. Although we might be able to reduce blood pressure in such persons, the problem exists of the side effects of antihypertensive agents. Unless some health benefit to the patients can be demonstrated, use of these antihypertensive agents would not be justified in people whose blood pressure is only minimally elevated.

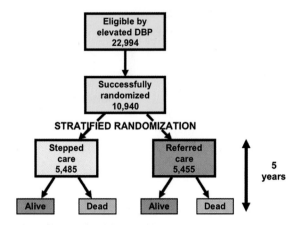

Figure 8-9. Design of the Hypertension Detection and Follow-up Program (HDFP).

The multicenter Hypertension Detection and Follow-up Program (HDFP) study was designed to investigate the benefits of treating mild to moderate hypertension. In this study, of 22,994 subjects who were eligible because they had elevated diastolic blood pressure, 10,940 were randomized either to the stepped care or to the referred care group (Fig. 8-9).

Stepped care meant treatment according to a precisely defined protocol, under which treatment was changed when a specified decrease in blood pressure had not been obtained during a certain period. The comparison group posed a problem: from the standpoint of study design, a group receiving no care for hypertension might have been desirable. However, the investigators believed it would be ethically unjustifiable to withhold antihypertensive care from known hypertensive subjects. So the subjects in the comparison group were referred back to their own physicians, and this group was therefore called the *referred care group.* Mortality in both groups over a 5-year period was then studied.[3]

Figure 8-10 shows that at every interval following entry into the study, the patients in the stepped care group had lower mortality than did those in the referred care group. In Figure 8-10 we see that the same pattern held in those with only mild increases in blood pressure.

The results are shown in greater detail in Table 8-6, in which the data are presented according to diastolic blood pressure at entry into the study. The right-hand column shows the percent reduction in mortality for the stepped care group: the greatest reduction occurred in those subjects with a minimal increase in diastolic pressure.

This study has had considerable impact in encouraging physicians to treat even mild to moderate elevations in blood pressure. It has been criticized, however, because of the absence of an untreated group for comparison. Not only were these patients referred back to their own physicians, but there was no monitoring of the care that was provided to them by their physicians. There is therefore some problem in interpreting these data. Even today, people differ on whether there was indeed a legitimate ethical

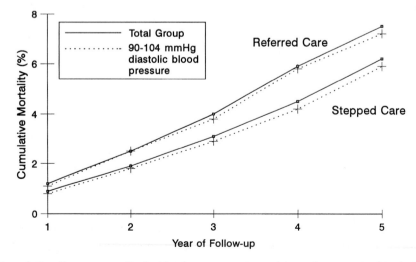

Figure 8-10. Cumulative all-cause mortality by blood pressure status and type of care received in the HDFP. (Adapted from Hypertension Detection and Follow-up Program Cooperative Group: Five-year findings of the Hypertension Detection and Follow-up Program: I. Reduction in mortality of persons with high blood pressure, including mild hypertension. JAMA 242:2562–2571, 1979.)

TABLE 8-6. **Mortality from All Causes during the Hypertension Detection and Follow-up Program**

Diastolic Blood Pressure at Entry (mm Hg)	Stepped Care (SC)	Referred Care (RC)	5-YR DEATH RATE		Mortality Reduction in SC Group (%)
			SC	RC	
90–104	3,903	3,922	5.9	7.4	20.3
105–114	1,048	1,004	6.7	7.7	13.0
≥115	534	529	9.0	9.7	7.2
Total	5,485	5,455	6.4	7.7	16.9

From Hypertension Detection and Follow-up Program Cooperative Group: Five-year findings of the Hypertension Detection and Follow-up Program: I. Reduction in mortality of persons with high blood pressure, including mild hypertension. JAMA 242:2562–2571, 1979.

objection to including an untreated placebo group in this study or whether there was an ethical problem in designing an expensive study that was difficult to mount and left so much uncertainty and difficulty in interpretation.

The Multiple Risk Factor Intervention Trial

A serious problem in large-scale trials that require the investment of tremendous resources, financial and otherwise, and take years to complete is that their interpretation is often clouded by a problem in design or methodology that may not have been appreciated at an early stage of the study. The Multiple Risk Factor Intervention Trial (MRFIT) was a randomized study designed to determine whether mortality from myocardial infarction could be reduced by changes in lifestyle and other measures. In this study, one group received special intervention (SI), consisting of stepped care for hypertension and intensive education and counseling about lifestyle changes. The comparison group received its usual care (UC) in the community. Over an average follow-up period of 7 years, levels of coronary heart disease (CHD) risk factors declined more in SI men than in UC men (Fig. 8-11).

However, by the end of the study, no statistically significant differences were evident between the groups in either CHD mortality or all-cause mortality (Fig. 8-12).

Serious problems complicated the interpretation of these results. First, the study was conducted at a time when mortality from coronary disease was declining in the United States. In addition, it was not clear whether the lack of difference found in this study was because lifestyle change made no difference or because the control group, on its own, had

made the same lifestyle changes as those made by many other people in the United States during this period. Widespread dietary changes, increases in exercise, and smoking cessation have taken place in much of the population, so the control group may have been "contaminated" with some of the behavior changes that had been encouraged in the study group in a formal and structured manner.

This study also shows the problem of using intermediate measures as endpoints of effectiveness in randomized trials. Because any effect on mortality may take years to manifest, it is tempting to use measures that might be affected sooner by the intervention. However, as seen here, although the intervention succeeded in reducing smoking, cholesterol levels, and diastolic blood pressure, one could not conclude on the basis of these changes that the intervention was effective, because the objective of the study was to determine whether the intervention could reduce CHD mortality, which it did not.

Because of these problems, which often lead to problems in interpretation of the findings in very large and expensive studies, some have advocated that the same funds invested in a number of smaller studies by different investigators in different populations might be a wiser choice: If the results were consistent, they might be more credible, despite the problems of smaller sample size that would be introduced in the individual studies.

Study of Breast Cancer Prevention Using Tamoxifen

The observation that women treated with tamoxifen for breast cancer had a lower incidence of cancer in the other breast suggested that tamoxifen might have value in preventing breast cancer. To test this

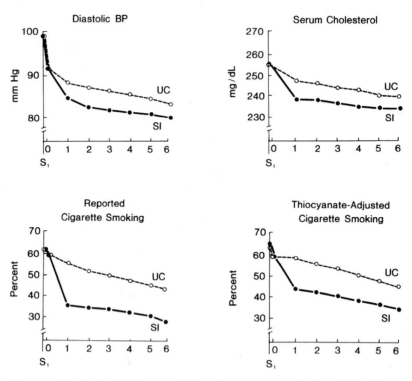

Figure 8-11. Mean risk factor levels by year of follow-up for Multiple Risk Factor Intervention Trial Research Group participants. BP, blood pressure; S_1, first screening visit; SI, special intervention; UC, usual care. (From Multiple Risk Factor Intervention Trial Research Group: Multiple Risk Factor Intervention Trial: Risk factor changes and mortality results. JAMA 248:1465–1477, 1982.)

hypothesis, a randomized trial was initiated in 1992. By September 1997, 13,388 women 35 years of age or older had been enrolled in the trial and had been randomly assigned to receive either placebo or 20 mg per day of tamoxifen for 5 years. In March 1998 an independent, data-monitoring committee decided that the evidence of a reduction in breast cancer risk was sufficiently strong to warrant stopping the study. As seen in Figure 8-13, cumulative rates of both invasive and noninvasive breast cancer were markedly reduced in women receiving tamoxifen. At the same time, as seen in Figure 8-14, rates of invasive endometrial cancer were increased in the tamoxifen group. Thus, when the decision is being made whether to use tamoxifen for breast cancer prevention, the potential benefits of tamoxifen must be weighed against the increased incidence of endometrial cancer. The picture is further complicated by the fact that at the time the results of this trial were published, two smaller studies in Europe did not find the reduction reported in the American study. Thus, the issue here is one of benefit versus harm; in addition, the question arises why other studies have not demonstrated the same marked effect on breast cancer incidence and

how the results of those studies should be taken into account in developing public policy in this area.

PHASES IN TESTING OF NEW DRUGS IN THE UNITED STATES

As new drugs are developed, the U.S. Food and Drug Administration follows a standard sequence in testing these new agents. *Phase I* studies are clinical pharmacologic studies—small studies of 20 to 80 patients that look at toxic and pharmacologic effects. If the drug passes these studies, it then undergoes *phase II* studies, clinical investigations of 100 to 200 patients for efficacy and relative safety. If the drug passes phase II studies, it is then tested in *phase III* studies—large-scale randomized controlled trials for effectiveness and relative safety, which are often multicentered. If the drug passes phase III testing, it can be licensed for marketing. It has been increasingly recognized, however, that certain adverse effects of drugs, such as carcinogenesis and teratogenesis, may not become manifest for many years, or that these effects may be so infrequent that they may not be detectable even in relatively large clinical trials but may become evident

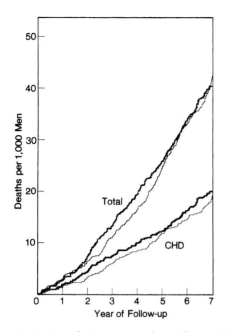

Figure 8-12. Cumulative coronary heart disease (CHD) and total mortality rates for Multiple Risk Factor Intervention Trial Research Group participants. The *heavy line* indicates men receiving usual care; the *thin line* indicates men receiving special intervention. (From Multiple Risk Factor Intervention Trial Research Group: Multiple Risk Factor Intervention Trial: Risk factor changes and mortality results. JAMA 248:1465–1477, 1982.)

only when the drug is in use by large populations. For this reason, *phase IV* studies, postmarketing surveillance, are important for monitoring new agents as they come into general use by the public.

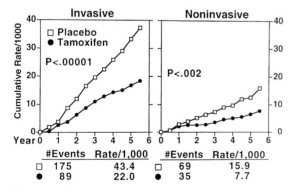

Figure 8-13. Cumulative rates of invasive and noninvasive breast cancer occurring in participants receiving placebo or tamoxifen. (From Fisher B, Constantino JP, Wickerham DL, et al: Tamoxifen for prevention of breast cancer: Report of the National Surgical Adjuvant Breast and Bowel Project P-1 Study. J Natl Cancer Inst 90:1371–1388, 1998.)

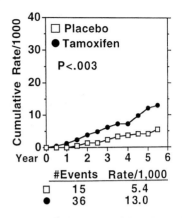

Figure 8-14. Cumulative rates of invasive endometrial cancer occurring in participants receiving placebo or tamoxifen. (From Fisher B, Constantino JP, Wickerham DL, et al: Tamoxifen for prevention of breast cancer: Report of the National Surgical Adjuvant Breast and Bowel Project P-1 Study. J Natl Cancer Inst 90:1371–1388, 1998.)

This rigorous sequence has protected the American public against many hazardous agents. In recent years, however, the pressure to speed up the processing of new agents for the treatment of AIDS has led to a reexamination of this approval process. It seems likely that whatever modifications are made in the approval process will not remain limited to drugs used against AIDS, but will in fact have extensive ramifications for the general process of approving new drugs and will therefore have major implications for the health of the public both in the United States and throughout the world.

ETHICAL CONSIDERATIONS

Many ethical issues arise in the context of clinical trials. These issues are discussed in detail in the excellent monographs listed at the end of this chapter.

One frequently raised question is whether randomization is ethical. How can we knowingly withhold a drug from patients, particularly those with serious and life-threatening diseases? Randomization is ethical only when we do not know whether drug A is better than drug B. We may have some indication that one treatment is better than the other (and, often, this is the rationale for conducting a trial in the first place), but we are not certain. Often, however, it is not clear at what point we "know" that drug A is better than drug B. The question may be better stated as, "When do we have adequate evidence to support the conclusion that drug A is better than drug B?"

One question that has received considerable attention in recent years is whether it is ethical to use a placebo.[4] Implicit in this question is the issue of whether it is ethical to withhold a treatment that has been shown to be effective.[5]

The question can also be posed in the reverse: "Is it ethical not to randomize?" When we are considering drugs, preventive measures, or systems of health care delivery that apply to large numbers of people, both in the United States and in other countries, the mandate may be to carry out a randomized trial to resolve the questions of benefit and harm, and not to continue to subject people to unnecessary toxic effects and raise false hopes, often at tremendous expense. Hence, the question about the ethics of randomization should be asked in both directions: randomizing and not randomizing.

Another important question is whether truly informed consent can be obtained. Many protocols for multicentered clinical trials require that patients be entered into the study immediately after diagnosis. The patient may be incapable of giving consent, and the family may be so shocked by the diagnosis and its implications that they have great difficulty in dealing with the notion of randomization. For example, much of the progress of recent decades in the treatment of childhood leukemia has been a result of the rigorous multicentered protocols that have required enrollment of the child immediately after the diagnosis of leukemia has been made. Clearly, at such a time the parents are so distressed that one may question whether they are capable of giving truly informed consent. Nevertheless, only through such rigorous trials has the progress been made that has saved the lives of so many children with acute leukemia.

Finally, under what circumstances should a trial be stopped earlier than originally planned? This is also a difficult issue and could arise because either harmful effects or beneficial effects of the agent become apparent early, before the full sample has been enrolled, or before subjects have been studied for the full follow-up period. In many studies, an outside data monitoring board monitors the data as they are received, and the board makes that decision, as seen, for example, in the Physicians' Health Study discussed in Chapter 7 in which the board decided that the findings for aspirin were sufficiently clear that the aspirin part of the study should be terminated but that the beta-carotene portion of the study should be continued.

RANDOMIZED TRIALS FOR EVALUATING WIDELY ACCEPTED INTERVENTIONS

Randomized controlled trials can be used for two major purposes: (1) to evaluate new forms of intervention before they are approved and recommended for general use and (2) to evaluate interventions that are highly controversial or that have been widely used or recommended without having been adequately evaluated. In assessing the impact that randomized controlled trials have on medical practice, the latter use demonstrates the challenge of changing approaches used in existing medical practice which may not have been well evaluated. Two examples of such use are presented in this section.

A Trial of Arthroscopic Knee Surgery for Osteoarthritis

About 6% of adults older than 30 years of age and 12% of adults older than 65 years of age have significant knee pain as a result of osteoarthritis. In the United States, a frequently performed operation for patients with knee pain and evidence of osteoarthritis has been arthroscopic surgery with lavage (washing out) or débridement (cleaning out) of the knee joint using an arthroscope. It has been estimated that the procedure has been performed on more than 225,000 middle-aged and older adults each year, at an annual cost of more than 1 billion dollars.

In a number of randomized controlled trials in which patients receiving débridement or lavage of the knee were compared with controls receiving no treatment, those who were treated reported more improvement in knee pain than those who were untreated. Other studies, however, in which only saline was injected into the knee, also reported improvement of knee symptoms. Thus, it became clear that the perceived benefits might be related more to patient expectations than to actual effectiveness, because the subjective improvements reported by patients were more likely when patients were not masked as to whether they received or did not receive surgical treatment. In order to resolve the question of whether arthroscopic lavage or débridement reduces symptoms of knee pain in patients with osteoarthritis, a randomized controlled trial was needed in which the controls would have a sham treatment. In July 2002, a beautifully conducted randomized trial of this procedure, using sham arthroscopy for the controls, was reported by Moseley and colleagues.[6]

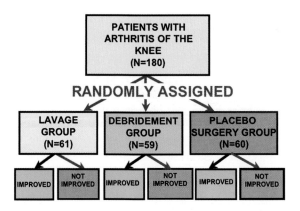

Figure 8-15. Design of a controlled trial of arthroscopic surgery for osteoarthritis of the knee. (Based on Moseley JB, O'Malley K, Petersen NJ, Menke TJ, et al: A controlled trial of arthroscopic surgery for osteoarthritis of the knee. N Engl J Med 347:81–88, 2002.)

The design of this study is shown in Figure 8-15. One hundred eighty veterans were randomized to a group receiving arthroscopic débridement (59), a group receiving arthroscopic lavage (61), or a placebo group receiving a sham (placebo) intervention (60). The sham intervention consisted of a skin incision and simulated débridement without insertion of an arthroscope. Outcomes that were measured included level of knee pain, as determined by self-reports, and physical function, as determined by both self-reports and direct observation. These were assessed over a 2-year period. Those who assessed pain and functional levels in the participants as well as the partici-

pants themselves were blinded to the treatment group assignment of each patient.

The results are shown in Figures 8-16 and 8-17. At no point did either arthroscopic intervention group have greater pain relief than the placebo group (Fig. 8-16). Moreover, at no point did either intervention group have significantly greater improvement in physical function than the placebo (sham intervention) group (Fig. 8-17).

The principal investigator of the study, Dr. Nelda Wray, of the Houston Veterans Affairs Medical Center, where the trial was performed, summarized the results by saying, "Our study shows that the surgery is no better than the placebo—the procedure itself is useless." One month after publication of this study, the Department of Veterans Affairs issued an advisory to its physicians, stating that the procedure should not be performed pending additional review. The advisory statement said that knee pain was not a sufficient indicator for the surgery unless there was also evidence of "anatomic or mechanical abnormalities," which presumably could be improved by such a procedure.

Effect of Group Psychosocial Support on Survival of Patients with Metastatic Breast Cancer

In 1989, a study was reported in which women with metastatic breast cancer were randomly assigned to supportive-expressive group therapy or to a control group. Supportive-expressive therapy is a standardized treatment for patients with life-threatening

Figure 8-16. Mean values (and 95% confidence intervals) on the Knee-Specific Pain Scale. Assessments were made before the procedure and 2 weeks, 6 weeks, 3 months, 6 months, 12 months, 18 months, and 24 months after the procedure. Higher scores indicate more severe pain.

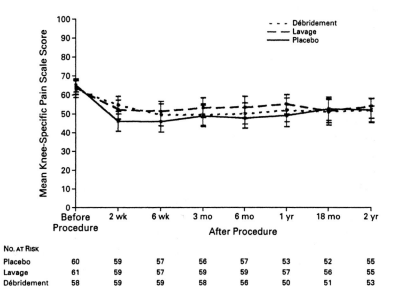

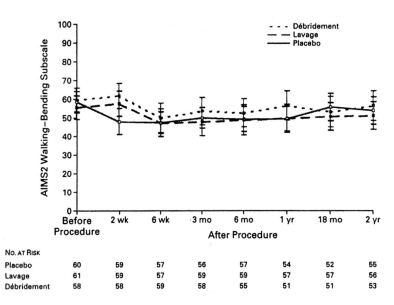

Figure 8-17. Mean values (and 95% confidence intervals) on the Walking-Bending Subscale of the Arthritis Impact Measurement Scales (AIMS2). Assessments were made before the procedure and 2 weeks, 6 weeks, 3 months, 6 months, 12 months, 18 months, and 24 months after the procedure. Higher scores indicate poorer functioning.

No. at Risk								
Placebo	60	59	57	56	57	54	52	55
Lavage	61	59	57	59	59	57	57	56
Débridement	58	58	59	58	55	51	51	53

illness that encourages a group of participants, led by a therapist, to express their feelings and concerns about their illness and its impact. This study showed a survival benefit, although a survival analysis had not been originally planned in the study. Other trials of other psychosocial interventions showed no survival benefit.

To clarify this issue, Goodwin and colleagues[7] conducted a multicenter randomized trial in which 235 women with metastatic breast cancer were randomized either to a group that received supportive-expressive therapy or to a control group that did not receive this intervention (Fig. 8-18). Of the 235 women, 158 were assigned to the intervention group and 77 to the control group.

Over the period of the study, survival was not prolonged in patients who received supportive-expressive therapy (Fig. 8-19). However, mood and pain perception were improved, particularly in women who were the most distressed. Although the findings in the literature are still mixed regarding survival and additional studies are being conducted, the results of this study suggest that there is no survival benefit from this intervention. Therefore, the wishes of women who choose to cope with their illness in different ways, including not sharing their feelings in a group, should be respected. Furthermore, it should not be suggested to women who prefer not to participate in such group therapy at this difficult time in their lives that their refusal may be hastening their own deaths.

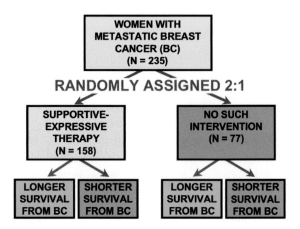

Figure 8-18. Design of a randomized, controlled trial of group psychosocial support on survival in patients with metastatic breast cancer. (Based on Huston P, Peterson R: Withholding proven treatment in clinical research. N Engl J Med 345:912–914, 2001.)

REGISTRATION OF CLINICAL TRIALS

It has long been recognized that not all results of clinical trials are published. This can pose a serious problem when the results from all published clinical trials are reviewed. For example, if clinical trials of a new drug are reviewed but only those that show beneficial results have been published and those showing negative results (for some reason) have not been published, an erroneous conclusion that *all* studies of the new drug have shown a clear benefit

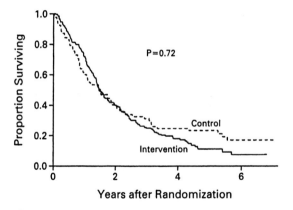

Figure 8-19. Kaplan-Meier survival curves for women assigned to the intervention group and the control group. There was no significant difference in survival between the two groups.

might be drawn from the published studies. This type of common problem is called *publication bias* or *non-publication bias*. For example, Liebeskind and colleagues[8] identified 178 controlled clinical trials of acute ischemic stroke reported in English over a 45-year period from 1955 to 1999 through a systematic search of several large databases. These trials enrolled a total of 73,949 subjects and evaluated 75 agents or other types of intervention. They found the issue of publication bias to be an important factor in reviewing the literature on trials of acute ischemic strokes. Trials in which the tested agent was shown to be harmful were substantially more likely **not** to be published than trials in which results indicated the tested agent was neutral or beneficial.

Several factors account for the problem of publication bias. Journals are more eager to publish results from studies showing dramatic effects than results from studies showing no benefit from a new drug. Both researchers and journals appear less excited about studies showing either that a new treatment is inferior to current treatment or that the findings are not clear one way or the other. An even more important issue is contributing to this problem: Companies that develop new drugs and fund studies of these drugs frequently want to keep the results unpublished when they show no benefits, or show serious side effects, or when the drug studied is shown to be less effective than currently available agents. The companies are clearly concerned that the results of such studies could adversely affect sales of the product and significantly impact the large potential profits

they anticipate from the new agent. The net result, however, is concealment of the data, giving a picture of the agent—including its effectiveness and safety—that is not complete, so that regulators, physicians, and the public are prevented from making an evidence-based decision, that is, a decision based on the total information generated through clinical trials.

The extent of the risk to public health from selective reporting of clinical trials and the frequency with which this selective reporting occurs led the International Committee of Medical Journal Editors to adopt a policy, which became effective in 2005, that *all* clinical trials of medical interventions must be registered in a public trials registry before any participants are enrolled in the study.[9] Medical interventions include drugs, surgical procedures, devices, behavioral treatments, and processes of health care. Registration in a registry accessible to the public at no charge is required before any clinical trial will be considered for publication by the major journals that have agreed to this policy.

CONCLUSION

The randomized trial is the gold standard for evaluating the efficacy of therapeutic, preventive, and other measures in both clinical medicine and public health. Chapters 7 and 8 have provided an overview of approaches to study design in randomized trials and the measures used to minimize or avoid selection and other types of bias. From a societal viewpoint, generalizability and ethical concerns are major considerations, and these issues have been discussed. For those who wish to explore further this important type of study, a list of selected monographs on randomized trials is provided at the end of this chapter.

EPILOGUE

We shall conclude this discussion of randomized trials by citing an article by Caroline and Schwartz which was published in the journal *Chest* in 1975. The article was entitled "Chicken Soup Rebound and Relapse of Pneumonia: Report of a Case."[10]

The authors introduced their topic by saying:

Chicken soup has long been recognized to possess unusual therapeutic potency against a wide variety of viral and bacterial agents. Indeed, as early as the 12th century, the theologian, philosopher and physician, Moses Maimonides wrote, "Chicken soup

. . . is recommended as an excellent food as well as medication." Previous anecdotal reports regarding the therapeutic efficacy of this agent, however, have failed to provide details regarding the appropriate length of therapy. What follows is a case report in which abrupt withdrawal of chicken soup led to a severe relapse of pneumonia.[10]

The authors then present a case report of a 47-year-old physician who was treated with chicken soup for pneumonia. Chicken soup administration was terminated prematurely, and the patient suffered a relapse. Chicken soup being unavailable, the relapse was treated with intravenous penicillin.

The authors' discussion is of particular interest. It reads in part:

The therapeutic efficacy of chicken soup was first discovered several thousand years ago when an epidemic highly fatal to young Egyptian males seemed not to affect an ethnic minority residing in the same area. Contemporary epidemiologic inquiry revealed that the diet of the group not afflicted by the epidemic contained large amounts of a preparation made by boiling chicken with various vegetables and herbs. It is notable in this regard that the dietary injunctions given to Moses on Mount Sinai, while restricting consumption of no less than 19 types of fowl, exempted chicken from the prohibition. Some scholars believe that the recipe for chicken soup was transmitted to Moses on the same occasion, but was relegated to the oral tradition when the scriptures were canonized. . . . While chicken soup is now widely employed against a variety of organic and functional disorders, its manufacture remains largely in the hands of private individuals and standardization has proved nearly impossible. Preliminary investigation into the pharmacology of chicken soup (Bohbymycetin) has shown that it is readily absorbed after oral administration. . . . Parenteral administration is not recommended.[10]

This report stimulated several letters to the editor. In one, Dr. Laurence F. Greene, Professor of Urology at the Mayo Clinic, wrote:

You may be interested to know that we have successfully treated male impotence with another chicken-derived compound, sodium cytarabine hexamethylacetyl lututria tetrazolamine (Schmaltz [Upjohn]). This compound, when applied in ointment form to the penis, not only cures impotence, but also increases libido and prevents premature ejaculation. . . . Preliminary studies indicate that its effects are dose related inasmuch as intercourse continues for 5 minutes when 5% ointment is applied, 15 minutes when 15% ointment is applied, and so forth.

We have received a grant in the sum of $650,000 from the National Scientific Foundation to carry out a prospective randomized, controlled double-blind study. Unfortunately, we are unable to obtain a suitable number of subjects inasmuch as each volunteer refuses to participate unless we assure him that he will be a subject rather than a control.[11]

REFERENCES

1. Gehan E: Clinical trials in cancer research. Environ Health Perspect 32:31, 1979.
2. Veterans Administration Cooperative Study Group on Hypertensive Agents: Effects of treatment on morbidity in hypertension: Results in patients with diastolic blood pressure averaging 115 through 129 mm Hg. JAMA 213:1028–1034, 1967.
3. Hypertension Detection and Follow-up Program Cooperative Group: Five year findings of the Hypertension Detection and Follow-up Program: I. Reduction of mortality of persons with high blood pressure, including mild hypertension. JAMA 242:2562, 1979.
4. Emanuel EJ, Miller FG: The ethics of placebo-controlled trials: A middle ground. N Engl J Med 345:915–919, 2001.
5. Huston P, Peterson R: Withholding proven treatment in clinical research. N Engl J Med 345:912–914, 2001.
6. Moseley JB, O'Malley K, Petersen NJ, et al: A controlled trial of arthroscopic surgery for osteoarthritis of the knee. N Engl J Med 347:81–88, 2002.
7. Goodwin PJ, Leszcz M, Ennis M, et al: The effect of group psychosocial support on survival in metastatic breast cancer. N Engl J Med 345:1719–1726, 2001.
8. Liebeskind DS, Kidwell CS, Sayre JW, Saver JL: Evidence of publication bias in reporting acute stroke clinical trials. Neurology 67:973–979, 2006.
9. DeAngelis CD, Drazen JM, Frizelle FA: Clinical trial registration: A statement from the International Committee of Medical Journal Editors. JAMA 292:1363–1364, 2004.
10. Caroline NL, Schwartz H: Chicken soup rebound and relapse of pneumonia: Report of a case. Chest 67:215–216, 1975.
11. Greene LF: The chicken soup controversy [letter]. Chest 68:605, 1975.

─────────────── **MONOGRAPHS ON RANDOMIZED TRIALS** ───────────────

Friedman LM, Furberg CD, DeMets DL: Fundamentals of Clinical Trials. Boston, PSG, 1982.

Johnson FN, Johnson S: Clinical Trials. Oxford, Blackwell Scientific, 1977.

Lavori PW, Kelsey JL (eds): Introduction and Overview. Epidemiol Rev 24:1–3, 2002.

Meinert CL: Clinical Trials: Design, Conduct, and Analysis. Monographs in Epidemiology, vol 8. New York, Oxford University Press, 1986.

Pocock SJ: Clinical Trials: A Practical Approach. New York, John Wiley & Sons, 1983.

Silverman WA: Human Experimentation: A Guided Step into the Unknown. New York, Oxford University Press, 1985.

REVIEW QUESTIONS FOR CHAPTERS 7 AND 8

1. The major purpose of random assignment in a clinical trial is to:
   a. Help ensure that study subjects are representative of the general population
   b. Facilitate double blinding (masking)
   c. Facilitate the measurement of outcome variables
   d. Ensure that the study groups have comparable baseline characteristics
   e. Reduce selection bias in the allocation of treatment

2. An advertisement in a medical journal stated that "2,000 subjects with sore throats were treated with our new medicine. Within 4 days, 94% were asymptomatic." The advertisement claims that the medicine was effective. Based on the evidence given above, the claim:
   a. Is correct
   b. May be incorrect because the conclusion is not based on a rate
   c. May be incorrect because of failure to recognize a long-term cohort phenomenon
   d. May be incorrect because no test of statistical significance was used
   e. May be incorrect because no control or comparison group was involved

3. The purpose of a *double blind* or *double masked* study is to:
   a. Achieve comparability of treated and untreated subjects
   b. Reduce the effects of sampling variation
   c. Avoid observer and subject bias
   d. Avoid observer bias and sampling variation
   e. Avoid subject bias and sampling variation

4. In many studies examining the association between estrogens and endometrial cancer of the uterus, a one-sided significance test was used. The underlying assumption justifying a one-sided rather than a two-sided test is:
   a. The distribution of the proportion exposed followed a "normal" pattern
   b. The expectation before doing the study was that estrogens cause endometrial cancer of the uterus
   c. The pattern of association could be expressed by a straight-line function
   d. Type II error was the most important potential error to avoid
   e. Only one control group was being used

5. In a randomized trial, a planned crossover design:
   a. Eliminates the problem of a possible order effect
   b. Must take into account the problem of possible residual effects of the first therapy
   c. Requires stratified randomization
   d. Eliminates the need for monitoring compliance and noncompliance
   e. Enhances the generalizability of the results of the study

6. A randomized trial comparing the efficacy of two drugs showed a difference between the two (with a P value $< .05$). Assume that in reality, however, the two drugs do not differ. This is therefore an example of:
   a. Type I error (α error)
   b. Type II error (β error)
   c. $1 - \alpha$
   d. $1 - \beta$
   e. None of the above

Number of Patients Needed in an Experimental and a Control Group for a Given Probability of Obtaining a Significant Result (Two-Sided Test)

Lower of the Two Cure Rates	DIFFERENCES IN THE CURE RATES BETWEEN THE TWO TREATMENT GROUPS					
	.05	.10	.15	.20	.25	.30
.05	420	130	69	44	36	31
.10	680	195	96	59	41	35
.15	910	250	120	71	48	39
.20	1,090	290	135	80	53	42
.25	1,250	330	150	88	57	44
.30	1,380	360	160	93	60	44
.35	1,470	370	170	96	61	44
.40	1,530	390	175	97	61	44

$\alpha = .05$; power $(1 - \beta) = .80$.
Data from Gehan E: Clinical trials in cancer research. Environ Health Perspect 32:31, 1979.

Question 7 is based on the above table:

7. A drug company maintains that a new drug G for a certain disease has a 50% cure rate as compared with drug H, which has only a 25% cure rate. You are asked to design a clinical trial comparing drugs G and H. Using the preceding table, estimate the number of patients needed in each therapy group to detect such a difference with $\alpha = .05$, two-sided, and $\beta = .20$.

The number of patients needed in each therapy group is _____.

8. All of the following are potential benefits of a randomized clinical trial, *except:*
   a. The likelihood that the study groups will be comparable is increased
   b. Self-selection for a particular treatment is eliminated
   c. The external validity of the study is increased
   d. Assignment of the next subject cannot be predicted
   e. The therapy that a subject receives is not influenced by either conscious or subconscious bias of the investigator

In Section I, we addressed the issues of defining and diagnosing disease and describing its transmission, acquisition, and natural history. We then discussed the use of randomized trials for evaluating and selecting pharmacologic agents or other interventions to modify the natural history of disease, through both disease prevention and effective treatment. In Section II, we turn to a different issue: How do we design and conduct studies to elucidate the etiology of and risk factors for human disease? Such studies are critically important in both clinical medicine and public health practice.

Why should a clinician be concerned with disease etiology? Has not the clinician's traditional role been to treat disease once it has become apparent? To answer this question, several points should be made. First, *prevention* is a major responsibility of the physician; both prevention and treatment should be viewed by the physician as essential elements of his or her professional role. Indeed, many patients take the initiative and ask their physicians questions about what measures to take to maintain health and prevent certain diseases. Most opportunities to prevent disease require an understanding of the *etiology* or *cause* of disease, so that exposure to a causative environmental factor can be reduced or the pathogenic chain leading from the causal factor to the development of clinical illness can be interrupted.

Second, patients and their families often ask the physician questions about the *risk* of disease. What is the risk that the disease will recur? What is the risk that other family members may develop the disease? For example,

A man who suffers a myocardial infarction at a young age may ask, "Why did it happen to me? Can I prevent my having a second infarction? Are my children also at high risk for having an infarction at a young age? If so, can anything be done to lower their risk?"

A woman who delivers a baby with a congenital malformation may ask, "Why did it happen? Is it because of something I did during the pregnancy? If I get pregnant again, is that child also likely to have a malformation?"

Third, in the course of doing clinical work and making bedside observations, a physician often "gets a hunch" regarding a possible relationship between a factor and the risk of a disease that is as yet not understood. For example, Alton Ochsner, the famous surgeon, noted that virtually all the patients on whom he

165

operated for lung cancer were cigarette smokers; this observation led him to suggest that smoking was causally related to the development of lung cancer and indicated the need to clarify the nature of this relationship by means of rigorously conducted studies in defined human populations.

Whereas clinical practice focuses on individuals, public health practice focuses on populations. In view of the tremendous potential impact of public health actions, which often affect entire communities, public health practitioners must understand how conclusions regarding health risks to a community are arrived at, and how a foundation for preventive measures and actions is developed on the basis of population-centered data that are properly interpreted in their biologic context. Only in this way can rational policies be adopted for preventing disease and for enhancing the health of populations at the lowest possible cost.

Alert and astute physicians and other public health practitioners in academic, clinical, and health department settings have many opportunities to conduct studies of disease etiology or disease risk to confirm or refute preliminary clinical or other impressions regarding the origins of diseases. The findings may be of critical importance in providing the rationale for preventing these diseases, for enhancing our understanding of their pathogenesis, and for suggesting directions for future laboratory and epidemiologic research. Consequently, an understanding of the types of study design that are used for investigating etiology and identifying risk factors, together with an appreciation of the methodologic problems involved in such studies, is fundamental to both clinical medicine and public health practice.

This section discusses the basic study designs that are used in etiologic studies (Chapters 9 and 10) and describes how the findings from such studies may be used to estimate the risks of disease associated with specific exposures (Chapters 11 and 12). Because we ultimately wish to answer questions about disease etiology or cause, the chapters that follow discuss how observed associations can be interpreted and how causal inferences are derived from them (Chapters 14 and 15). Finally, this section closes with a discussion of how epidemiology can be used to assess the relative contributions of genetic and environmental factors to the causation of human disease, an assessment that has major clinical and public health policy implications (Chapter 16).

Chapter 9

Cohort Studies

In this chapter, and in the following chapters in Section II, we turn to the uses of epidemiology in elucidating etiologic or causal relationships. The two steps that underlie the study designs that are discussed in Chapters 9 and 10 are shown schematically in Figure 9-1.

1. First, we determine whether there is an association between a factor or a characteristic and the development of a disease. This can be accomplished by studying the characteristics of groups, by studying the characteristics of individuals, or both (see Chapters 9 through 12).
2. Second, we derive appropriate inferences regarding a possible causal relationship from the patterns of association that have been found (see Chapters 14 and 15).

Chapters 9 and 10 describe the study designs used for step 1. In this chapter, cohort studies are discussed; case-control and cross-sectional studies are discussed in Chapter 10.

DESIGN OF A COHORT STUDY

In a cohort study, the investigator selects a group of exposed individuals and a group of nonexposed individuals and follows up both groups to compare the incidence of disease (or rate of death from disease) in the two groups (Fig. 9-2). The design may include more than two groups, although only two groups are shown for diagrammatic purposes.

If a positive association exists between the exposure and the disease, we would expect that the proportion of the exposed group in whom the disease develops (incidence in the exposed group) would be greater than the proportion of the nonexposed group in whom the disease develops (incidence in the nonexposed group).

The calculations involved are seen in Table 9-1. We begin with an exposed group and a nonexposed group. Of the $a + b$ exposed persons the disease develops in a but not in b. Thus the incidence of the disease among the exposed is $\dfrac{a}{a+b}$. Similarly,

in the $c + d$ nonexposed persons in the study, the disease develops in c but not in d. Thus the incidence of the disease among the nonexposed is $\dfrac{c}{c+d}$.

The use of these calculations is seen in a hypothetical example of a cohort study shown in Table 9-2. In this cohort study, the association of smoking with coronary heart disease (CHD) is investigated by selecting for study a group of 3,000 smokers (exposed) and a group of 5,000 nonsmokers (nonexposed) who are free of heart disease at baseline. Both groups are followed for the development of CHD, and the *incidence* of CHD in both groups is compared. CHD develops in 84 of the smokers and in 87 of the nonsmokers. The result is an incidence of CHD of 28.0/1,000 in the smokers and 17.4/1,000 in the nonsmokers.

Note that because we are identifying *new* (incident) cases of disease as they occur, we can determine whether a temporal relationship exists between the exposure and the disease, that is, whether the expo-

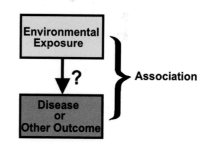

Figure 9-1. If we observe an association between an exposure and a disease or another outcome, the question is: Is the association causal?

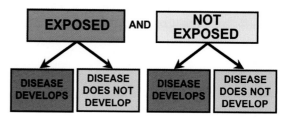

Figure 9-2. Design of a cohort study.

TABLE 9-1. Design of a Cohort Study

		Then Follow to See Whether		Totals	Incidence Rates of Disease
		Disease Develops	*Disease Does Not Develop*		
First Select	Exposed	a	b	$a + b$	$\dfrac{a}{a + b}$
	Not exposed	c	d	$c + d$	$\dfrac{c}{c + d}$

sure preceded the onset of the disease. Clearly, such a temporal relationship must be established if we are to consider the exposure a possible cause of the disease in question.

COMPARING COHORT STUDIES WITH RANDOMIZED TRIALS

At this point, it is useful to compare the observational cohort study just described with the randomized trial (experimental cohort) design described previously, in Chapters 7 and 8 (Fig. 9-3).

Both types of studies compare exposed with non-exposed groups (or a group with a certain exposure to a group with another exposure). Because, for ethical and other reasons, we cannot randomize people to receive a putatively harmful substance, such as a suspected carcinogen, the "exposure" in most randomized trials is a treatment or preventive measure. In cohort studies investigating etiology, the "exposure" is often to a possibly toxic or carcinogenic agent. In both types of design, however, an exposed group is compared with a nonexposed group or with a group with another exposure.

The difference between these two designs—the presence or absence of randomization—is critical with regard to interpreting the study findings. The advantages of randomization were discussed in Chapters 7 and 8. In a nonrandomized study, when we observe an association of an exposure with a disease, we are left with uncertainty as to whether the association may be a result of the fact that people were not randomized to the exposure; perhaps it is not the exposure, but rather the factors that led people to be exposed, that are associated with the disease. For example, if an increased risk of a disease is found in workers at a certain factory, and if most of the workers at this factory live in a certain area, the increased risk of disease could result from an exposure associated with their place of residence rather than with their occupation or place of work. This issue is discussed in Chapters 13 and 14.

SELECTION OF STUDY POPULATIONS

The essential characteristic in the design of cohort studies is the comparison of outcomes in an exposed group and in a nonexposed group (or, a group with a certain characteristic and a group without that characteristic). There are two basic ways to generate such groups:

1. We can create a study population by selecting groups for inclusion in the study on the basis of whether or not they were exposed (e.g., occupationally exposed cohorts) (Fig. 9-4).
2. Or we can select a defined population before any of its members become exposed or before their

TABLE 9-2. Results of a Hypothetical Cohort Study of Smoking and Coronary Disease (CHD)

		Then Follow to See Whether		Totals	Incidence per 1,000 per Year
		CHD Develops	*CHD Does Not Develop*		
First Select	Smoke cigarettes	84	2,916	3,000	28.0
	Do not smoke cigarettes	87	4,913	5,000	17.4

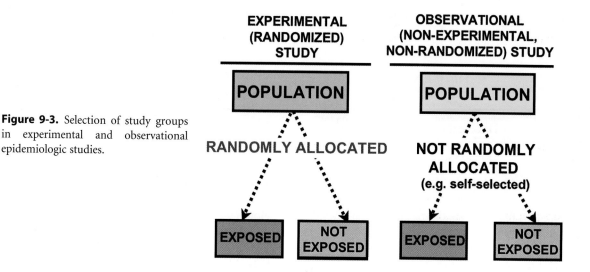

Figure 9-3. Selection of study groups in experimental and observational epidemiologic studies.

exposures are identified. We could select a population on the basis of some factor not related to exposure (such as community of residence) (Fig. 9-5) and take histories of, or perform blood tests or other assays on, the entire population. Using the results of the histories or the tests, one can separate the population into *exposed* and *nonexposed* groups (or those who have and those who do not have certain biologic characteristics), such as was done in the Framingham Study, described later in this chapter.

Cohort studies, in which we wait for an outcome to develop in a population, often require a long follow-up period, lasting until enough events (outcomes) have occurred. When the second approach is used—in which a population is identified for study based on some characteristic unrelated to the exposure in question—the exposure of interest may not take place for some time, even for many years after the population has been defined. Consequently, the length of follow-up required is even greater with the second approach than it is with the first. Note that

with either approach the cohort study design is fundamentally the same: *we compare exposed and nonexposed persons.* This comparison is the hallmark of the cohort design.

TYPES OF COHORT STUDIES

A major problem with the cohort design just described is that the study population often must be followed up for a long period to determine whether the outcome of interest has developed. Consider as an example a hypothetical study of the relationship of smoking to lung cancer. We identify a population of elementary school students and follow them up; 10 years later, when they are teenagers, we identify those who smoke and those who do not. We then follow up both groups—smokers and nonsmokers—to see who develops lung cancer and who does not.

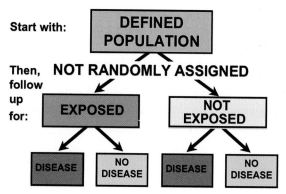

Figure 9-5. Design of a cohort study beginning with a defined population.

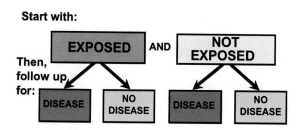

Figure 9-4. Design of a cohort study beginning with exposed and nonexposed groups.

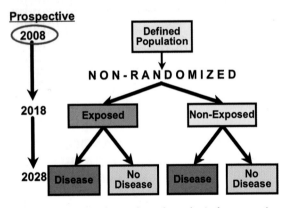

Figure 9-6. Time frame for a hypothetical prospective cohort study begun in 2008.

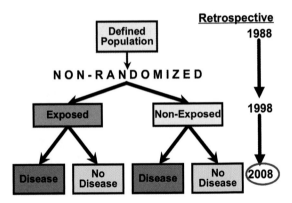

Figure 9-7. Time frame for a hypothetical retrospective cohort study begun in 2008.

For purposes of this example, let us assume that the latent period from beginning smoking to development of lung cancer is 10 years. Let us say that we begin our study in 2008 (Fig. 9-6). Because the interval from the time of identification of the elementary school children to the time of identification of their smoking status as teenagers or college students is 10 years, exposure status (smoker or nonsmoker) will not be ascertained until the year 2018. Development of lung cancer will not be ascertained until 10 years later, in 2028.

This type of study design is called a *prospective cohort study* (also a *concurrent cohort* or *longitudinal study*). It is *concurrent* because the investigator identifies the original population at the beginning of the study and, in effect, accompanies the subjects concurrently through calendar time until the point at which the disease develops or does not develop.

What is the problem with this approach? The difficulty is that, as just described, the study will take at least 20 years to complete. Several problems can result. If one is fortunate enough to obtain a research grant, such funding is generally limited to a maximum of only 3 to 5 years. In addition, with a study of this length, there is the risk that the study subjects will outlive the investigator, or at least that the investigator may not survive to the end of the study. Given these issues, the prospective cohort study often proves unattractive to investigators who are contemplating new research.

Do these problems mean that the cohort design is not practical? Is there any way to shorten the time period needed to conduct a cohort study? Let us consider an alternate approach using the cohort design (Fig. 9-7). Suppose that we again begin our study in 2008, but now we find that an old roster of elementary schoolchildren from 1988 is available in our community, and that they had been surveyed regarding their smoking habits in 1998. Using these data resources in 2008, we can begin to determine who in this population has developed lung cancer and who has not. This is called a *retrospective cohort* or *historical cohort study* (also called a *nonconcurrent prospective study*). Note, however, that the study design does not differ from that of the prospective cohort design—we are still comparing exposed and nonexposed groups; what we have done in the retrospective cohort design is to use historical data from the past so that we can telescope the frame of calendar time for the study and obtain our results sooner. It is no longer a prospective design, because we are beginning the study with a preexisting population to reduce the duration of the study. But, as shown in Figure 9-8, the *designs for both the prospective cohort*

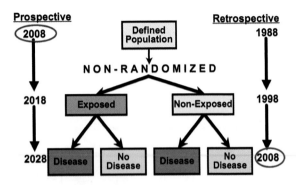

Figure 9-8. Time frames for a hypothetical prospective cohort study and a hypothetical retrospective cohort study begun in 2008.

study and the retrospective or *historical cohort study* are identical: we are comparing exposed and nonexposed populations. The only difference between them is calendar time. In a *prospective cohort design*, exposure and nonexposure are ascertained as they occur during the study; the groups are then followed up for several years into the future and incidence is measured. In a *retrospective cohort design*, exposure is ascertained from past records and outcome (development or no development of disease) is ascertained at the time the study is begun.

It is also possible to conduct a study that is a combination of prospective cohort and retrospective cohort designs. With this approach, exposure is ascertained from objective records in the past (as in a historical cohort study), and follow-up and measurement of outcome continue into the future.

EXAMPLES OF COHORT STUDIES

Example 1: The Framingham Study

One of the most important and best-known cohort studies is the Framingham Study of cardiovascular disease, which was begun in 1948.[1] Framingham is a town in Massachusetts, about 20 miles from Boston. It was thought that the characteristics of its population (just under 30,000) would be appropriate for such a study and would facilitate follow-up of participants.

Residents were considered eligible if they were between 30 and 62 years of age. The rationale for using this age range was that people younger than 30 years would generally be unlikely to manifest the cardiovascular endpoints being studied during the proposed 20-year follow-up period. Many persons older than 62 years would already have established coronary disease, and it would therefore not be rewarding to study persons in this age group for incidence of coronary disease.

The investigators sought a sample size of 5,000. Table 9-3 shows how the final study population was derived. It consisted of 5,127 men and women who were between 30 and 62 years of age at the time of study entry and were free of cardiovascular disease at that time. In this study, many "exposures" were defined, including smoking, obesity, elevated blood pressure, elevated cholesterol levels, low levels of physical activity, and other factors.

New coronary events were identified by examining the study population every 2 years and by daily surveillance of hospitalizations at the only hospital in Framingham.

TABLE 9-3. Derivation of the Framingham Study Population

	Number of Men	Number of Women	Total
Random sample	3,074	3,433	6,507
Respondents	2,024	2,445	4,469
Volunteers	312	428	740
Respondents free of CHD	1,975	2,418	4,393
Volunteers free of CHD	307	427	734
Total free of CHD: The Framingham Study Group	2,282	2,845	5,127

CHD, coronary heart disease.
From Dawber TR, Kannel WB, Lyell LP: An approach to longitudinal studies in a community: The Framingham Study. Ann NY Acad Sci 107:539–556, 1993.

The study was designed to test the following hypotheses:

- The incidence of CHD increases with age. It occurs earlier and more frequently in males.
- Persons with hypertension develop CHD at a greater rate than those who are normotensive.
- Elevated blood cholesterol level is associated with an increased risk of CHD.
- Tobacco smoking and habitual use of alcohol are associated with an increased incidence of CHD.
- Increased physical activity is associated with a decrease in the development of CHD.
- An increase in body weight predisposes a person to the development of CHD.
- An increased rate of development of CHD occurs in patients with diabetes mellitus.

When we examine this list today, we might wonder why such obvious and well-known relationships should have been examined in such an extensive study. The danger of this "hindsight" approach should be kept in mind; it is primarily *because* of the Framingham Study, a classic cohort study that made fundamental contributions to our understanding of the epidemiology of cardiovascular disease, that these relationships are well known today.

This study used the second method described earlier in the chapter for selecting a study population for a cohort study: A defined population was selected on the basis of location of residence or other factors not related to the exposure(s) in question. The population was then observed over time to determine which individuals developed or already had the "exposure(s)" of interest and, later on, to determine which ones developed the cardiovascular outcome(s) of interest. This approach offered an important advantage: It permitted the investigators to study multiple "exposures," such as hypertension, smoking, obesity, cholesterol levels, and other factors, as well as the complex interactions among the exposures, by using multivariable techniques. Thus, whereas a cohort study that begins with an exposed and a non-exposed group focuses on the specific exposure, a cohort study that begins with a defined population can explore the roles of many exposures.

Example 2: Incidence of Breast Cancer and Progesterone Deficiency

It has long been recognized that breast cancer is more common in women who are older at the time of their first pregnancy. A difficult question is raised by this observation: Is the relationship between late age at first pregnancy and increased risk of breast cancer related to the finding that early first pregnancy protects against breast cancer (and therefore such protection is missing in women who have a later pregnancy or no pregnancy), or are both a delayed first pregnancy and an increased risk of breast cancer the result of some third factor, such as an underlying hormonal abnormality?

It is difficult to tease apart these two interpretations. However, in 1978, Cowan and coworkers[2] carried out a study designed to determine which of these two explanations was likely to be the correct one (Fig. 9-9). The researchers identified a population of women who were patients at the Johns Hopkins Hospital Infertility Clinic in Baltimore, Maryland, from 1945 to 1965. Because they were patients at this clinic, the subjects, by definition, all had a late age at first pregnancy. In the course of their diagnostic evaluations, detailed hormonal profiles were developed for each woman. The researchers were therefore able to separate the women with an underlying hormonal abnormality, including progesterone deficiency (exposed), from those without such a hormonal abnormality (nonexposed) who had another cause of infertility, such as a problem with tubal patency or a husband's low sperm count. Both groups of women were then followed for subsequent development of breast cancer.

How could the results of this study design clarify the relationship between late age at first pregnancy

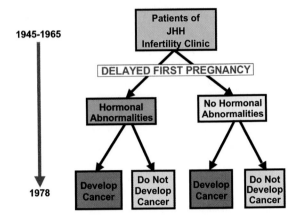

Figure 9-9. Design of Cowan's retrospective cohort study of breast cancer. (Data from Cowan LD, Gordis L, Tonascia JA, Jones GS: Breast cancer incidence in women with progesterone deficiency. Am J Epidemiol 114:209–217, 1981.)

and increased risk of breast cancer? If the explanation for the association of late age at first pregnancy and increased risk of breast cancer is that an early first pregnancy protects against breast cancer, we would not expect any difference in the incidence of breast cancer between the women who have a hormonal abnormality and those who do not. However, if the explanation for the increased risk of breast cancer is that the underlying hormonal abnormality predisposes these women to breast cancer, we would expect to find a higher incidence of breast cancer in women with the hormonal abnormality than in those without this abnormality.

The study found that, when the development of breast cancer was considered for the entire group, the incidence was 1.8 times greater in women with hormonal abnormalities than in women without such abnormalities, but the finding was not statistically significant. However, when the occurrence of breast cancer was divided into categories of premenopausal and postmenopausal incidence, women with hormonal abnormalities had a 5.4 times greater risk of premenopausal occurrence of breast cancer; no difference was seen for postmenopausal occurrence of breast cancer. It is not clear whether this lack of a difference in the incidence of postmenopausal breast cancer represents the true absence of a difference or whether it can be attributed to the small number of women in this population who had reached menopause at the time the study was conducted.

What type of study design is this? Clearly, it is a cohort design, because it compares exposed and nonexposed persons. Furthermore, because the study was carried out in 1978 and the investigator used a roster of patients who had been seen at the Infertility Clinic from 1945 to 1965, it is a retrospective cohort design.

COHORT STUDIES FOR INVESTIGATING CHILDHOOD HEALTH AND DISEASE

A particularly appealing use of the cohort design is for long-term cohort studies of childhood health and disease. In recent years, there has been increasing recognition that experiences and exposures during fetal life may have long-lasting effects, even into adult life. Infections during pregnancy, as well as exposures to environmental toxins, hormonal abnormalities, or the use of drugs (either medications taken during pregnancy or substances abused during pregnancy), may have potentially damaging effects on the fetus and child, and these agents might have possible effects that last even into adult life. David Barker and his colleagues concluded from their studies that adult chronic disease is biologically programmed in intrauterine life or early infancy.[3] The importance of including a life course approach to the epidemiologic study of chronic disease throughout life has been emphasized.

In this chapter, we have discussed two types of cohort studies; both have applicability to the study of childhood health. In the first type of cohort study, we start with exposed and nonexposed groups. For example, follow-up studies of fetuses exposed to radiation from atomic bombs in Hiroshima and Nagasaki during World War II have provided much information about cancer and other health problems resulting from intrauterine exposure to radiation.[4] The exposure dose was calibrated for the survivors on the basis of how far the person was from the point of the bomb drop at the time the bomb was dropped and the nature of the barriers between that person and the point of the bomb drop. It was then possible to relate the risk of adverse outcome to the radiation dose that each person received. Another example is the cohort of pregnancies during the Dutch Famine in World War II.[5] Because the Dutch kept excellent records, it was possible to identify cohorts who were exposed to the severe famine at different times in gestation and to compare them with each other and with a nonexposed group.

As discussed earlier in this chapter, in the second type of cohort study, we identify a group before any

of its members become exposed or before the exposure has been identified. For example, infants born during a single week in 1946 in Great Britain were followed into childhood and later into adult life. The Collaborative Perinatal Study, begun in the United States in the 1950s, was a multicenter cohort study that followed more than 58,000 children from birth to age 7 years.[6]

Although the potential knowledge to be gained by such studies is very attractive, several challenging questions arise when such large cohort studies of children are envisioned, and when such long-term follow-up is planned. Among the questions are the following:

1. At what point should the individuals in the cohort first be identified? When a cohort is initiated at birth and then followed (Fig. 9-10A), data on prenatal exposures can be obtained only retrospectively by interview and from relevant records. Therefore, some cohort studies have begun in the prenatal period, when the pregnancy is first identified. However, even when this is done, preconceptual and periconceptual data that may be needed to answer certain questions may only be obtained retrospectively. Therefore, a cohort initiated at the time of conception (Fig. 9-10B) is desirable for answering many questions because it permits concurrent gathering of data about conception and early pregnancy. However, this is generally a logistically difficult and expensive challenge.

2. Should the cohort be drawn from one center or from a few centers, or should it be a national sample drawn in an attempt to make the cohort representative of a national population? Will the findings of studies based on the cohort be broadly generalizable only if the cohort is drawn from a national sample?

3. For how long should a cohort be followed? Eaton urged that a cohort should be established at the time of conception and followed into adult life or until death.[7] This approach would help to test Barker's hypothesis regarding the early origins of many chronic diseases.

4. What hypotheses and how many hypotheses should be tested in the cohort that will be established? A major problem associated with long-term follow-up of large cohorts is that, by the time the cohort has been established and followed for a number of years, the hypotheses that originally led to the establishment of the cohort may no longer be of sufficient interest or relevance because

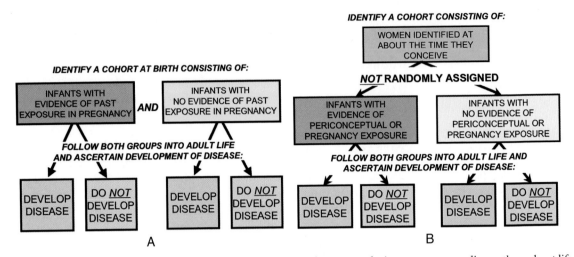

Figure 9-10. Design of a cohort study to investigate the effects of exposures during pregnancy on disease throughout life. **A,** Study beginning at birth. **B,** Study beginning at about the time of conception.

scientific and health knowledge has changed over time. Furthermore, as new knowledge leads to new hypotheses and to questions that were not originally anticipated when the study was initiated, data on the variables needed to test such new hypotheses and to answer such new questions may not be available in the data originally collected.

POTENTIAL BIASES IN COHORT STUDIES

A number of potential biases must be either avoided or taken into account in conducting cohort studies. The major biases include the following:

1. *Bias in assessment of the outcome:* If the person who decides whether disease has developed in each subject also knows whether that subject was exposed, and if that person is aware of the hypothesis being tested, that person's judgment as to whether the disease developed may be biased by that knowledge. This problem can be addressed by masking the person who is making the disease assessment and also by determining whether this person was, in fact, aware of each subject's exposure status.

2. *Information bias:* If the quality and extent of information obtained is different for exposed persons than for nonexposed persons, a significant bias can be introduced. This is particularly likely to occur in historical cohort studies, in which information is obtained from past records. As we discussed with regard to randomized trials,

in any cohort study, it is essential that the quality of the information obtained be comparable in both exposed and nonexposed individuals.

3. *Biases from nonresponse and losses to follow-up:* As was discussed in connection with randomized trials, nonparticipation and nonresponse can introduce major biases that can complicate the interpretation of the study findings. Similarly, loss to follow-up can be a serious problem: If people with the disease are selectively lost to follow-up, the incidence rates calculated in the exposed and nonexposed groups will clearly be difficult to interpret.

4. *Analytic bias:* As in any study, if the epidemiologists and statisticians who are analyzing the data have strong preconceptions, they may unintentionally introduce their biases into their data analyses and into their interpretation of the study findings.

WHEN IS A COHORT STUDY WARRANTED?

Figure 9-11 reviews the basic steps in a cohort study, beginning with identifying an exposed group and an unexposed group (Fig. 9-11A). We then ascertain the rate of development of disease (incidence) in both the exposed and the nonexposed groups (Fig. 9-11B). If the exposure is associated with disease, we would expect to find a greater rate of development of disease in the exposed group than in the nonexposed group, as shown schematically in Fig. 9-11C.

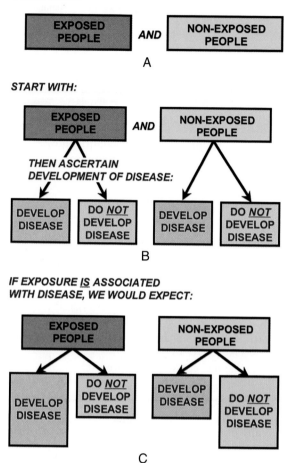

START WITH:

A

START WITH:

THEN ASCERTAIN DEVELOPMENT OF DISEASE:

B

IF EXPOSURE IS ASSOCIATED WITH DISEASE, WE WOULD EXPECT:

C

Figure 9-11. Design of a cohort study. **A,** Starting with exposed and nonexposed groups. **B,** Measuring the development of disease in both groups. **C,** Expected findings if the exposure is associated with disease.

Clearly, to carry out a cohort study, we must have some idea of which exposures are suspected as possible causes of a disease and are therefore worth investigating. Consequently, a cohort study is indicated when good evidence suggests an association of a disease with a certain exposure or exposures (evidence obtained from either clinical observations or case-control or other types of studies).

Because cohort studies often involve follow-up of populations over a long period, the cohort approach is particularly attractive when we can minimize attrition (losses to follow-up) of the study population. Consequently, such studies are generally easier to conduct when the interval between the exposure and the development of disease is short. An example of an association in which the interval between exposure and outcome is short is the relationship between rubella infection during pregnancy and the development of congenital malformations in the offspring.

Several considerations can make the cohort design impractical. Often, strong evidence does not exist to justify mounting a large and expensive study for in-depth investigation of the role of a specific risk factor in the etiology of a disease. Even when such evidence is available, a cohort of exposed and nonexposed persons often cannot be identified. Generally, we do not have appropriate past records or other sources of data that enable us to conduct a retrospective cohort study; as a result, a long study is required because of the need for extended follow-up of the population after exposure. Furthermore, many of the diseases that are of interest today occur at very low rates. Consequently, very large cohorts must be enrolled in a study to ensure that enough cases develop by the end of the study period to permit valid analysis and conclusions.

In view of these considerations, an approach other than a cohort design is often needed—one that will surmount many of these difficulties. Chapter 10 presents such a study design—the case-control study and other study designs that are being increasingly used. Chapters 11 and 12 discuss the use of these study designs in estimating increased risk associated with an exposure, and the characteristics of both cohort and case-control studies are reviewed in Chapter 13.

REFERENCES

1. Kannel WB: CHD risk factors: A Framingham Study update. Hosp Pract 25:93–104, 1990.
2. Cowan LD, Gordis L, Tonascia JA, Jones GS: Breast cancer incidence in women with progesterone deficiency. Am J Epidemiol 114:209–217, 1981.
3. Barker DJP (ed): Fetal and Infant Origins of Adult Disease. London, BMJ Books, 1992.
4. Yoshimoto Y, Kato H, Schull WJ: Cancer risk among in utero exposed survivors: A review of 45 years of study of Hiroshima and Nagasaki atomic bomb survivors. J Radiat Res (Tokyo)

32(Suppl):231–238, 1991. Also available as RERF Technical Report 4–88, and in Lancet 2:665–669, 1988.

5. Susser E, Hoek HW, Brown A: Neurodevelopmental disorders after prenatal famine: The story of the Dutch Famine Study. Am J Epidemiol 147:213–216, 1998.

6. Broman S: The Collaborative Perinatal Project: An overview. In Mednick SA, Harway M, Pinello KM (eds): Handbook of Longitudinal Research, vol I. New York, Praeger, 1984.

7. Eaton WW: The logic for a conception-to-death cohort study. Ann Epidemiol 12:445–451, 2002.

REVIEW QUESTIONS FOR CHAPTER 9

1. In cohort studies of the role of a suspected factor in the etiology of a disease, it is essential that:
   a. There be equal numbers of persons in both study groups
   b. At the beginning of the study, those with the disease and those without the disease have equal risks of having the factor
   c. The study group with the factor and the study group without the factor be representative of the general population
   d. The exposed and nonexposed groups under study be as similar as possible with regard to possible confounding factors
   e. Both *b* and *c*

2. Which of the following is *not* an advantage of a prospective cohort study?
   a. It usually costs less than a case-control study
   b. Precise measurement of exposure is possible
   c. Incidence rates can be calculated
   d. Recall bias is minimized compared with a case-control study
   e. Many disease outcomes can be studied simultaneously

3. Retrospective cohort studies are characterized by all of the following *except:*
   a. The study groups are exposed and non-exposed
   b. Incidence rates may be computed
   c. The required sample size is smaller than that needed for a prospective cohort study

   d. The required sample size is similar to that needed for a prospective cohort study
   e. They are useful for rare exposures

4. A major problem resulting from the lack of randomization in a cohort study is:
   a. The possibility that a factor that led to the exposure, rather than the exposure itself, might have caused the disease
   b. The possibility that a greater proportion of people in the study may have been exposed
   c. The possibility that a smaller proportion of people in the study may have been exposed
   d. That, without randomization, the study may take longer to carry out
   e. Planned crossover is more likely

5. In a cohort study, the advantage of starting by selecting a defined population for study before any of its members become exposed, rather than starting by selecting exposed and nonexposed individuals, is that:
   a. The study can be completed more rapidly
   b. A number of outcomes can be studied simultaneously
   c. A number of exposures can be studied simultaneously
   d. The study will cost less to carry out
   e. *a* and *d*

Chapter 10

Case-Control Studies and Other Study Designs

Suppose you are a clinician and you have seen a few patients with a certain type of cancer, almost all of whom report that they have been exposed to a particular chemical. You hypothesize that the exposure is related to the risk of developing this type of cancer. How would you go about confirming or refuting your hypothesis?

Consider two real-life examples:

In the early 1940s, Alton Ochsner, a surgeon in New Orleans, observed that virtually all of the patients on whom he was operating for lung cancer gave a history of cigarette smoking.[1] Although this relationship is accepted and well recognized today, it was relatively new and controversial at the time that Ochsner made his observation. He hypothesized that cigarette smoking was linked to lung cancer. Based only on his observations in cases of lung cancer, was this conclusion valid?

A second example:

Again in the 1940s, Sir Norman Gregg, an Australian ophthalmologist, observed a number of infants and young children in his ophthalmology practice who presented with an unusual form of cataract.[2] Gregg noted that these children had been in utero during the time of a rubella (German measles) outbreak. He suggested that there was an association between prenatal rubella exposure and the development of the unusual cataracts. Keep in mind that at that time there was no knowledge that a virus could be teratogenic. Thus, he proposed his hypothesis solely on the basis of observational data, the equivalent of data from ambulatory or bedside practice today.

Let us suppose that Gregg had observed that 90% of these infants had been in utero during the rubella outbreak. Would he have been justified in concluding that rubella was associated with the cataracts? Clearly, the answer is no. For although such an observation would be interesting, it would be difficult to interpret without data for a comparison group of children without cataracts. It is possible, for example, that 90% of *all* mothers in that community—both mothers of children with the cataracts and mothers of children with no cataracts—had been pregnant during the outbreak of rubella. In such a case, the exposure history would be no different for mothers of children with cataracts than for mothers of controls. The question was, therefore, whether the prevalence of rubella exposure (i.e., having been in utero during the outbreak) was greater in children with cataracts than in a group of children without cataracts.

To determine the significance of such observations in a group of cases, a comparison or control group is needed. Without such a comparison, Ochsner's or Gregg's observations would only constitute a case series. The observations would have been intriguing, but no conclusion is possible without comparative observations in a series of *noncases*. Comparison is an essential component of epidemiologic investigation and is well exemplified by the case-control study design.

DESIGN OF A CASE-CONTROL STUDY

Figure 10-1 shows the design of a *case-control study*. To examine the possible relation of an exposure to a certain disease, we identify a group of individuals with that disease (called *cases*) and, for purposes of comparison, a group of people without that disease (called *controls*). We determine what proportion of the cases were exposed and what proportion were not. We also determine what proportion of the controls were exposed and what proportion were not. In the example of the children with cataracts, the cases would consist of children with cataracts and the controls would consist of children without cataracts. For

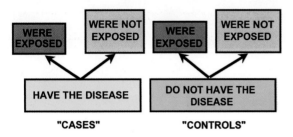

Figure 10-1. Design of a case-control study.

each child, it would then be necessary to ascertain whether or not the mother was exposed to rubella during her pregnancy with that child. We anticipate that if the exposure (rubella) is in fact related to the disease (cataracts), the prevalence of history of exposure among the cases—children with cataracts—will be greater than that among the controls—children with no cataracts. Thus, in a case-control study, if there is an association of an exposure with a disease, the prevalence of history of exposure should be higher in persons who have the disease (cases) than in those who do not (controls).

Table 10-1 presents a hypothetical schema of how a case-control study is conducted. We begin by selecting cases with the disease and controls without the disease, and then measure past exposure by interview and by review of medical or employee records or of results of chemical or biologic assays of blood, urine, or tissues. If exposure is dichotomous, that is, exposure has either occurred (yes) or not occurred (no), breakdown into four groups is possible: There are a

cases who were exposed and c cases who were not exposed. Similarly, there are b controls who were exposed and d controls who were not exposed. Thus the total number of cases is $a + c$ and the total number of controls is $b + d$. If exposure is associated with disease, we would expect the proportion of the cases who were exposed, or or $\dfrac{a}{a+c}$, to be greater than the proportion of the controls who were exposed, or $\dfrac{b}{b+d}$.

A hypothetical example of a case-control study is seen in Table 10-2. We are conducting a case-control study of the relationship of smoking to coronary heart disease (CHD). We start with 200 people with CHD (cases) and compare them to 400 people without CHD (controls). If there is a relationship between smoking and CHD, we would anticipate that a greater proportion of the CHD cases than of the controls would have been smokers (exposed). We find that of the 200 CHD cases, 112 were smokers and 88 were nonsmokers. Of the 400 controls, 176 were smokers and 224 were nonsmokers. Thus 56% of CHD cases were smokers compared to 44% of the controls. This calculation is only a first step. Further calculations to determine whether or not there is an association of the exposure with the disease will be discussed in Chapters 11 and 12. This chapter focuses on issues of design in case-control studies.

Parenthetically, it is of interest to note that if we use only the data from a case-control study, we cannot estimate the prevalence of the disease. In this example we had 200 cases and 400 controls, but this does not imply that the prevalence is 33%, or $\dfrac{200}{200+400}$. The decision as to the number of controls to select per case in a case-control study is

---

TABLE 10-1. Design of Case-Control Studies

	First Select	
	Cases (With Disease)	Controls (Without Disease)
Then Measure Past Exposure		
Were exposed	a	b
Were not exposed	c	d
Total	$a + c$	$b + d$
Proportions exposed	$\dfrac{a}{a+c}$	$\dfrac{b}{b+d}$

TABLE 10-2. Hypothetical Example of a Case-Control Study of Coronary Heart Disease and Cigarette Smoking

	CHD Cases	Controls
Smoke cigarettes	112	176
Do not smoke cigarettes	88	224
Total	200	400
% Smoking cigarettes	56.0	44.0

in the hands of the investigator, and does not reflect the prevalence of disease in the population. In this example, the investigator could have selected 200 cases and 200 controls (1 control per case), or 200 cases and 800 controls (4 controls per case). Because the proportion of the entire study population that consists of cases is determined by the ratio of controls per case, and this proportion is determined by the investigator, it clearly does not reflect the true prevalence of the disease in the population.

At this point, we should emphasize that the hallmark of the case-control study is that it begins with people with the disease (cases) and compares them to people without the disease (controls). This is in contrast to the design of a cohort study, discussed in Chapter 9, which begins with a group of exposed people and compares them to a nonexposed group. Some people have the erroneous impression that the distinction between the two types of study design is that cohort studies go forward in time and case-control studies go backward in time. Such a distinction is not correct; in fact, it is unfortunate that the term retrospective has been used for case-control studies, as the term incorrectly implies that calendar time is the characteristic that distinguishes case-control from cohort design. As was shown in the previous chapter, a retrospective cohort study also uses data obtained in the past. Thus, calendar time is not the characteristic that distinguishes a case-control from a cohort study. What distinguishes the two study designs is whether the study begins with diseased and nondiseased people (case-control study) or with exposed and nonexposed people (cohort study).

Table 10-3 presents the results of a case-control study of the use of artificial sweeteners and bladder cancer. This study included 3,000 cases with bladder cancer and 5,776 controls without bladder cancer. Why the unusual number of controls? The most likely explanation is that the investigation planned for two controls per case (i.e., 6,000 controls), and that some of the controls did not participate. Of the 3,000 cases, 1,293 had used artificial sweeteners (43.1%), and of the 5,776 controls, 2,455 had used artificial sweeteners (42.5%). The proportions are very close, and the investigators in this study did not confirm the findings that had been reported in animal studies, which had caused considerable controversy and had major policy implications for government regulation.

TABLE 10-3. **History of Use of Artificial Sweeteners in Bladder Cancer Cases and Controls**

Artificial Sweetener Use	Cases	Controls
Ever	1,293	2,455
Never	1,707	3,321
Total	3,000	5,776

From Hoover RN, Strasser PH: Artificial sweeteners and human bladder cancer: Preliminary results. Lancet 1:837–840, 1980.

One of the earliest studies of cigarette smoking and lung cancer was conducted by Sir Richard Doll and Bradford Hill. (Sir Richard Doll is an internationally known epidemiologist who was knighted for his scientific work, an honor that comes all too infrequently to epidemiologists!) Table 10-4 presents data from this study for 1,357 males with lung cancer and 1,357 controls according to the average number of cigarettes smoked per day in the 10 years preceding the present illness.[3]

We see that there are fewer heavy smokers among the controls and very few nonsmokers among the

TABLE 10-4. **Distribution of 1,357 Male Lung Cancer Patients and a Male Control Group According to Average Number of Cigarettes Smoked Daily Over the 10 Years Preceding Onset of the Current Illness**

Average Daily Cigarettes	Lung Cancer Patients	Control Group
0	7	61
1–4	55	129
5–14	489	570
15–24	475	431
25–49	293	154
50+	38	12
Total	1,357	1,357

From Doll R, Hill AB: A study of the aetiology of carcinoma of the lung. BMJ 2:1271–1286, 1952.

lung cancer cases, a finding strongly suggestive of an association between smoking and lung cancer. In contrast to the previous example, exposure in this study is not just dichotomized (exposed or not exposed), but the exposure data are further stratified in terms of dose, as measured by the number of cigarettes smoked per day. Because many of the environmental exposures about which we are concerned today are not all-or-nothing exposures, the possibility of doing a study and analysis that takes into account the dose of the exposure is very important.

SELECTION OF CASES AND CONTROLS

Selection of Cases

In a case-control study, cases can be selected from a variety of sources, including hospital patients, patients in physicians' practices, or clinic patients. Many communities maintain registries of patients with certain diseases, such as cancer, and such registries can serve as valuable sources of cases for such studies.

Several problems must be kept in mind in selecting cases for a case-control study. If cases are selected from a single hospital, any risk factors that are identified may be unique to that hospital as a result of referral patterns or other factors, and the results may not be generalizable to all patients with the disease. Consequently, if hospitalized cases are to be used, it is desirable to select the cases from several hospitals in the community. Furthermore, if the hospital from which the cases are drawn is a tertiary care facility, which selectively admits severely ill patients, any risk factors identified in the study may be risk factors only in persons with severe forms of the disease. In any event, it is essential that in case-control studies, just as in randomized trials, the criteria for eligibility be carefully specified in writing.

Incident or Prevalent Cases

An important consideration in case-control studies is whether to use incident cases of a disease (newly diagnosed cases) or prevalent cases of the disease (people who may have had the disease for some time). The problem with use of incident cases is that we must often wait for new cases to be diagnosed; whereas if we use prevalent cases, which have already been diagnosed, a larger number of cases is often available for study. Despite this practical advantage

of using prevalent cases, however, it is generally preferable to use incident cases of the disease in case-control studies of disease etiology. The reason is that any risk factors we may identify in a study using prevalent cases may be related more to *survival* with the disease than to the development of the disease *(incidence)*. If, for example, most people who develop the disease die soon after diagnosis, they will be underrepresented in a study that uses prevalent cases, and such a study is more likely to include longer-term survivors. This would constitute a highly nonrepresentative group of cases, and any risk factors identified with this nonrepresentative group may not be a general characteristic of all patients with the disease, but only of survivors.

Even if we include only *incident* cases (patients who have been newly diagnosed with the disease) in a case-control study, we will of course be excluding any patients who may have died before the diagnosis was made. There is no easy solution to this problem or to certain other problems in case selection, but it is important that we keep these issues in mind when we finally interpret the data and derive conclusions from the study. At that time, it is critical to take into account possible selection biases that may have been introduced by the study design and by the manner in which the study was conducted.

Selection of Controls

In 1929, Raymond Pearl, Professor of Biostatistics at Johns Hopkins University, Baltimore, conducted a study to test the hypothesis that tuberculosis protected against cancer.[4] From 7,500 consecutive autopsies at Johns Hopkins Hospital, Pearl identified 816 cases of cancer. He then selected a control group of 816 from among the others on whom autopsies had been carried out at Johns Hopkins and determined the percent of the cases and of the controls who had findings of tuberculosis on autopsy. Pearl's findings are seen in Table 10-5.

Of the 816 autopsies of patients with cancer, 54 had tuberculosis (6.6%), whereas of the 816 controls with no cancer, 133 had tuberculosis (16.3%). From the finding that the prevalence of tuberculosis was considerably higher in the control group (no cancer findings) than in the case group (cancer diagnoses), Pearl concluded that tuberculosis had an antagonistic or protective effect against cancer.

Was Pearl's conclusion justified? The answer to this question depends on the adequacy of his control

TABLE 10-5. **Summary of Data from Pearl's Study of Cancer and Tuberculosis**		
	Cases (With Cancer)	Controls (Without Cancer)
Total number of autopsies	816	816
Number (%) of autopsies with tuberculosis	54 (6.6)	133 (16.3)

From Pearl R: Cancer and tuberculosis. Am J Hyg 9:97–159, 1929.

group. If the prevalence of tuberculosis in the *non-cancer* patients was similar to that of all people who were free of cancer, his conclusion would be valid. But that was not the case. At the time of the study, tuberculosis was one of the major reasons for hospitalization at Johns Hopkins Hospital. Consequently, what Pearl had inadvertently done in choosing the cancer-free control group was to select a group in which many of the patients had been diagnosed with and hospitalized for tuberculosis. Pearl thought that the control group's rate of tuberculosis would represent the level of tuberculosis expected in the general population; but because of the way he selected the controls, they came from a pool that was heavily weighted with tuberculosis patients, which did not represent the general population. He was, in effect, comparing the prevalence of tuberculosis in a group of patients with cancer with the prevalence of tuberculosis in a group of patients in which many had already been diagnosed with tuberculosis. Clearly, his conclusion was not justified on the basis of these data.

How could Pearl have overcome this problem in his study? Instead of comparing his cancer patients with a group selected from all other autopsied patients, he could have compared the patients with cancer to a group of patients admitted for some specific diagnosis other than cancer (and not tuberculosis). In fact, Carlson and Bell[5] repeated Pearl's study but compared the patients who died of cancer to patients who died of heart disease at Johns Hopkins. They found no difference in the prevalence of tuberculosis at autopsy between the two groups. (It is of interest, however, that despite the methodologic

limitations of Pearl's study, bacille Calmette-Guérin [BCG] is used today as a form of immunotherapy in several types of cancer.)

The problem with Pearl's study exemplifies the challenge of selecting appropriate controls for case-control studies. This is one of the most difficult problems in epidemiology. The challenge is this: If we conduct a case-control study and find more exposure in the cases than in the controls, we would like to be able to conclude that there is an association between the exposure and the disease in question. The way the controls are selected is a major determinant of whether such a conclusion is valid.

A fundamental conceptual issue relating to selection of controls is whether the controls should be similar to the cases in all respects other than having the disease in question, or whether they should be representative of all persons without the disease in the population from which the cases are selected. This question has stimulated considerable discussion, but in actuality, the characteristics of the nondiseased people in the population from which the cases are selected are often not known, because the reference population may not be well defined.

Consider, for example, a case-control study using hospitalized cases. We want to identify the reference population that is the source of the cases so that we can then sample this reference population to select controls. Unfortunately, it is usually either not easy or not possible to identify such a reference population for hospitalized patients. Patients admitted to a hospital may come from the surrounding neighborhood, may live farther away in the same city, or may, through a referral process, come from another city or another country. Under these circumstances it is virtually impossible to define a specific reference population from which the cases emerged and from which we might select controls. Nevertheless, we want to design our study so that when it is finished, we can be reasonably certain that if we find a difference in exposure history between cases and controls, there are not likely to be any other important differences between them that might limit the inferences we may derive.

Sources of Controls

Controls may be selected from nonhospitalized persons living in the community or from hospitalized patients admitted for diseases other than that for which the cases were admitted.

Nonhospitalized Persons as Controls

Nonhospitalized controls may be selected from several sources in the community. Ideally, a probability sample of the total population might be selected, but as a practical matter, this is rarely possible. Other sources include school rosters, selective service lists, and insurance company lists. Another option is to select, as a control for each case, a resident of a defined area, such as the neighborhood in which the case lives. Such *neighborhood controls* have been used for many years. In this approach, interviewers are instructed to identify the home of a case as a starting point, and from there walk past a specified number of houses in a specified direction and seek the first household that contains an eligible control. Because of increasing problems of security in urban areas of the United States, however, many people will no longer open their doors to interviewers. Nevertheless, in many other countries, particularly in developing countries, the door-to-door approach to obtaining controls may be ideal.

Because of the difficulties in many cities in the United States in obtaining neighborhood controls using the door-to-door approach, an alternate method for selecting such controls is to use random-digit dialing. Because telephone exchanges generally match neighborhood boundaries, a case's seven-digit telephone number, of which the first three digits are the exchange, can be used to select a control telephone number, in which the terminal four digits of the phone number are randomly selected and the same three-digit exchange is used. In many developing countries this approach is impractical, as only government offices and business establishments are likely to have telephones.

Another approach to control selection is to use a *best friend control*. A case is asked for the name of a best friend who, in principle, is more likely to participate in the study knowing that his or her friend is also participating. A control obtained in this fashion may be likely to be similar to the case in age and in many other demographic and social characteristics. Sometimes a spouse or sibling control may be useful; a sibling may provide some control over genetic differences between cases and controls.

Hospitalized Patients as Controls

Hospital inpatients are often selected as controls because of the extent to which they are a "captive population" and are clearly identified; it should therefore be relatively more economical to carry out

a study using such controls. However, as just discussed, they represent a sample of an ill-defined reference population that generally cannot be characterized. Moreover, hospital patients differ from people in the community. For example, the prevalence of cigarette smoking is known to be higher in hospitalized patients than in community residents; many of the diagnoses for which people are admitted to the hospital are smoking related.

Given that we generally cannot characterize the reference population from which hospitalized cases come, there is a conceptual attractiveness to comparing hospitalized cases to hospitalized controls from the same institution, who presumably would tend to come from the same reference population (Fig. 10-2); that is, whatever selection factors in the referral system affected the cases' admission to a particular hospital would also pertain to the controls. However, referral patterns at the same hospital may differ for various clinical services, and such an assumption may be questionable.

In using hospital controls the question arises of whether to use a sample of all other patients admitted to the hospital (other than those with the cases' diagnosis) or whether to select a specific "other diagnosis." If we wish to choose specific diagnostic groups, on what basis do we select those groups, and on what basis do we exclude others? The problem is that

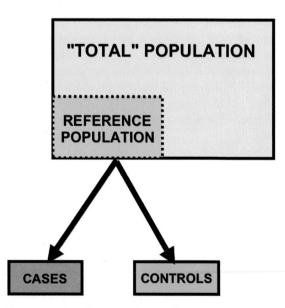

Figure 10-2. Whatever selection factors in the referral system affected admissions of cases to a certain hospital would also affect the admission of hospital controls.

although it is attractive to choose as hospitalized controls a disease group that is obviously unrelated to the putative causative factor under investigation, such controls are unlikely to be representative of the general reference population. As a result, it will not be clear whether it is the cases or the controls who differ from the general population.

The issue of which diagnostic groups would be eligible for use as controls and which would be ineligible (and therefore excluded) is very important. Let us say we are conducting a case-control study of lung cancer and smoking: we select as cases patients who have been hospitalized with lung cancer, and as controls we select patients who have been hospitalized with emphysema. What problem would this present? Because we know that there is a strong relationship between smoking and emphysema, our controls, the emphysema patients, would include a high number of smokers. Consequently, any relationship of smoking to lung cancer would not be detectable in this study, because we would have selected as controls a group of persons in which there is a greater-than-expected prevalence of smoking. We might therefore want to exclude from our control group those persons who have other smoking-related diagnoses, such as coronary heart disease, bladder cancer, pancreatic cancer, and emphysema. Such exclusions might yield a control group with a lower-than-expected prevalence of smoking and the exclusion process becomes complex. One alternative is to not exclude any groups from selection as controls in the design of the study, but to analyze the study data separately for different diagnostic subgroups that constitute the control group.

PROBLEMS IN CONTROL SELECTION

The following example demonstrates the problem of exclusions in the process of control selection:

In 1981, MacMahon and coworkers[6] reported a case-control study of cancer of the pancreas. The cases were patients with a histologically confirmed diagnosis of pancreatic cancer in 11 Boston and Rhode Island hospitals from 1974 to 1979. Controls were selected from all patients who were hospitalized at the same time as the cases; and they were selected from other inpatients hospitalized by the attending physicians who had hospitalized the cases. One finding in this study was an apparent dose–response relationship between coffee consumption and cancer of the pancreas, particularly in women (Table 10-6).

When such a relationship is observed, it is difficult to know whether the disease is *caused* by the coffee consumption or by some factor closely related to the coffee consumption. Because smoking is a known risk factor for cancer of the pancreas, and because coffee consumption is closely related to cigarette smoking (it is rare to find a smoker who does not drink coffee), did MacMahon and others observe an association of coffee consumption with pancreatic cancer because the coffee caused the pancreatic cancer, or because coffee consumption is related to cigarette smoking, and cigarette smoking is known to be a risk factor for cancer of the pancreas? Recognizing this problem, the authors analyzed the data after stratifying for smoking history. The relationship with coffee consumption held both for current smokers and for those who had never smoked (Table 10-7).

This report aroused great interest in both the scientific and lay communities, particularly among coffee manufacturers. Given the widespread exposure of human beings to coffee, if the reported relationship were true, it would have major public health implications.

Let us examine the design of this study. The cases were white patients with cancer of the pancreas at 11 Boston and Rhode Island hospitals. The controls are of particular interest: They were patients with other diseases who were hospitalized by the same physicians who had hospitalized the cases. That is, when a case had been identified, the attending physician was asked if another of his or her patients who was hospitalized at the same time for another condition could be interviewed as a control. This unusual method of control selection had a practical advantage: One of the major obstacles in obtaining participation of hospital controls in case-control studies is that permission to contact the patient is requested of the attending physician. The physicians are often not motivated to have their patients serve as controls, because the patients do not have the disease that is the focus of the study. By asking physicians who had already given permission for patients with pancreatic cancer to participate, the likelihood was increased that permission would be granted for patients with other diseases to participate as controls.

Did that practical decision introduce any problems? The underlying question that the investigators wanted to answer was whether patients with cancer of the pancreas drank more coffee than did people without cancer of the pancreas in the same population (Fig. 10-3). What MacMahon and coworkers

TABLE 10-6. **Distribution of Cases and Controls by Coffee-Drinking Habits and Estimates of Risk Ratios**

Sex	Category	Coffee Consumption (Cups/Day)				Total
		0	1–2	3–4	≥5	
M	Number of cases	9	94	53	60	216
	Number of controls	32	119	74	82	307
	Adjusted relative risk*	1.0	2.6	2.3	2.6	2.6
	95% Confidence interval	–	1.2–5.5	1.0–5.3	1.2–5.8	1.2–5.4
F	Number of cases	11	59	53	28	151
	Number of controls	56	152	80	48	336
	Adjusted relative risk*	1.0	1.6	3.3	3.1	2.3
	95% Confidence interval	–	0.8–3.4	1.6–7.0	1.4–7.0	1.2–4.6

*Chi-square (Mantel extension) with equally spaced scores, adjusted over age in decades: 1.5 for men, 13.7 for women. Mantel-Haenszel estimates of risk ratios, adjusted over categories of age in decades. In all comparisons, the referent category was subjects who never drank coffee.
From MacMahon B, Yen S, Trichopoulos D, et al: Coffee and cancer of the pancreas. N Engl J Med 304(11):630–633, 1981.

found was that the level of coffee consumption in cases was greater than the level of coffee consumption in controls.

The investigators would like to be able to establish that the level of coffee consumption observed in the controls is what would be expected in the general population without pancreatic cancer and that cases therefore demonstrate *excessive* coffee consumption (Fig. 10-4). But the problem is this: Which physicians are most likely to admit patients with cancer of the pancreas to the hospital? Gastroenterologists are often the admitting physicians. Many of their other hospitalized patients (who served as controls) also have gastrointestinal problems, such as esophagitis and peptic ulcer. So in this study, the persons who served as controls may very well have reduced their intake of coffee, either because of a physician's instructions or because of their own realization that reducing their coffee intake could relieve their symptoms. We cannot assume that the controls' levels of coffee consumption are representative of the level of coffee consumption expected in the general popula-

TABLE 10-7. **Estimates of Relative Risk* of Cancer of the Pancreas Associated with Use of Coffee and Cigarettes**

Cigarette Smoking Status	Coffee Drinking (Cups/Day)			Total†
	0	1–2	≥3	
Never smoked	1.0	2.1	3.1	1.0
Ex-smokers	1.3	4.0	3.0	1.3
Current smokers	1.2	2.2	4.6	1.2 (0.9–1.8)
Total*	1.0	1.8 (1.0–3.0)	2.7 (1.6–4.7)	

*The referent category is the group that uses neither cigarettes nor coffee. Estimates are adjusted for sex and age in decades.
†Values are adjusted for the other variables, in addition to age and sex, and are expressed in relation to the lowest category of each variable. Values in parentheses are 95% confidence intervals of the adjusted estimates.
From MacMahon B, Yen S, Trichopoulos D, et al: Coffee and cancer of the pancreas. N Engl J Med 304(11):630–633, 1981.

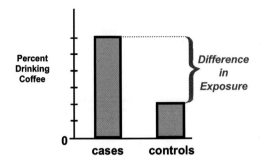

Figure 10-3. Interpreting the results of a case-control study of coffee drinking and pancreatic cancer.

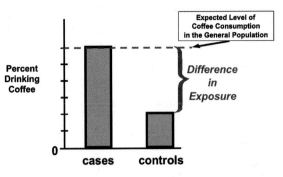

Figure 10-5. Interpreting the results of case-control studies: Is the higher level the expected level of exposure?

tion; their rate of coffee consumption may be abnormally low. Thus, the observed difference in coffee consumption between pancreatic cancer cases and controls may not necessarily have been the result of cases drinking more coffee than expected, but rather of the controls drinking less coffee than expected (Fig. 10-5).

MacMahon and his colleagues subsequently repeated their analysis but separated controls with gastrointestinal illness from controls with other conditions. They found that the risk associated with coffee consumption was indeed higher when the comparison was with controls with gastrointestinal illness but that the relationship between coffee consumption and pancreatic cancer persisted, albeit at a lower level, even when the comparison was with controls with other illnesses. Several years later, Hsieh and coworkers reported a new study that attempted to replicate these results; it did not support the original findings.[7]

In summary, when a difference in exposure is observed between cases and controls, we must ask

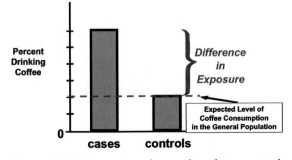

Figure 10-4. Interpreting the results of case-control studies: Is the lower level the expected level of exposure?

whether the level of exposure observed in the controls is really the level expected in the population in which the study was carried out or whether—perhaps given the manner of selection—the controls may have a particularly high or low level of exposure that might not be representative of the level in the population in which the study was carried out.

MATCHING

A major concern in conducting a case-control study is that cases and controls may differ in characteristics or exposures other than the one that has been targeted for study. If more cases than controls are found to have been exposed, we may be left with the question of whether the observed association could be due to differences between the cases and controls in factors other than the exposure being studied. For example, if more cases than controls are found to have been exposed, and if most of the cases are poor and most of the controls are affluent, we would not know whether the factor determining development of disease is exposure to the factor being studied or another characteristic associated with being poor. To avoid such a situation, we would like to ensure that the distribution of the cases and controls by socioeconomic status is similar, so that a difference in exposure will likely constitute the critical difference, and the presence or absence of disease is not likely to be attributable to a difference in socioeconomic status.

One approach to dealing with this problem in the design and conduct of the study is to match the cases and controls for factors about which we may be concerned, such as income, as in the preceding example. *Matching* is defined as the process of selecting the controls so that they are similar to the cases in certain characteristics, such as age, race, sex, socioeconomic status, and occupation. Matching may be of two types: (1) group matching and (2) individual matching.

Group Matching

Group matching (or *frequency matching*) consists of selecting the controls in such a manner that the proportion of controls with a certain characteristic is identical to the proportion of cases with the same characteristic. Thus, if 25% of the cases are married, the controls will be selected so that 25% of that group is also married. This type of selection generally requires that all of the cases be selected first. After calculations are made of the proportions of certain characteristics in the group of cases, then a control group, in which the same characteristics occur in the same proportions, is selected.

Individual Matching

A second type of matching is *individual matching* (or *matched pairs*). In this approach, for each case selected for the study, a control is selected who is similar to the case in terms of the specific variable or variables of concern. For example, if the first case enrolled in our study is a 45-year-old white woman, we will seek a 45-year-old white female control. If the second case is a 24-year-old black man, we will select a control who is also a 24-year-old black man. This type of control selection yields matched case-control pairs; that is, each case is individually matched to a control. The implications of this method of control selection for the estimation of excess risk are discussed in Chapter 11.

Individual matching is often used in case-control studies that use hospital controls. The reason for this is more practical than conceptual. Let us say that sex and age are considered important variables, and it is thought to be important that the cases and the controls be comparable in terms of these two characteristics. There is generally no practical way to dip into a pool of hospital patients to select a group with certain sex and age characteristics. Rather, it is easier to identify a case and then to choose the next hospital admission that matches the case for sex and age. Thus individual matching is most expedient in studies using hospital controls.

What are the problems with matching? The problems with matching are of two types: practical and conceptual.

1. *Practical Problems with Matching:* If an attempt is made to match according to too many characteristics, it may prove difficult or impossible to identify an appropriate control. For example, suppose that it is decided to match each case for race, sex, age, marital status, number of children, zip code of residence, and occupation. If the case is a 48-year-old black woman who is married, has four children, lives in Zip code 21209, and works in a photo-processing plant, it may prove difficult or impossible to find a control who is similar to the case in all of these characteristics. Therefore, the more variables that we choose to match, the more difficult it will be to find a suitable control.

2. *Conceptual Problems with Matching:* Perhaps a more important problem is the conceptual one: Once we have matched controls to cases according to a given characteristic, we cannot study that characteristic. For example, suppose we are interested in studying marital status as a risk factor for breast cancer. If we match the cases (breast cancer) and the controls (no breast cancer) for marital status, we can no longer study whether or not marital status is a risk factor for breast cancer. Why not? Because in matching according to marital status we have artificially established an identical proportion in cases and controls: if 35% of the cases are married, and through matching we create a control group in which 35% are also married, we have artificially ensured that the proportion of married subjects will be identical in both groups. By using matching to impose comparability for a certain factor, we ensure the same prevalence of that factor in the cases and the controls. Clearly, we will not be able to ask whether cases differ from controls in the prevalence of that factor. We would therefore not want to match on the variable of marital status in this study. Indeed, we do not want to match on any variable that we may wish to explore in our study.

It is also important to recognize that unplanned matching may inadvertently occur in case-control studies. For example, if we use neighborhood controls, we are in effect matching for socioeconomic status as well as for cultural and other characteristics of a neighborhood. If we use best-friend controls, it is likely that the case and his or her best friend share many lifestyle characteristics, which in effect produces a match for these characteristics. For example, in a study of oral contraceptive use and cancer in which best-friend controls were considered, there was concern that if the case used oral contraceptives it might well be that her best friend would also be likely to be an oral contraceptive user. The result would be an unplanned matching on oral contraceptive use, so that this variable could no longer be investigated in this study.

In carrying out a case-control study, therefore, we only match on variables that we are convinced are risk factors for the disease, which we are therefore not interested in investigating in this study. Matching on variables other than these, in either a planned or inadvertent manner, is called *overmatching*.

PROBLEMS OF RECALL

A major problem in case-control studies is that of recall. Recall problems are of two types: limitations in recall and recall bias.

Limitations in Recall

Much of the information relating to exposure in case-control studies often involves collecting data from subjects by interviews. Because virtually all human beings are limited to varying degrees in their ability to recall information, limitations in recall are an important issue in such studies. A related issue that is somewhat different from limitations in recall is that persons being interviewed may simply not have the information being requested.

This was demonstrated years ago in a study carried out by Lilienfeld and Graham published in 1958.[8] At that time, considerable interest centered on the observation that cancer of the cervix was highly unusual in two groups of women: Jewish women and nuns. This observation suggested that an important risk factor for cervical cancer could be sexual intercourse with an uncircumcised man, and a number of studies were carried out to confirm this hypothesis. However, the authors were skeptical about the validity of the responses regarding circumcision status. To address this question they asked a group of men whether or not they had been circumcised. The men were then examined by a physician. As seen in Table 10-8, of the 56 men who stated they were circumcised, 19, or 33.9%, were found to be uncircumcised. Of the 136 men who stated they were not circumcised, 47, or 34.6%, were found to be cir-

cumcised. These data demonstrate that the findings from studies using interview data may not always be clear-cut.

Table 10-9 shows more recent data (2002) regarding the relationship of self-reported circumcision to

TABLE 10-8. Comparison of Patients' Statements with Examination Findings Concerning Circumcision Status, Roswell Park Memorial Institute, Buffalo, New York

	PATIENTS' STATEMENTS REGARDING CIRCUMCISION			
	Yes		No	
Examination Finding	*Number*	*%*	*Number*	*%*
Circumcised	37	66.1	47	34.6
Not circumcised	19	33.9	89	65.4
Total	56	100.0	136	100.0

Adapted from Lilienfeld AM, Graham S: Validity of determining circumcision status by questionnaire as related to epidemiologic studies of cancer of the cervix. J Natl Cancer Inst 21:713–720, 1958.

TABLE 10-9. Comparison of Patients' Statements with Physicians' Examination Findings Concerning Circumcision Status in the Study of Circumcision, Penile HPV, and Cervical Cancer

	PATIENTS' STATEMENTS REGARDING CIRCUMCISION			
	Yes		No	
Physician Examination Findings	*Number*	*%*	*Number*	*%*
Circumcised	282	98.3	37	7.4
Not circumcised	5	1.7	466	92.6
Total	287	100.0	503	100.0

Adapted from Castellsague X, Bosch FX, Munoz N, et al: Male circumcision, penile human papillomavirus infection, and cervical cancer in female partners. N Engl J Med 346(15):1105–1112, 2002.

actual circumcision status. These data suggest that men have improved in their knowledge and reporting of their circumcision status, or the differences observed may be due to the studies having been conducted in different countries. There may also have been methodological differences, which could have accounted for the different results between the two studies.

If a limitation of recall regarding exposure affects all subjects in a study to the same extent, regardless of whether they are cases or controls, a misclassification of exposure status may result. Some of the cases or controls who were actually exposed will be erroneously classified as unexposed, and some who were actually not exposed will be erroneously classified as exposed. This generally leads to an underestimate of the true risk of the disease associated with the exposure.

Recall Bias

A more serious potential problem in case-control studies is that of recall bias. Suppose that we are studying the possible relationship of congenital malformations to prenatal infections. We conduct a case-control study and interview mothers of children with congenital malformations (cases) and mothers of children without malformations (controls). Each mother is questioned about infections she may have had during the pregnancy.

A mother who has had a child with a birth defect often tries to identify some unusual event that occurred during her pregnancy with that child. She wants to know whether the abnormality was caused by something she did. Why did it happen? Such a mother may even recall an event, such as a mild respiratory infection, that a mother of a child without a birth defect may not even notice or may have forgotten entirely. This type of bias is known as *recall bias*; Ernst Wynder, a well-known epidemiologist, also called it "rumination bias."

In the study just mentioned, let us assume that the true infection rate during pregnancy in mothers of malformed infants and in mothers of normal infants is 15%; that is, there is no difference in infection rates. Suppose that mothers of malformed infants recall 60% of any infections they had during pregnancy, and mothers of normal infants recall only 10% of infections they had during pregnancy. As seen in Table 10-10, the *apparent* infection rate estimated from this case-control study using interviews

TABLE 10-10. Example of Artificial Association Resulting from Recall Bias: A Study of Maternal Infections during Pregnancy and Congenital Malformations

	Cases (With Congenital Malformations)	Controls (Without Congenital Malformations)
Assume that:		
True incidence of infection (%)	15	15
Infections recalled (%)	60	10
Result will be:		
Infection rate as ascertained by interview (%)	9.0	1.5

would be 9% for mothers of malformed infants and 1.5% for mothers of control infants. Thus the *differential recall* between cases and controls introduces a recall bias into the study that could artifactually suggest a relation of congenital malformations and prenatal infections. Although a potential for recall bias is self-evident in case-control studies, in point of fact, few actual examples demonstrate that recall bias has, in fact, been a major problem in case-control studies and has led to erroneous conclusions regarding associations. The small number of examples available could reflect infrequent occurrence of such bias, or the fact that the data needed to clearly demonstrate the existence of such bias in a certain study are frequently not available. Nevertheless, the potential problem cannot be disregarded, and the possibility for such bias must always be kept in mind.

USE OF MULTIPLE CONTROLS

Early in this chapter, we noted that the investigator can determine how many controls will be used per case in a case-control study and that multiple controls for each case are frequently used. Such controls may be either (1) *controls of the same type*, or (2) *controls of different types*, such as hospital and neighborhood controls, or controls with different diseases.

Controls of the Same Type

Multiple controls of *the same type*, such as two controls or three controls for each case, are used to increase the power of the study. Practically speaking, a noticeable increase in power is gained only up to a ratio of about 1 case to 4 controls. One might ask, Why use multiple controls for each case? Why not keep the ratio of controls to cases at 1 : 1 and just increase the number of cases? The answer is that for many of the relatively infrequent diseases we study, there may be a limit to the number of potential cases available for study. A clinic may see only a certain number of patients with a given cancer or with a certain connective tissue disorder each year. Because the number of cases cannot be increased without either extending the study in time to enroll more cases or developing a collaborative multicentered study, the option of increasing the number of controls per case is often chosen. These controls are of the same type; only the ratio of controls to cases has changed.

Multiple Controls of Different Types

In contrast, we may choose to use *multiple controls of different types*. For example, we may be concerned that the exposure of the hospital controls used in our study may not represent the rate of exposure that is "expected" in a population of nondiseased persons; that is, the controls may be a highly selected subset of nondiseased individuals and may have a different exposure experience. We mentioned earlier that hospitalized patients smoke more than people living in the community, and we are concerned because we do not know what the prevalence level of smoking in hospitalized controls represents or how to interpret a comparison of these rates with those of the cases. To address this problem, we may choose to use an additional control group, such as neighborhood controls. The hope is that the results obtained when cases are compared with hospital controls will be similar to the results obtained when cases are compared with neighborhood controls. If the findings differ, the reason for the discrepancy should be sought. In using

multiple controls of different types, the investigator should ideally decide which comparison will be considered the "gold standard of truth" before embarking on the actual study.

In 1979, Gold and coworkers published a case-control study of brain tumors in children.[9] They used two types of controls: children with no cancer (called *normal controls*) and children with cancers other than brain tumors (called *cancer controls*) (Fig. 10-6). What was the rationale for using these two control groups?

Let us consider the question, "Did mothers of children with brain tumors have more prenatal radiation exposure than control mothers?" Some possible results are seen in Figure 10-7.

If the radiation exposure of mothers of children with brain tumors is found to be greater than that of mothers of normal controls, and the radiation exposure of mothers of children with other cancers is also found to be greater than that of mothers of normal children, what are the possible explanations? One conclusion might be that prenatal radiation is a risk factor both for brain tumors and for other cancers; that is, its effect is that of a carcinogen that is not site specific. Another explanation to consider is that the findings could have resulted from recall bias and that mothers of children with any type of cancer recall prenatal radiation exposure better than mothers of normal children.

Consider another possible set of findings, shown in Figure 10-8.

If mothers of children with brain tumors have a greater radiation exposure history than do both mothers of normal controls and mothers of children with other cancers, the findings might suggest that prenatal radiation is a specific carcinogen for the brain. These findings would also reduce the likeli-

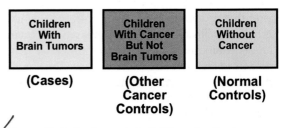

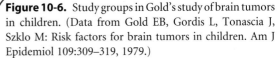

Figure 10-6. Study groups in Gold's study of brain tumors in children. (Data from Gold EB, Gordis L, Tonascia J, Szklo M: Risk factors for brain tumors in children. Am J Epidemiol 109:309–319, 1979.)

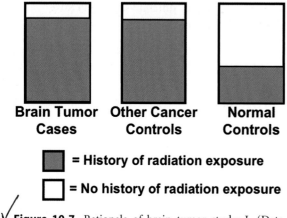

Figure 10-7. Rationale of brain tumor study: I. (Data from Gold EB, Gordis L, Tonascia J, Szklo M: Risk factors for brain tumors in children. Am J Epidemiol 109:309–319, 1979.)

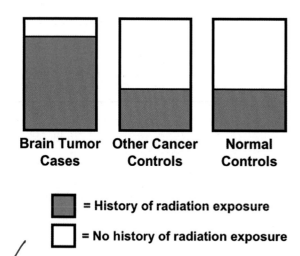

Figure 10-8. Rationale of brain tumor study: II. (Data from Gold EB, Gordis L, Tonascia J, Szklo M: Risk factors for brain tumors in children. Am J Epidemiol 109:309–319, 1979.)

hood that recall bias is playing a role, as it would seem implausible that mothers of children with brain tumors would recall prenatal radiation better than mothers of children with other cancers. Thus, multiple controls of different types can be valuable for exploring alternate hypotheses and for taking into account possible potential biases, such as recall bias.

Despite the issues raised in this chapter, case-control studies are invaluable in exploring the etiology of disease. For example, in October 1989, three patients with eosinophilia and severe myalgia who had been taking L-tryptophan were reported to the Health Department in New Mexico. This led to recognition of a distinct entity, the eosinophilia-myalgia syndrome (EMS). To confirm the apparent association of EMS with L-tryptophan ingestion, a case-control study was conducted.[10] Eleven cases and 22 matched controls were interviewed for information on symptoms and other clinical findings and on use of L-tryptophan-containing products. All 11 cases were found to have used L-tryptophan, compared to only 2 of the controls. These findings led to a nationwide recall of over-the-counter L-tryptophan preparations in November 1989.

A subsequent case-control study in Oregon compared the brand and source of L-tryptophan used by 58 patients with EMS with the brand and source of L-tryptophan used by 30 asymptomatic controls.[11] A single brand and lot of L-tryptophan manufactured by a single Japanese petrochemical company was used by 98% of the cases, compared with 44% of the controls. In a case-control study in Minnesota, 98% of cases had ingested L-tryptophan from that manufacturer compared with 60% of the controls.[12] The findings of both studies indicated that a contaminant introduced during the manufacturing of L-tryptophan or some alteration of L-tryptophan in the manufacturing process was responsible for the outbreak of EMS.

WHEN IS A CASE-CONTROL STUDY WARRANTED?

A case-control study is useful as a first step when searching for a cause of an adverse health outcome, as seen in the two examples at the beginning of this chapter. At an early stage in our search for an etiology, we may suspect any one of several exposures, but we may not have evidence, and certainly no strong evidence, to suggest an association of any one of the suspect exposures with the disease in question. Using the case-control design, we compare people with the disease (cases) and people without the disease (controls) (Fig. 10-9A). We can then explore the possible roles of a variety of exposures or characteristics in causing the disease (Fig. 10-9B). If the exposure is associated with the disease, we would expect the proportion of cases who have been exposed to be greater than the proportion of controls who have been exposed (Fig. 10-9C). When such an association is documented in a case-control study, the next step is often to carry out a cohort study to further elucidate the relationship. Because case-control studies are generally less expensive than cohort studies and can

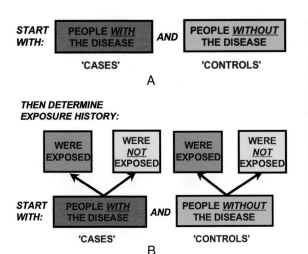

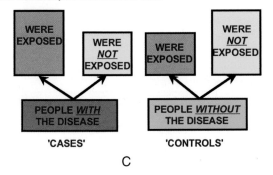

Figure 10-9. Design of a case-control study. **A,** Starting with cases and controls. **B,** Measuring exposure in both groups. **C,** Expected findings if the exposure is associated with disease.

CASE-CONTROL STUDIES BASED IN A DEFINED COHORT

In Chapter 9 we discussed cohort studies. Up to this point in the present chapter we have discussed case-control studies. These discussions have addressed the attributes of these two types of study designs. In recent years, considerable attention has focused on whether it is possible to take advantage of the benefits of both types of study by combining some elements of both the cohort and case-control approaches into a single study. The resulting combined study is in effect a hybrid design in which a case-control study is initiated within a cohort study. The general design is shown schematically in Figure 10-10.

In this type of study, a population is identified and followed over time. At the time the population is identified, baseline data are obtained from records or interviews, from blood or urine tests, and in other ways. The population is then followed for a period of years. For most of the diseases that are studied, a small percentage of study participants manifest the disease, whereas most do not. As seen in Figure 10-10, a case-control study is then carried out using as cases persons in whom the disease developed and using as controls a sample of those in whom the disease did not develop.

Such cohort-based case-control studies can be divided into two types largely on the basis of the approach used for selecting the controls. These two types of studies are called *nested case-control studies* and *case-cohort studies*.

be carried out more quickly, they are often the first step in determining whether an exposure is linked to an increased risk of disease.

Case-control studies are also valuable when the disease being investigated is rare. It is often possible to identify cases for study from disease registries, hospital records, or other sources. In contrast, if we conduct a cohort study for a rare disease, an extremely large study population may be needed in order to observe a sufficient number of individuals in the cohort develop the disease in question. In addition, depending on the length of the interval between exposure and development of disease, a cohort design may involve many years of follow-up of the cohort and considerable logistical difficulty and expense in maintaining and following the cohort over the study period.

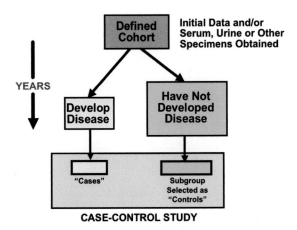

Figure 10-10. Design of a case-control study initiated within a cohort.

Nested Case-Control Studies

In *nested case-control studies* the controls are a sample of individuals who are at risk for the disease *at the time each case of the disease develops*. This is shown schematically in Figure 10-11A–I.

Figure 10-11A shows the starting point as a defined cohort of individuals. Some of them develop the disease in question but most do not. In this hypothetical example, the cohort is observed over a 5-year period. During this time, 5 cases develop—1 case

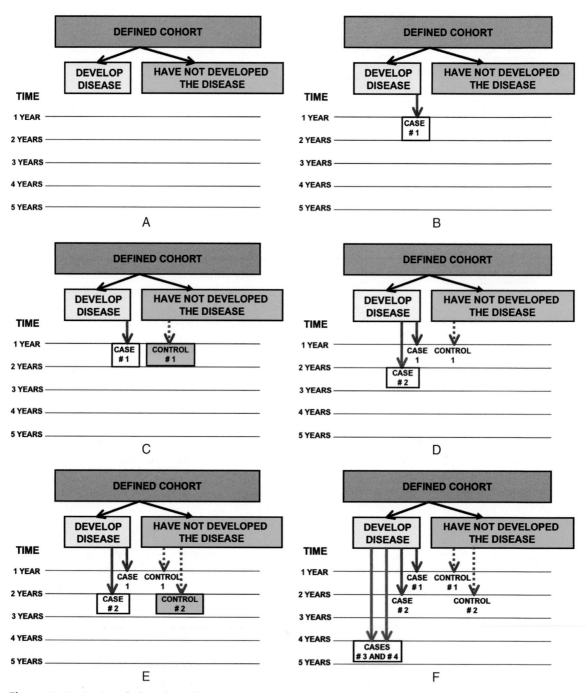

Figure 10-11. Design of a hypothetical nested case-control study: Steps in selecting cases and controls (see text).

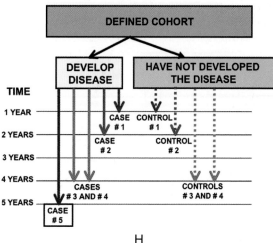

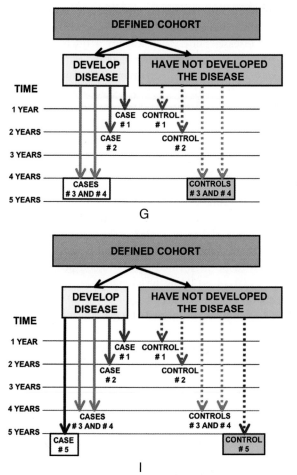

Figure 10-11, cont'd

after 1 year, 1 after 2 years, 2 after 4 years, and 1 after 5 years.

Let us follow the sequence of steps over time. Figures 10-11B–I show the time sequence in which the cases develop after the start of observations. At the time each case or cases develop, the same number of controls is selected. The solid arrows on the left side of the figure denote the appearance of cases of the disease, and the dotted arrows on the right side denote the selection of controls who are disease-free but who are at risk of developing the disease in question at the time the case develops the disease. Figure 10-11B shows case #1 developing after 1 year and Figure 10-11C shows control #1 being selected at that time. Figure 10-11D shows case #2 developing after 2 years and Figure 10-11E shows control #2 being selected at that time. Figure 10-11F shows cases #3 and #4 developing after 4 years and Figure 10-11G shows controls #3 and #4 being selected at that time.

Finally, Figure 10-11H shows the final case (#5) developing after 5 years and Figure 10-11I shows control #5 being selected at this point.

Figure 10-11I is also a summary of the design and the final study populations used in the nested case-control study. At the end of 5 years, 5 cases have appeared and at the times the cases appeared a total of 5 controls were selected for study. In this way, the cases and controls are, in effect, matched on calendar time and length of follow-up. Because a control is selected each time a case develops, a control who is selected early in the study could later develop the disease and become a case in the same study.

Case-Cohort Studies

The second type of cohort-based case-control study is the *case-cohort design* seen in Figure 10-12. In the hypothetical case-cohort study seen here, cases develop at the same times that were seen in the nested

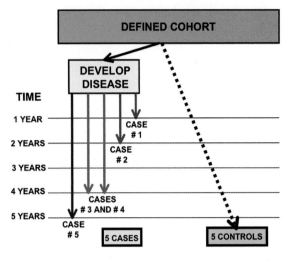

Figure 10-12. Design of a hypothetical case-cohort study: Steps in selecting cases and controls (see text).

case-control design just discussed, but the controls are randomly chosen from the defined cohort with which the study began. This subset of the full cohort is called the subcohort. An advantage of this design is that because controls are not individually matched to each case, it is possible to study different diseases (different sets of cases) in the same case-cohort study using the same cohort for controls. In this design, in contrast to the nested case-control design, cases and controls are not matched on calendar time and length of follow-up; instead, exposure is characterized for the subcohort. This difference in study design needs to be taken into account in analyzing the study results.

Advantages of Embedding a Case-Control Study in a Defined Cohort

What are the advantages of conducting a case-control study in a defined cohort? First, because interviews are completed or certain blood or urine specimens are obtained at the beginning of the study (at baseline), the data are obtained before any disease has developed. Consequently, the problem of possible recall bias discussed earlier in this chapter is eliminated. Second, if abnormalities in biologic characteristics such as laboratory values are found, because the specimens were obtained years before the development of clinical disease, it is more likely that these findings represent risk factors or other premorbid characteristics than a manifestation of early, subclinical disease. When such abnormalities are found

in the traditional case-control study, we do not know whether they preceded the disease or were a result of the disease. Third, such a study is often more economical to conduct. One might ask, why perform a nested case-control study? Why not perform a regular prospective cohort study? The answer is that in a cohort study of, say, 10,000 people, laboratory analyses of all the specimens obtained would have to be carried out, often at great cost, to define *exposed and nonexposed* groups. In a nested case-control study, however, the specimens obtained initially are frozen or otherwise stored. Only after the disease has developed in some subjects is a case-control study begun and the specimens from the relatively small number of people who are included in the case-control study are thawed and tested. But laboratory tests would not need to be performed on all 10,000 people in the original cohort. Thus the laboratory burden and costs are dramatically reduced.

Finally, in both nested case-control and case-cohort designs, cases and controls are derived from the same original cohort, so there is likely to be greater comparability between the cases and the controls than one might ordinarily find in a traditional case-control study. For all of these reasons, the cohort-based case-control study is an extremely valuable type of study design.

OTHER STUDY DESIGNS

Case-Crossover Design

The *case-crossover design* is primarily used for studying the etiology of acute outcomes such as myocardial infarctions or deaths from acute events in situations where the suspected exposure is transient and its effect occurs over a short time. This type of design has been used in studying exposures such as air pollution characterized by rapid and transient increases in particulate matter. In this type of study, a case is identified (for example, a person who has suffered a myocardial infarction) and the level of the environmental exposure, such as level of particulate matter, is ascertained for a short time period preceding the event (the at-risk period). This level is compared with the level of exposure in a control time period that is more remote from the event. Thus, each person who is a case serves as his own control, with the period immediately before his adverse outcome being compared with a "control" period at a prior time when no adverse outcome occurred. The question being asked is: Was there any difference in exposure between the time period immediately preceding the outcome and a time period in the more remote past which was not immediately followed by any adverse health effect?

Let us look at a very small hypothetical 4-month case-crossover study of air pollution and myocardial infarction (Fig. 10-13A–E).

Figure 10-13A shows that over a 4-month period, January–April, four cases of myocardial infarction (MI) were identified, symbolized by the small red hearts in the diagrams. The vertical dotted lines delineate 2-week intervals during the 4-month period. For the same 4-month period, levels of air pollution were measured. Three periods of high levels of air pollution of different lengths of time were identified and are shown by the pink areas in Figure 10-13B.

For each person with an MI in this study, an "at-risk" period (also called a hazard period) was defined as the 2 weeks immediately prior to the event. These at-risk periods are indicated by the red brackets in Figure 10-13C. If an exposure has a short-term effect on risk of an MI, we would expect that exposure to have occurred during that 2-week at-risk period. The critical element, however, in a case-crossover design is that for each subject in the study, we compare the level of exposure in that at-risk period with a control period (also called a referent period) that is unlikely to be relevant to occurrence of the event (the MI) because it is too far removed in time from the occurrence. In this example, the control period selected for each subject is a 2-week period beginning 1 month before the at-risk period, and these control periods are indicated by the blue brackets in Figure 10-13D. Thus, as shown by the yellow arrows in Figure 10-13E, for each subject, we are comparing the air pollution level in the at-risk period to the air pollution level in the control period. In order to demonstrate an association of MI with air pollution, we would expect to see greater exposure to high levels of air pollution during the at-risk period than during the control period.

In this example, we see that for subject 1 both the at-risk period and the control period were in low pollution times. For subjects 2 and 3, the at-risk periods were in high pollution times and the control periods in low pollution times. For subject 4, both the at-risk and control periods were in high pollution times.

Thus, in the case-crossover design, each subject serves as his or her own control. In this sense the case-crossover design is similar to the planned cross-over design discussed in Chapter 7. In this type of design, we are not concerned about other differences between the characteristics of the cases and those of a separate group of controls. This design also eliminates the additional cost that would be associated with identifying and interviewing a separate control population.

Attractive as this design is, unanswered questions remain. For example, the case-crossover design can be used to study people with heart attacks in regard to whether there was an episode of severe grief or anger during the period immediately preceding the attack. In this study design, the frequency of such emotionally charged events during that time interval would be compared, for example, with the frequency of such events during a period a month earlier, which was not associated with any adverse health event. Information on such events in both periods is often obtained by interviewing the subject. The question arises, however, whether there could be recall bias, in that a person may recall an emotionally charged episode that occurred shortly before his coronary event, while a comparable episode a month earlier in the absence of any adverse health event may remain forgotten. Thus, recall bias may be a problem not only when we compare cases and controls as discussed earlier in this chapter but also when we compare the same individual in two different time periods. Further discussion of case-crossover is provided by Maclure and Mittleman.[13]

Cross-Sectional Studies

Another study design used in investigating etiology of disease is *cross-sectional studies.* Let us assume we are interested in the possible relationship of increased serum cholesterol level (the *exposure*) to electrocardiographic (ECG) evidence of CHD (the *disease*). We survey a population; for each participant we determine the serum cholesterol level and perform an ECG for evidence of CHD. This type of study design is called a *cross-sectional study* because both exposure and disease outcome are determined *simultaneously* for each subject; it is as if we were viewing a snapshot of the population at a certain point in time. Another way to describe a cross-sectional study is to imagine that we have sliced through the population, capturing levels of cholesterol *and* evidence of CHD at the same time. Note that in this type of approach, the cases of disease that we identify are *prevalent* cases of the disease in question, because we know that they existed at the time of the study but do not know their duration. For this reason, this design is also called a *prevalence study.*

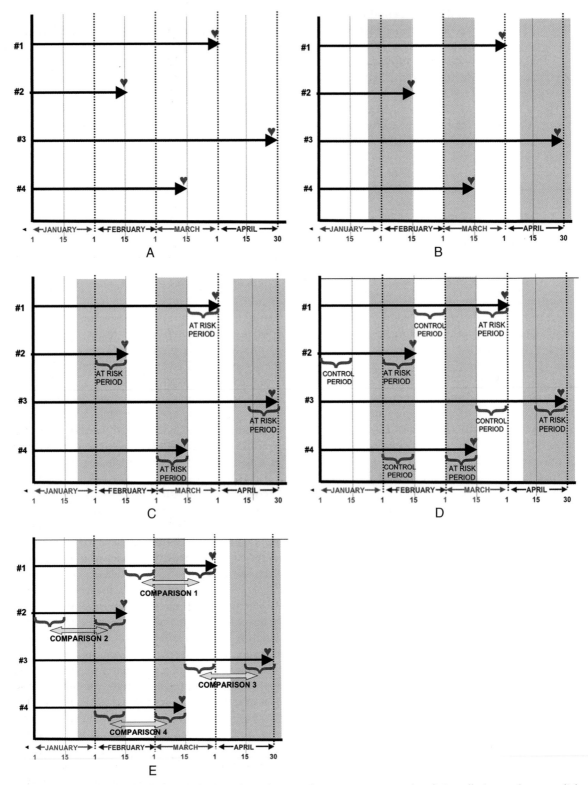

Figure 10-13. Design and findings of a hypothetical 4-month case-crossover study of air pollution and myocardial infarction (MI) (see text). **A,** Times of development of MI cases. **B,** Periods of high air pollution (shown by the colored bands). **C,** Defining at-risk periods (red brackets). **D,** Defining control periods (blue brackets). **E,** Comparisons made of air pollution levels in at-risk and in control periods for each MI case in the study (yellow arrows).

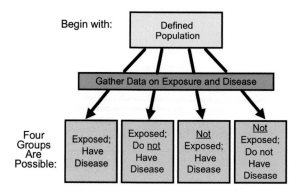

Figure 10-14. Design of a cross-sectional study: I.

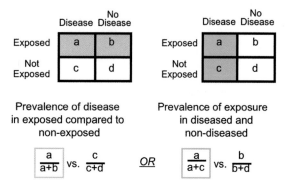

Figure 10-16. Design of a cross-sectional study: III.

The general design of such a cross-sectional or prevalence study is seen in Figure 10-14. We define a population and determine the presence or absence of exposure and the presence or absence of disease for each individual. Each subject then can be categorized into one of four possible subgroups.

The findings can be viewed in a 2 × 2 table, as seen in Figures 10-15 and 10-16, which also show the two approaches to interpreting the findings from such studies.

We identify a population of *n* persons for study, and determine presence or absence of exposure and disease for each subject. As seen in Figures 10-15 and 10-16, there will be *a* persons, who have been exposed and have the disease; *b* persons, who have been exposed but do not have the disease; *c* persons, who have the disease but have not been exposed; and *d* persons, who have neither been exposed nor have the disease. To determine whether there is an association between exposure and disease, we have two choices: (1) We can calculate the *prevalence of disease*

in $\left(\dfrac{a}{a+b}\right)$ and compare it with the prevalence of disease in persons without the exposure $\left(\dfrac{c}{c+d}\right)$, or (2) we can compare the *prevalence of exposure* in persons with the disease $\left(\dfrac{a}{a+c}\right)$ to the prevalence of exposure in persons without the disease $\left(\dfrac{b}{b+d}\right)$.

If we determine in such a study that there appears to be an association between increased cholesterol level and CHD, we are left with several problems. First, in this cross-sectional study, we are identifying prevalent cases of CHD rather than incident (new) cases; such prevalent cases may not be representative of all cases of CHD that have developed in this population. For example, identifying only prevalent cases would exclude those who died after the disease developed but before the study was carried out. Therefore, even if an association of exposure and disease is observed, the association may be with *survival* after CHD rather than with the risk of *developing* CHD. Second, because the presence or absence of both exposure and disease was determined at the same time in each subject in the study, it is often not possible to establish a temporal relationship between the exposure and the onset of disease. Thus, in the example given at the beginning of this section, it is not possible to tell whether or not the increased cholesterol level *preceded* the development of CHD. Without information on temporal relationships, it is conceivable that the increased cholesterol level could have occurred as a result of the coronary heart disease, or perhaps both may have occurred as a result of another factor. If it turns out that the exposure did not precede the development of the disease, the association cannot reflect a causal relationship.

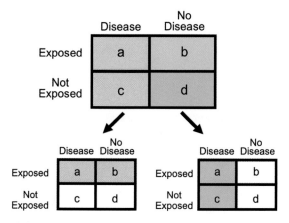

Figure 10-15. Design of a cross-sectional study: II.

TABLE 10-11. **Finding Your Way in the Terminology Jungle**

Case-control study		=		Retrospective study
Cohort study	=	Longitudinal study	=	Prospective study
Prospective cohort study	=	Concurrent cohort study	=	Concurrent prospective study
Retrospective cohort study	=	Historical cohort study	=	Nonconcurrent prospective study
Randomized trial		=		Experimental study
Cross-sectional study		=		Prevalence survey

Consequently, although a cross-sectional study can be very suggestive of a possible risk factor or risk factors for a disease, when an association is found in such a study, given the limitations in establishing a temporal relationship between exposure and outcome, we rely on cohort and case-control studies to establish etiologic relationships.

CONCLUSION

We have now reviewed the basic study designs used in epidemiologic investigations and clinical research.

Unfortunately, a variety of different terms are used in the literature to describe different study designs, and it is important to be familiar with them. Table 10-11 is designed to help guide you through the often confusing terminology.

The purpose of all of these types of studies is to identify associations between exposures and diseases. If such associations are found, the next step is to determine whether they are likely to be causal. These topics, starting with estimating risk, are addressed in Chapters 11 through 16.

REFERENCES
---

1. Ochsner A, DeBakey M: Carcinoma of the lung. Arch Surg 42:209–258, 1941.
2. Gregg NM: Congenital cataract following German measles in the mother. Trans Ophthalmol Soc Aust 3:35–46, 1941.
3. Doll R, Hill AB: A study of the aetiology of carcinoma of the lung. BMJ 2:1271–1286, 1952.
4. Pearl R: Cancer and tuberculosis. Am J Hyg 9:97–159, 1929.
5. Carlson HA, Bell ET: Statistical study of occurrence of cancer and tuberculosis in 11,195 postmortem examinations. J Cancer Res 13:126–135, 1929.
6. MacMahon B, Yen S, Trichopoulos D, et al: Coffee and cancer of the pancreas. N Engl J Med 304:630–633, 1981.
7. Hsieh CC, MacMahon B, Yen S, et al: Coffee and pancreatic cancer (Chapter 2) [letter]. N Engl J Med 315:587–589, 1986.
8. Lilienfeld AM, Graham S: Validity of determining circumcision status by questionnaire as related to epidemiologic studies of cancer of the cervix. J Natl Cancer Inst 21:713–720, 1958.
9. Gold EB, Gordis L, Tonascia J, Szklo M: Risk factors for brain tumors in children. Am J Epidemiol 109:309–319, 1979.
10. Edison M, Philen RM, Sewell CM, et al: L-Tryptophan and eosinophilia-myalgia syndrome in New Mexico. Lancet 335:645–648, 1990.
11. Slutsker L, Hoesly FC, Miller L, et al: Eosinophilia-myalgia syndrome associated with exposure to tryptophan from a single manufacturer. JAMA 264:213–217, 1990.
12. Belongia EZ, Hedberg CW, Gleich GJ, et al: An investigation of the cause of the eosinophilia-myalgia syndrome associated with tryptophan use. N Engl J Med 232:357–365, 1990.
13. Maclure M, Mittleman MA: Should we use a case-crossover design? Annu Rev Public Health 21:193–221, 2000.

REVIEW QUESTIONS FOR CHAPTER 10

1. A case-control study is characterized by all of the following *except:*
   a. It is relatively inexpensive compared with most other epidemiologic study designs
   b. Patients with the disease (cases) are compared with persons without the disease (controls)
   c. Incidence rates may be computed directly
   d. Assessment of past exposure may be biased
   e. Definition of cases may be difficult

2. Residents of three villages with three different types of water supply were asked to participate in a survey to identify cholera carriers. Because several cholera deaths had occurred recently, virtually everyone present at the time underwent examination. The proportion of residents in each village who were carriers was computed and compared. What is the proper classification for this study?

a. Cross-sectional study
b. Case-control study
c. Concurrent cohort study
d. Nonconcurrent cohort study
e. Experimental study

3. Which of the following is a case-control study?
    a. Study of past mortality or morbidity trends to permit estimates of the occurrence of disease in the future
    b. Analysis of previous research in different places and under different circumstances to permit the establishment of hypotheses based on cumulative knowledge of all known factors
    ✓ c. Obtaining histories and other information from a group of known cases and from a comparison group to determine the relative frequency of a characteristic or exposure under study
    d. Study of the incidence of cancer in men who have quit smoking
    e. Both *a* and *c*

4. In a study begun in 1965, a group of 3,000 adults in Baltimore were asked about alcohol consumption. The occurrence of cases of cancer between 1981 and 1995 was studied in this group. This is an example of:
    a. A cross-sectional study
    b. A concurrent cohort study
    c. A retrospective cohort study
    d. A clinical trial
    e. A case-control study

5. In a small pilot study, 12 women with endometrial cancer (cancer of the uterus) and 12 women with no apparent disease were contacted and asked whether they had ever used estrogen. Each woman with cancer was matched by age, race, weight, and parity to a woman without disease. What kind of study design is this?

a. Concurrent cohort
b. Retrospective cohort
✓ c. Case-control
d. Cross-sectional
e. Experimental

6. The physical examination records of the entire incoming freshman class of 1935 at the University of Minnesota were examined in 1977 to see if their recorded height and weight at the time of admission to the university was related to the development of coronary heart disease by 1986. This is an example of:
    a. A cross-sectional study
    b. A case-control study
    c. A concurrent cohort study
    d. A retrospective cohort study
    e. An experimental study

7. In a case-control study, which of the following is true?
    a. The proportion of cases with the exposure is compared with the proportion of controls with the exposure
    b. Disease rates are compared for people with the factor of interest and for people without the factor of interest
    c. The investigator may choose to have multiple comparison groups
    d. Recall bias is a potential problem
    ✓ e. *a, c,* and *d*

8. In which one of the following types of study designs does a subject serve as his own control?
    a. Prospective cohort study
    b. Retrospective cohort study
    c. Case-cohort study
    d. Case-crossover study
    e. Case-control study

Chapter 11

Estimating Risk: Is There an Association?

In the four previous chapters, we discussed the three basic study designs that are used in epidemiologic investigations. These are shown diagrammatically in Figures 11-1 through 11-3.

Recall that the fundamental difference between a randomized trial and a cohort study is that, in a cohort study, subjects are not randomly assigned to be exposed or to remain nonexposed, because randomization to exposure to possibly toxic or carcinogenic agents clearly would not be acceptable. Consequently, cohort studies are used in many studies of etiology, because this study design enables us to capitalize on populations that have had a certain exposure and to compare them with populations that have not had that exposure. Case-control studies are also used to address questions of etiology. Regardless of which design is used, the objective is to determine whether there is an excess risk (incidence), or perhaps a reduced risk, of a certain disease in association with a certain exposure or characteristic. In Chapter 3, we stated that incidence is a measure of risk of disease. Risk can be defined as the probability of an event (such as developing a disease) occurring.

Before describing these comparative approaches, we will introduce the concept of absolute risk.

ABSOLUTE RISK

The incidence of a disease in a population is termed the *absolute risk.* Absolute risk can indicate the magnitude of the risk in a group of people with a certain exposure, but because it does not take into consideration the risk of disease in non-exposed individuals, it does not indicate whether the exposure is associated with an increased risk of the disease. Comparison is fundamental to epidemiology. Nevertheless, absolute risk may have important implications in both clinical and public health policy: For example, a woman who contracts rubella in the first trimester of pregnancy and asks her physician, "What is the risk that my child will be malformed?" is given a certain number as an answer. On the basis of this information, she may decide to abort her pregnancy. She is not explicitly given comparative data, but an implicit comparison is generally being made: The woman is wondering not only what her risk is, but she is wondering how that risk compares with what it would have been had she not contracted rubella. So although absolute risk does not stipulate any explicit comparison, an implicit comparison is often made whenever we look at the incidence of a disease. However, to

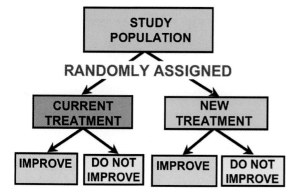

Figure 11-1. Design of a randomized clinical trial.

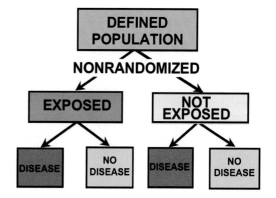

Figure 11-2. Design of a cohort study.

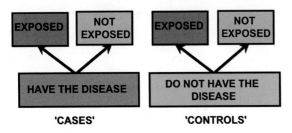

Figure 11-3. Design of a case-control study.

Food	Ate (% Sick)	Did Not Eat (% Sick)
	TABLE 11-1. A Foodborne Disease Outbreak: I. Percent of People Sick among Those Who Ate and Those Who Did Not Eat Specific Foods	
Egg salad	83	30
Macaroni	76	67
Cottage cheese	71	69
Tuna salad	78	50
Ice cream	78	64
Other	72	50

address the question of association, we must use approaches that involve explicit comparisons.

HOW DO WE DETERMINE WHETHER A CERTAIN DISEASE IS ASSOCIATED WITH A CERTAIN EXPOSURE?

To determine whether such an association exists, we must determine, using data obtained in case-control and cohort studies, whether there is an excess risk of the disease in persons who have been exposed to a certain agent. Let us consider the results of a hypothetical investigation of a foodborne disease outbreak. The suspect foods were identified, and for each food, the attack rate (or incidence rate) of the disease was calculated for those who ate the food (exposed) and for those who did not eat the food (nonexposed), as shown in Table 11-1.

How can we determine whether an excess risk is associated with each of the food items? One approach, shown in column C of Table 11-2, is to calculate the *ratio* of the attack rate in those who ate each food to the attack rate in those who did not eat the food. An alternate approach for identifying any excess risk in exposed individuals is shown in column D. We can subtract the risk in those who did not eat the food from the risk in those who did eat the food. The *dif-*

ference represents the excess risk in those who were exposed.

Thus, as seen in this foodborne outbreak, to determine whether a certain exposure is associated with a certain disease, we must determine whether there is an excess risk of disease in exposed populations by comparing the risk of disease in exposed populations to the risk of disease in nonexposed populations. We have just seen that such an excess risk can be calculated in the two following ways:

1. The *ratio* of the risks (or of the incidence rates):

$$\frac{\text{Disease risk in exposed}}{\text{Disease risk in nonexposed}}$$

2. The *difference* in the risks (or in the incidence rates):

$$\left(\begin{array}{c}\text{Disease risk}\\\text{in exposed}\end{array}\right) - \left(\begin{array}{c}\text{Disease risk}\\\text{in non exposed}\end{array}\right)$$

Does the method that we choose to calculate excess risk make any difference? Let us consider a

TABLE 11-2. Foodborne Disease Outbreak: II. Ways of Calculating Excess Risk

Food	(A) Ate (% Sick)	(B) Did Not Eat (% Sick)	(C) (A)/(B)	(D) (A)–(B) (%)
Egg salad	83	30	2.77	53
Macaroni	76	67	1.13	9
Cottage cheese	71	69	1.03	2
Tuna salad	78	50	1.56	28
Ice cream	78	64	1.21	14
Other	72	50	1.44	22

TABLE 11-3. **An Example Comparing Two Ways of Calculating Excess Risk**

	POPULATION	
	A	**B**
Incidence (%)		
In exposed	40	90
In nonexposed	10	60
Difference in incidence rates (%)	30	30
Ratio of incidence rates	4.0	1.5

TABLE 11-4. **Interpreting Relative Risk (RR) of a Disease**

If RR = 1	Risk in exposed equal to risk in nonexposed (no association)
If RR > 1	Risk in exposed greater than risk in nonexposed (positive association; possibly causal)
If RR < 1	Risk in exposed less than risk in nonexposed (negative association; possibly protective)

hypothetical example of two communities, A and B, seen in Table 11-3.

In community A, the incidence of a disease in exposed persons is 40% and the incidence in nonexposed persons is 10%. Is there an excess risk associated with exposure? As in the food poisoning example, we can calculate the ratio of the rates or the difference between the rates. The *ratio* of the incidence rates it 4.0. If we calculate the *difference* in incidence rates, it is 30%. In community B, the incidence in exposed persons is 90% and the incidence in nonexposed persons is 60%. If we calculate the *ratio* of the incidence of exposed to nonexposed persons in population B, it is 90/60, or 1.5. If we calculate the *difference* in the incidence in exposed and nonexposed persons in community B it is, again, 30%.

What do these two measures tell us? Is there a difference in what we learn from the ratio of the incidence rates compared to the difference in the incidence rates? This question is the theme of this chapter and of Chapter 12.

RELATIVE RISK

The Concept of Relative Risk

Both case-control and cohort studies are designed to determine whether there is an association between exposure to a factor and development of a disease. If an association exists, how strong is it? If we carry out a cohort study, we can put the question another way: "What is the ratio of the risk of disease in exposed individuals to the risk of disease in nonexposed individuals?" This ratio is called the *relative risk*:

$$\text{Relative risk} = \frac{\text{Risk in exposed}}{\text{Risk in nonexposed}}$$

The relative risk can also be defined as the probability of an event (developing a disease) occurring in exposed people compared to the probability of the event in nonexposed people, or as the ratio of the two probabilities.

Interpreting the Relative Risk

How do we interpret the value of a relative risk?

There are three possibilities (Table 11-4):

1. If the relative risk is equal to 1, the numerator equals the denominator, and the risk in exposed persons equals the risk in nonexposed persons. Therefore, no evidence exists for any increased risk in exposed individuals or for any association of the disease with the exposure in question.
2. If the relative risk is greater than 1, the numerator is greater than the denominator, and the risk in exposed persons is greater than the risk in nonexposed persons. This is evidence of a positive association, and may be causal (this is discussed in Chapter 14).
3. If the relative risk is less than 1, the numerator is less than the denominator, and the risk in exposed persons is less than the risk in nonexposed persons. This is evidence of a negative association, and it may be indicative of a protective effect. Such a finding can be observed in people who are given an effective vaccine ("exposed" to the vaccine).

Calculating the Relative Risk in Cohort Studies

In a *cohort* study, the relative risk can be calculated *directly*. Recall the design of a cohort study seen in Table 11-5.

In this table, we see that the incidence in exposed individuals is

$$\frac{a}{a+b}$$

TABLE 11-5. Risk Calculations in a Cohort Study

		Then Follow to See Whether			
		Disease Develops	*Disease Does Not Develop*	*Totals*	Incidence Rates of Disease
First Select	Exposed	*a*	*b*	*a + b*	$\dfrac{a}{a+b}$
	Not exposed	*c*	*d*	*c + d*	$\dfrac{c}{c+d}$
	$\dfrac{a}{a+b}$ = Incidence in exposed		$\dfrac{c}{c+d}$ = Incidence in nonexposed		

and the incidence in nonexposed individuals is

$$\frac{c}{c+d}$$

We calculate the relative risk as follows:

$$\text{Relative risk} = \frac{\text{Incidence in exposed}}{\text{Incidence in nonexposed}} = \frac{\left(\dfrac{a}{a+b}\right)}{\left(\dfrac{c}{c+d}\right)}$$

Table 11-6 shows a hypothetical cohort study of 3,000 smokers and 5,000 nonsmokers to investigate the relation of smoking to the development of coronary heart disease (CHD) over a 1-year period.

In this example:

$$\text{Incidence among the exposed} = \frac{84}{3,000}$$
$$= 28.0 \text{ per } 1,000$$

and

$$\text{Incidence among the nonexposed} = \frac{87}{5,000}$$
$$= 17.4 \text{ per } 1,000$$

Consequently,

$$\text{Relative risk} = \frac{\text{Incidence in exposed}}{\text{Incidence in nonexposed}} = \frac{28.0}{17.4} = 1.61$$

A similar expression of risks is seen in Table 11-7, which shows data from the first 12 years of the Framingham Study relating risk of coronary disease to age, sex, and cholesterol level.

First, direct your attention to the upper part of the table, which shows incidence rates per 1,000 by age, sex, and serum cholesterol level. In men, the relation of risk to cholesterol level seems dose related; risk increases for both age groups with increases in cholesterol level. The relationship is not as consistent in women.

In the lower half of the table, the values have been converted to relative risks. The authors have taken the incidence rate of 38.2 in younger men with low cholesterol levels and assigned it a risk of 1.0; these subjects are considered "nonexposed." All other risks in the table are expressed in relation to this risk of 1.0. For example, the incidence of 157.5 in younger men with a cholesterol level greater than 250 mg/dL is compared to the 38.2 incidence rate; by dividing 157.5 by 38.2 we obtain a relative risk of 4.1. Using these relative risks, it is easier to compare the risks and to identify any trends. Although the lowest risk

TABLE 11-6. Smoking and Coronary Heart Disease (CHD): A Hypothetical Cohort Study of 3,000 Cigarette Smokers and 5,000 Nonsmokers

	CHD Develops	CHD Does Not Develop	Totals	Incidence per 1,000 per Year
Smoke cigarettes	84	2,916	3,000	28.0
Do not smoke cigarettes	87	4,913	5,000	17.4

TABLE 11-7. **Relationship between Serum Cholesterol Levels and Risk of Coronary Heart Disease by Age and Sex: Framingham Study during First 12 Years**

	MEN		WOMEN	
Serum Cholesterol (mg/dL)	**30–49 yrs**	**50–62 yrs**	**30–49 yrs**	**50–62 yrs**
	Incidence Rates (per 1,000)			
<190	38.2	105.7	11.1	155.2
190–219	44.1	187.5	9.1	88.9
220–249	95.0	201.1	24.3	96.3
250+	157.5	267.8	50.4	121.5
	*Relative Risks**			
<190	1.0	2.8	0.3	4.1
190–219	1.2	4.9	0.2	2.3
220–249	2.5	5.3	0.6	2.5
250+	4.1	7.0	1.3	3.2

*Incidence for each subgroup is compared with that of males 30 to 49 years of age, with serum cholesterol levels less than 190 mg/dL (risk = 1.0).
From Truett J, Cornfield J, Kannel W: A multivariate analysis of the risk of coronary heart disease in Framingham. J Chronic Dis 20:511–524, 1967.

in men has been chosen as the standard and set at 1.0, the authors could have chosen to set any of the values in the table at 1.0 and to make all others relative to it. One reason for choosing a low value as the standard is that most of the other values will be above 1.0; for most people, the table is easier to read when few values are completely to the right of the decimal.

Figure 11-4 shows data on 2,282 middle-aged men followed up for 10 years in the Framingham Study and 1,838 middle-aged men followed up for 8 years in Albany, New York. The data relate smoking, cholesterol level, and blood pressure to risk of myocardial infarction and death from CHD. The authors have assigned a value of 1 to the lowest of the risks in each of the two parts of the figure, and the other risks are calculated relative to this value. On the left is shown the risk in nonsmokers with low cholesterol

levels (which has been set at 1) and the risk in non-smokers with high cholesterol levels; risks for smokers with low and high cholesterol levels are each calculated relative to risks for nonsmokers with low cholesterol levels. Note that the risk is higher with high cholesterol levels, and that this holds both in smokers and in nonsmokers (although the risk is higher in smokers even when cholesterol levels are low). Thus both smoking and elevated cholesterol levels contribute to the risk of myocardial infarction and death from CHD. A comparable analysis with blood pressure and smoking is shown on the right.

THE ODDS RATIO (RELATIVE ODDS)

We have seen that in order to calculate a relative risk, we must have values for the incidence of the disease

Figure 11-4. Relative risk for myocardial infarction and death from coronary heart disease in men aged 30 to 62 years by serum cholesterol *(left)* and blood pressure levels *(right)* in relation to cigarette smoking. High cholesterol levels are defined as 220 mg/dL or greater. (Data from Doyle JT, Dawber TR, Kannel WB, et al: The relationship of cigarette smoking to coronary heart disease. JAMA 190:886, 1964.)

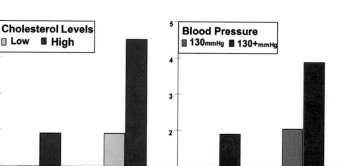

in the exposed and the incidence in the nonexposed, as can be obtained from a cohort study. In a *case-control* study, however, we do not know the incidence in the exposed population or the incidence in the nonexposed population because we start with diseased people (cases) and nondiseased people (controls). Hence, in a case-control study we *cannot* calculate the relative risk directly. In this section we shall see how another measure of association, the *odds ratio*, can be obtained from either a cohort or a case-control study and can be used instead of the relative risk. We will also see that even though we cannot calculate a relative risk from a case-control study, under many conditions, we can obtain a very good *estimate* of the relative risk from a case-control study using the odds ratio.

Defining the Odds Ratio in Cohort and in Case-Control Studies

In previous chapters we discussed the *proportion* of the exposed population in whom disease develops and the *proportion* of the nonexposed population in whom disease develops in a cohort study. Similarly, in case-control studies, we have discussed the *proportion* of the cases who were exposed and the *proportion* of the controls who were exposed (Table 11-8).

An alternate approach is to use the concept of *odds*. Suppose we are betting on a horse named Epi Beauty, which has a 60% probability of winning the race (*P*). Epi Beauty therefore has a 40% probability of losing (1 − *P*). If these are the probabilities, what are the *odds* that the horse will win the race? To answer this we must keep in mind that *the odds of an event can be defined as the ratio of the number of ways the event can occur to the number of ways the event cannot occur.* Consequently, the odds of Epi Beauty winning, as defined above, are as follows:

$$\text{Odds} = \frac{\text{Probability that Epi Beauty will win the race}}{\text{Probability that Epi Beauty will lose the race}}$$

Recall that, if *P* is the probability that Epi Beauty will win the race, 1 − *P* equals the probability that Epi Beauty will lose the race. Consequently, the odds of Epi Beauty winning are:

$$\text{Odds} = \frac{P}{1-P} \quad \text{or} \quad \frac{60\%}{40\%} = 1.5:1 = 1.5$$

It is important to keep in mind the distinction between probability and odds. In the above example:

$$\text{Probability of winning} = 60\%$$

and

$$\text{Odds of winning} = \frac{60\%}{40\%} = 1.5$$

The Odds Ratio in Cohort Studies

Let us examine how the concept of odds can be applied to both cohort and case-control studies. Let us first consider the cohort study design shown in Figure 11-5A. Our first question is, What is the *probability (P)* that the disease will develop in an exposed person? The answer to this is the incidence of the disease in the top row (exposed persons), which equals $\frac{a}{a+b}$. Next let us ask, "What are the *odds* that the disease will develop in an exposed person?" Again, looking only at the top row in Figure 11-5, we see that there are *a* + *b* exposed persons; the odds that the disease will develop in them are *a:b* or $\frac{a}{b}$. (Recall $\frac{P}{1-P}$ from the Epi Beauty example.) Similarly, looking only at the bottom row of this table, there are *c* + *d* nonexposed persons; the probability

---

TABLE 11-8. Calculation of Proportions Exposed in a Case-Control Study

		First Select	
		Cases (With Disease)	Controls (Without Disease)
Then Measure Past Exposure	Were exposed	*a*	*b*
	Were not exposed	*c*	*d*
	Totals	*a* + *c*	*b* + *d*
	Proportions exposed	$\dfrac{a}{a+c}$	$\dfrac{b}{b+d}$

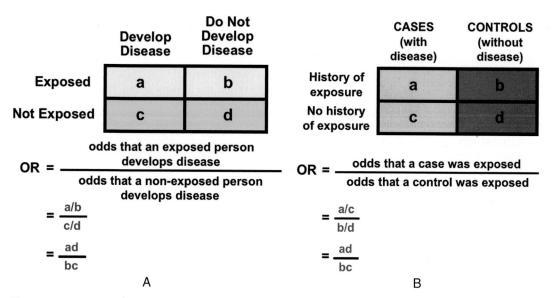

Figure 11-5. A, Odds ratio (OR) in a cohort study. **B,** Odds ratio (OR) in a case-control study.

that the disease will develop in nonexposed persons is $\dfrac{c}{c+d}$ and the odds of the disease developing in these nonexposed persons are $c{:}d$ or $\dfrac{c}{d}$.

Just as the ratio of the incidence in the exposed to the incidence in the nonexposed can be used to measure an association of exposure and disease, we can also look at the ratio of the odds that the disease will develop in an exposed person to the odds that it will develop in a nonexposed person. Either measure of association is valid in a cohort study.

In a cohort study, to answer the question of whether there is an association between the exposure and the disease, we can either use the relative risk discussed in the previous section or we can use the odds ratio (also called the *relative odds*). In a *cohort study*, the odds ratio is defined as the *ratio of the odds of development of disease in exposed persons to the odds of development of disease in nonexposed persons,* and it can be calculated as follows:

$$\frac{\left(\dfrac{a}{b}\right)}{\left(\dfrac{c}{d}\right)} = \frac{ad}{bc}$$

The Odds Ratio in a Case-Control Study

As just discussed, in a *case-control study*, we cannot calculate the relative risk directly to determine whether there is an association between the exposure and the disease. This is because, having started with

cases and controls rather than with exposed and non-exposed persons, we do not have information about the incidence of disease in exposed versus nonexposed persons. However, we can use the odds ratio as a measure of the association between exposure and disease in a case-control study, but we ask different questions: "What are the odds that a case was exposed?" Looking at the left-hand column in Figure 11-5B, we see that the *odds* of a case having been exposed are $a{:}c$ or $\dfrac{a}{c}$. Next, we ask, "What are the odds that a control was exposed?" Looking at the right-hand column, we see that the *odds* of a control having been exposed are $b{:}d$ or $\dfrac{b}{d}$.

We can then calculate the odds ratio, which in a case-control study, is defined as the ratio of the odds that the cases were exposed to the odds that the controls were exposed. This is calculated as follows:

$$\frac{\left(\dfrac{a}{c}\right)}{\left(\dfrac{b}{d}\right)} = \frac{ad}{bc}$$

Thus, interestingly, $\dfrac{ad}{bc}$ represents the odds ratio (or relative odds) in *both* cohort (Fig. 11-5A) and case-control (Fig. 11-5B) studies. In both types of studies, the odds ratio is an excellent measure of whether a certain exposure is associated with a specific disease. The *odds ratio* is also known as the *cross-products ratio*, because it can be obtained by multiplying both diagonal cells in a 2 × 2 table and then dividing $\dfrac{ad}{bc}$, as seen in Figures 11-5A and B.

As Dr. Lechaim Naggan has pointed out (personal communication), the odds ratio or the cross-products ratio can be viewed as the ratio of the product of the two cells that support the hypothesis of an association (cells *a* and *d*—diseased people who were exposed and nondiseased people who were not exposed), to the product of the two cells that negate the hypothesis of an association (cells *b* and *c*—nondiseased people who were exposed and diseased people who were not exposed).

Interpreting the Odds Ratio

We interpret the odds ratio just as we interpreted the relative risk. If the exposure is not related to the disease, the odds ratio will equal 1. If the exposure is positively related to the disease, the odds ratio will be greater than 1. If the exposure is negatively related to the disease, the odds ratio will be less than 1.

When Is the Odds Ratio a Good Estimate of the Relative Risk?

In a case-control study, only the odds ratio can be calculated as a measure of association, whereas in a cohort study, either the relative risk or the odds ratio is a valid measure of association. However, many people are more comfortable using the relative risk, and this is the most frequently used measure of association reported in the literature when results of cohort studies are published. Even when the odds ratio is used, people are often interested in knowing how well it approximates the relative risk. Even prestigious clinical journals have been known to publish reports of case-control studies and to label a column of results as *relative risks*. Having read the discussion in this chapter, you are aghast to see such a presentation, because you now know that relative risks cannot be calculated directly from a case-control study! Clearly, what is meant is an *estimate* of relative risks based on the odds ratios that are obtained in the case-control studies.

When is the odds ratio (relative odds) obtained in a case-control study a good approximation of the relative risk in the population? When the following three conditions are met:

1. When the *cases* studied are representative, with regard to history of exposure, of all people with the disease in the population from which the cases were drawn.

2. When the *controls* studied are representative, with regard to history of exposure, of all people without the disease in the population from which the cases were drawn.

3. When the disease being studied does not occur frequently.

The third condition (that the disease occurrence is not frequent) can be intuitively explained as follows:

Recall that there are $a + b$ exposed persons. Because most diseases with which we are dealing occur infrequently, very few persons in an exposed population will actually develop the disease; consequently, a is very small compared to b, and one can approximate $a + b$ as b, or $(a + b) \cong b$. Similarly, very few nonexposed persons $(c + d)$ develop the disease, and we can approximate $c + d$ as d, or $(c + d) \cong d$. Therefore, we may calculate a relative risk as follows:

$$\frac{\left(\dfrac{a}{a+b}\right)}{\left(\dfrac{c}{c+d}\right)} \cong \frac{\left(\dfrac{a}{b}\right)}{\left(\dfrac{c}{d}\right)}$$

From performing this calculation, we obtain $\dfrac{ad}{bc}$, which is the odds ratio. For the committed reader, a neater and more sophisticated derivation is provided in the appendix to this chapter.

Figures 11-6 and 11-7 show two examples of cohort studies that demonstrate how the odds ratio provides a good approximation of the relative risk when the occurrence of a disease is infrequent, but not when it is frequent. In Figure 11-6, the occur-

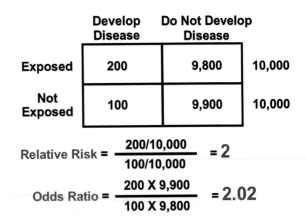

	Develop Disease	Do Not Develop Disease	
Exposed	200	9,800	10,000
Not Exposed	100	9,900	10,000

$$\text{Relative Risk} = \frac{200/10,000}{100/10,000} = 2$$

$$\text{Odds Ratio} = \frac{200 \times 9,900}{100 \times 9,800} = 2.02$$

Figure 11-6. Example: The odds ratio is a good estimate of the relative risk when a disease is infrequent.

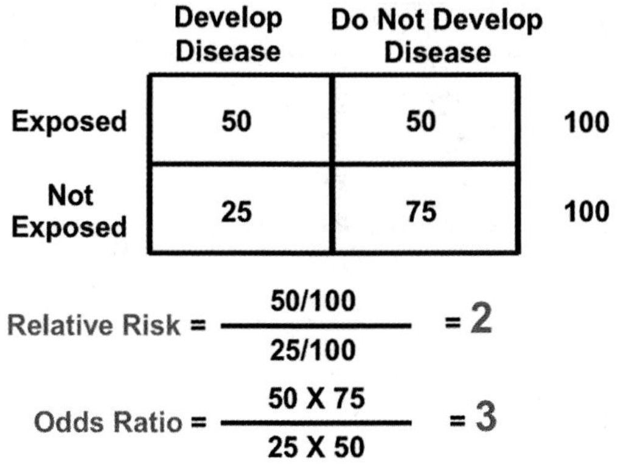

	Develop Disease	Do Not Develop Disease	
Exposed	50	50	100
Not Exposed	25	75	100

$$\text{Relative Risk} = \frac{50/100}{25/100} = 2$$

$$\text{Odds Ratio} = \frac{50 \times 75}{25 \times 50} = 3$$

Figure 11-7. Example: The odds ratio is *not* a good estimate of the relative risk when a disease is *not* infrequent.

CASES	CONTROLS
E	N
E	E
N	N
E	N
N	E
N	N
E	N
E	E
E	N
N	N

E = Exposed
N = Not Exposed

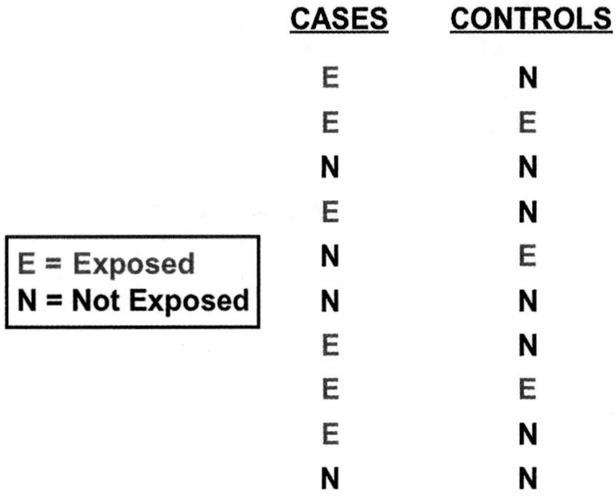

Figure 11-8. A case-control study of 10 cases and 10 unmatched controls.

rence of disease is infrequent and we see that the relative risk is 2. If we now calculate an odds (cross-products) ratio, we find it to be 2.02, which is a very close approximation.

Now, let us examine Figure 11-7, in which the occurrence of disease is frequent. Although the relative risk is again 2.0, the odds ratio is 3.0, which is considerably different from the relative risk.

We therefore see that the odds ratio is in itself a valid measure of association without even considering relative risk. If, however, you choose to use the relative risk as the index of association, when the disease occurrence is infrequent, the odds ratio is a very good approximation of the relative risk.

Remember
- The relative odds (odds ratio) is a useful measure of association, in and of itself, in both case-control and cohort studies.
- In a cohort study, the relative risk can be calculated directly.
- In a case-control study, the relative risk cannot be calculated directly, so that the relative odds or odds ratio (cross-products ratio) is used as an estimate of the relative risk when the risk of the disease is low.

Examples of Calculating Odds Ratios in Case-Control Studies

In this section, we will calculate odds ratios in two case-control studies (one in which the controls were *not* matched to the cases, and the other in which they *were* matched). For purposes of these examples, let us assume the following: our research budget is small, so we have carried out a case-control study of only 10 cases and 10 controls. *N* indicates a *nonexposed* individual, and *E* indicates an *exposed* individual.

Calculating the Odds Ratio in an Unmatched Case-Control Study

Let us assume that this case-control study is done without any matching of controls to cases, and that we obtain the results seen in Figure 11-8. Thus, 6 of the 10 cases were exposed and 3 of the 10 controls were exposed. If we arrange these data in a 2 × 2 table, we obtain the following:

	Cases	Controls
Exposed	6	3
Nonexposed	4	7
Total	10	10

The odds ratio in this *unmatched* study equals the ratio of the cross-products:

$$\text{Odds ratio} = \frac{ad}{bc}$$

$$\text{Odds ratio} = \frac{6 \times 7}{4 \times 3} = \frac{42}{12} = 3.5$$

Table 11-9 shows data from a hypothetical unmatched case-control study of smoking and CHD. The letters *a*, *b*, *c*, and *d* have been inserted to identify the cells of the 2 × 2 table that are used for the calculation. The odds ratio, as calculated from these data, is as follows:

$$\text{Odds ratio} = \frac{ad}{bc} = \frac{112 \times 224}{176 \times 88} = 1.62$$

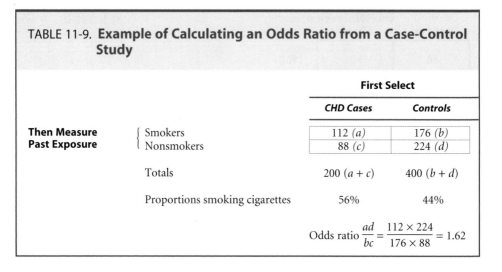

TABLE 11-9. **Example of Calculating an Odds Ratio from a Case-Control Study**

		First Select	
		CHD Cases	*Controls*
Then Measure Past Exposure	Smokers	112 *(a)*	176 *(b)*
	Nonsmokers	88 *(c)*	224 *(d)*
	Totals	200 *(a + c)*	400 *(b + d)*
	Proportions smoking cigarettes	56%	44%

$$\text{Odds ratio } \frac{ad}{bc} = \frac{112 \times 224}{176 \times 88} = 1.62$$

Calculating the Odds Ratio in a Matched-Pairs Case-Control Study

As discussed in the previous chapter, in selecting the study population in case-control studies, controls are often selected by matching each one to a case according to variables that are known to be related to disease risk, such as sex, age, or race (individual matching or matched pairs). The results are then analyzed in terms of case-control pairs rather than for individual subjects.

What types of case-control combinations are possible in regard to exposure history? Clearly, if exposure is dichotomous (a person is either exposed or not exposed), only the following four types of case-control pairs are possible:

Concordant pairs
1. Pairs in which *both* the case and the control were exposed
2. Pairs in which *neither* the case nor the control was exposed

Discordant pairs
3. Pairs in which the case was exposed but the control was not
4. Pairs in which the control was exposed and the case was not

Note that the case-control pairs that had the same exposure experience are termed *concordant pairs*, and those with different exposure experience are termed *discordant pairs*. These possibilities are shown schematically in the following 2 × 2 table. Note that unlike other 2 × 2 tables that we have examined previously, the figure in each cell represents pairs of subjects

(i.e., *case-control pairs*), *not* individual subjects. Thus, the following table contains *a* pairs—in which both the case and the control were exposed; *b* pairs—in which the case was exposed and the control was not; *c* pairs—in which the case was not exposed and the control was exposed; and *d* pairs—in which neither the case nor the control was exposed.

		Control	
		Exposed	*Not Exposed*
Case	*Exposed*	*a*	*b*
	Not Exposed	*c*	*d*

Calculation of the odds ratio in such a matched-pair study is based on the *discordant pairs* only (*b* and *c*). The concordant pairs (*a* and *d*, in which cases and controls were either both exposed or both not exposed) are ignored, because they do not contribute to our knowledge of how cases and controls differ in regard to past history of exposure.

The *odds ratio for matched pairs* is therefore the ratio of the discordant pairs (i.e., *the ratio of the number of pairs in which the case was exposed and the control was not, to the number of pairs in which the control was exposed and the case was not*). The odds ratio for the preceding 2 × 2 table is as follows:

$$\text{Odds ratio (matched pairs)} = \frac{b}{c}$$

Again, as Dr. Lechaim Naggan pointed out (personal communication), the matched-pairs odds ratio can be viewed as the ratio of the number of pairs that support the hypothesis of an association (pairs in

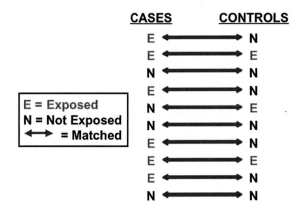

Figure 11-9. A case-control study of 10 cases and 10 matched controls.

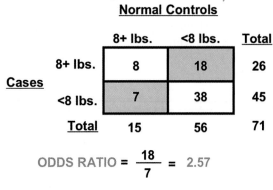

Figure 11-10. Birth weight of index child: Matched-pairs comparison of cases and normal controls (≥8 lbs vs. <8 lbs). (Data from Gold E, Gordis L, Tonascia J, Szklo M: Risk factors for brain tumors in children. Am J Epidemiol 109:309–319, 1979.)

which the case was exposed and the control was not) to the number of pairs that negate the hypothesis of an association (pairs in which the control was exposed and the case was not).

Let us now look at an example of an odds ratio calculation in a matched-pairs case-control study (Fig. 11-9). Let us return to our low-budget study, which included only 10 cases and 10 controls: now our study is designed so that each control has been individually matched to a case, resulting in 10 case-control *pairs* (the horizontal arrows indicate the matching of pairs). If we use these findings to construct a 2 × 2 table for *pairs*, we obtain the following:

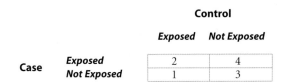

		Control	
		Exposed	**Not Exposed**
Case	**Exposed**	2	4
	Not Exposed	1	3

Note that there are two pairs in which *both* the case and the control were exposed and three pairs in which *neither* the case *nor* the control was exposed. These concordant pairs are ignored in the analysis of matched pairs.

There are four pairs in which the case was exposed and the control was not and one pair in which the control was exposed and the case was not.

Hence, the odds ratio for matched pairs is as follows:

$$\text{Odds ratio} = \frac{b}{c} = \frac{4}{1} = 4$$

Figures 11-10 and 11-11 present data selected from the case-control study of brain tumors in chil-

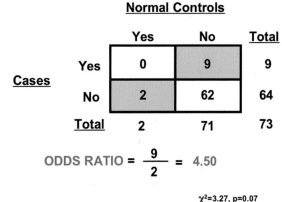

Figure 11-11. Exposure of index child to sick pets: Matched-pairs comparison of cases and normal controls. (Data from Gold E, Gordis L, Tonascia J, Szklo M: Risk factors for brain tumors in children. Am J Epidemiol 109:309–319, 1979.)

dren that was referred to in the previous chapter. Data are shown for two variables. Figure 11-10 presents a matched-pairs analysis for birth weight. A number of studies have suggested that children with higher birth weights are at increased risk for certain childhood cancers. In this analysis, *exposure* is defined as birth weight greater than 8 lbs. The result is an odds ratio of 2.57.

In Figure 11-11, a matched-pairs analysis is presented for exposure to sick pets. Many years ago, the Tri-State Leukemia Study found that more cases of leukemia than controls had family pets. Recent interest in oncogenic viruses has stimulated an interest in exposure to sick pets as a possible source of such agents. Gold and coworkers explored this question in their case-control study,[1] and the results are shown in Figure 11-11. Although the odds ratio was 4.5, the number of discordant pairs was very small.

CONCLUSION

This chapter has introduced the concepts of absolute risk, relative risk, and odds ratio. In Chapter 12 we turn to another important aspect of risk: the attributable risk. We will then review the study designs and indices of risk that have been discussed (see Chapter 13) before addressing the use of these concepts in deriving causal inferences (see Chapters 14 and 15).

REFERENCE

1. Gold E, Gordis L, Tonascia J, Szklo M: Risk factors for brain tumors in children. Am J Epidemiol 109:309–319, 1979.

REVIEW QUESTIONS FOR CHAPTER 11

1. Of 2,872 persons who had received radiation treatment in childhood because of an enlarged thymus, cancer of the thyroid developed in 24 and a benign thyroid tumor developed in 52. A comparison group consisted of 5,055 children who had received no such treatment (brothers and sisters of the children who had received radiation treatment). During the follow-up period, none of the comparison group developed thyroid cancer, but benign thyroid tumors developed in 6. Calculate the relative risk for benign thyroid tumors: _____

2. In a study of a disease in which all cases that developed were ascertained, if the relative risk for the association between a factor and the disease is *equal to or less than 1.0*, then:
   a. There is no association between the factor and the disease
   b. The factor protects against development of the disease
   c. Either matching or randomization has been unsuccessful
   d. The comparison group used was unsuitable, and a valid comparison is not possible
   e. There is either no association or a negative association between the factor and the disease

Questions 3 and 4 are based on the information given in the following table.

In a small pilot study, 12 women with uterine cancer and 12 with no apparent disease were contacted and asked whether they had ever used estrogen. Each woman with cancer was matched by age, race, weight, and parity to a woman without disease. The results are shown below:

Pair No.	Women with Uterine Cancer	Women without Uterine Cancer
1	Estrogen user	Estrogen nonuser
2	Estrogen nonuser	Estrogen nonuser
3	Estrogen user	Estrogen user
4	Estrogen user	Estrogen user
5	Estrogen user	Estrogen nonuser
6	Estrogen nonuser	Estrogen nonuser
7	Estrogen user	Estrogen nonuser
8	Estrogen user	Estrogen nonuser
9	Estrogen nonuser	Estrogen user
10	Estrogen nonuser	Estrogen user
11	Estrogen user	Estrogen nonuser
12	Estrogen user	Estrogen nonuser

3. What is the *estimated* relative risk of cancer when analyzing this study as a matched-pairs study?
   a. 0.25
   b. 0.33
   c. 1.00
   d. 3.00
   e. 4.20

4. Unmatch the pairs. What is the *estimated* relative risk of cancer when analyzing this study as an *unmatched* study design?
   a. 0.70
   b. 1.43
   c. 2.80
   d. 3.00
   e. 4.00

Questions 5 through 7 are based on the following information.

Talbot and colleagues carried out a study of sudden unexpected death in women. Data on smoking history are shown in the following table.

Smoking History for Cases of ASHD Sudden Death and Controls (Current Smoker, 1+ Pack/Day) [Matched Pairs], Allegheny County, 1980

	CONTROLS		
Cases	Smoking 1+ Pack/ Day	Smoking <1 Pack/ Day	Total
Smoking 1+ pack/day	2	36	38
Smoking <1 pack/day	8	34	42
Total	10	70	80

5. Calculate the matched-pairs odds ratio for these data. _____

6. Using data from the table, unmatch the pairs and calculate an unmatched odds ratio. _____

7. What are the odds that the controls smoke 1+ pack/day? _____

Questions 8 and 9 are based on the information given in the table at the bottom of this page.

8. The relative risk for developing ASHD subsequent to entering this study *in men as compared to women* is:
   a. Approximately equal in all age groups
   b. Highest in the oldest age group
   c. Lowest in the youngest and oldest age groups, and highest at ages 35–44 and 45–54 years
   d. Highest in the youngest and oldest age groups, and lowest at ages 35–44 and 45–54 years
   e. Lowest in the oldest age group

9. The most likely explanation for the differences in rates of ASHD between the *initial* examination and the yearly *follow-up* examinations in men is:
   a. The prevalence and incidence of ASHD increase with age in men
   b. Case-fatality rates of ASHD are higher at younger ages in men
   c. A classic cohort effect explains these results
   d. The case-fatality rate in ASHD is highest in the first 24 hours following a heart attack
   e. The initial examination measures the prevalence of ASHD, whereas the subsequent examinations primarily measure the incidence of ASHD

Rates of Atherosclerotic Heart Disease (ASHD) per 10,000 Population, By Age and Sex, Framingham, Massachusetts

	MEN		WOMEN	
Age at Beginning of Study (yr)	ASHD Rates at Initial Exam	Yearly Follow-up Exams (Mean Annual Incidence)	ASHD Rates at Initial Exam	Yearly Follow-up Exams (Mean Annual Incidence)
29–34	76.7	19.4	0.0	0.0
35–44	90.7	40.0	17.2	2.1
45–54	167.6	106.5	111.1	29.4
55–62	505.4	209.1	211.1	117.8

APPENDIX TO CHAPTER 11

Derivation of the relationship of the odds ratio and the relative risk can be demonstrated by the following algebra. Recall that:

$$\text{Relative risk (RR)} = \dfrac{\left(\dfrac{a}{a+b}\right)}{\left(\dfrac{c}{c+d}\right)}$$

$$\text{The odds ratio (OR)} = \dfrac{ad}{bc}$$

The relationship of the relative risk to the odds ratio can therefore be expressed as the ratio of the RR to the OR:

(1)

$$\dfrac{\text{RR}}{\text{OR}} = \dfrac{\left(\dfrac{a}{a+b}\right) \div \left(\dfrac{c}{c+d}\right)}{\left(\dfrac{ad}{bc}\right)}$$

$$= \dfrac{\left(\dfrac{a}{a+b}\right)}{\left(\dfrac{c}{c+d}\right)} \times \dfrac{bc}{ad}$$

$$= \dfrac{\left(\dfrac{abc}{a+b}\right)}{\left(\dfrac{cad}{c+d}\right)} = \dfrac{\left(\dfrac{b}{a+b}\right)}{\left(\dfrac{d}{c+d}\right)}$$

Since

$$\dfrac{b}{a+b} = \dfrac{a+b-a}{a+b} = \dfrac{a+b}{a+b} - \dfrac{a}{a+b} = 1 - \dfrac{a}{a+b}$$

and

$$\dfrac{d}{c+d} = \dfrac{c+d-c}{c+d} = \dfrac{c+d}{c+d} - \dfrac{c}{c+d} = 1 - \dfrac{c}{c+d}$$

The relationship of the relative risk to the odds ratio can therefore be reduced to the following equation:

$$\dfrac{\text{RR}}{\text{OR}} = \dfrac{1 - \left(\dfrac{a}{a+b}\right)}{1 - \left(\dfrac{c}{c+d}\right)}$$

Or, by multiplying through by the OR:

$$\text{RR} = \dfrac{1 - \left(\dfrac{a}{a+b}\right)}{1 - \left(\dfrac{c}{c+d}\right)} \times \text{OR}$$

If the disease is rare, both $\dfrac{a}{a+b}$ and $\dfrac{c}{c+d}$ will be very small, so that the term in parentheses in formula (1) will be approximately 1, and the odds ratio will then approximate the relative risk.

It also is of interest to examine this relationship in a different form. Recall the definition of *odds*—that is, the ratio of the number of ways the event can occur to the number of ways the event cannot occur:

$$O = \dfrac{P}{1-P}$$

where O is the *odds* that the disease will develop and P is the *risk* that the disease will develop. Note that, as P becomes smaller, the denominator $1 - P$ approaches 1, with the result that:

$$\dfrac{P}{1-P} \cong \dfrac{P}{1} = P$$

that is, the *odds* become a good approximation of the *risk*. Thus, if the risk is low (the disease is rare), the *odds* that the disease will develop are a good approximation of the *risk* that it will develop.

Now, consider an exposed group and a nonexposed group. If the risk of a disease is very low, the *ratio* of the *odds* in the exposed group to the *odds* in the nonexposed group closely approximates the *ratio* of the *risk* in the exposed group to the *risk* in the nonexposed group *(the relative risk):*

That is, when P is very small:

$$\dfrac{O_{\text{exp}}}{O_{\text{nonexp}}} \cong \dfrac{P_{\text{exp}}}{P_{\text{nonexp}}}$$

where:

O_{exp} is the odds of the disease developing in the exposed population,

O_{nonexp} is the odds of the disease developing in the nonexposed population,

P_{exp} is the probability (or risk) of the disease developing in the exposed population, and

P_{nonexp} is the probability (or risk) of the disease developing in the nonexposed population.

This ratio of odds is the odds ratio or relative odds.

Chapter 12

More on Risk: Estimating the Potential for Prevention

ATTRIBUTABLE RISK

Our discussion in the previous chapter focused on the relative risk and on the odds ratio, which is often used as a surrogate for the relative risk in a case-control study. The *relative risk* is important as a measure of the *strength of the association*, which (as Chapter 14 will demonstrate) is a major consideration in deriving causal inferences. In this chapter, we turn to a different question: *How much of the disease that occurs can be attributed to a certain exposure?* This is answered by another measure of risk, the *attributable risk*, which is defined as the amount or proportion of disease incidence (or disease risk) that can be attributed to a specific exposure. For example, how much of the lung cancer risk experienced by smokers can be attributed to smoking? Whereas the relative risk is important in establishing etiologic relationships, the attributable risk is in many ways more important in clinical practice and public health, because it addresses a different question: How much of the risk (incidence) of disease can we hope to prevent if we are able to eliminate exposure to the agent in question?

We can calculate the attributable risk for exposed persons (e.g., the attributable risk of lung cancer in smokers) or the attributable risk for the total population, which includes both exposed and nonexposed persons (e.g., the attributable risk of lung cancer in a total population, which consists of both smokers and non-smokers). These calculations and their uses and interpretations are discussed in this chapter.

Attributable Risk for the Exposed Group

Figure 12-1 offers a schematic introduction to this concept. Consider two groups: one exposed and the other not exposed. In Figure 12-1A, the total risk of the disease in the exposed group is indicated by the full height of the bar on the left, and the total risk of disease in the nonexposed group is indicated by the full height of the bar on the right. As seen here, the total risk of the disease is higher in the exposed group

than in the nonexposed group. We can ask the following question: In the exposed persons, how much of the total risk of disease is actually due to exposure (e.g., in a group of smokers, how much of the risk of lung cancer is due to smoking)?

How can this question be answered? Let us consider nonexposed persons, designated by the bar on the right. Although they are not exposed, they have some risk of disease (albeit at a much lower level than that of the exposed persons). That is, the risk of the disease is not zero even in nonexposed persons. For instance, in this example of smoking and lung cancer, even non-smokers have some risk (albeit a low risk) of lung cancer, possibly due to environmental chemical carcinogens or other factors. This risk is termed *background risk*. Every person shares the background risk regardless of whether or not he or she has had the specific exposure in question (in this case, smoking) (see Fig. 12-1B). Thus, both nonexposed and exposed persons have this background risk. Therefore, the total risk of the disease in exposed individuals is the sum of the background risk that any person has and the additional risk due to the exposure in question. If we want to know how much of the total risk in *exposed* persons is *due to the exposure*, we should subtract the background risk from the total risk (see Fig. 12-1C). Because the risk in the nonexposed group is equal to the background risk, we can calculate the risk in the exposed group that is a result of the specific exposure by subtracting the risk in the nonexposed group (the background risk) from the total risk in the exposed group.

Thus, the incidence of a disease that is attributable to the exposure in the exposed group can be calculated as follows:

Formula 12-1

$$\left(\begin{array}{c}\text{Incidence in} \\ \text{exposed group}\end{array}\right) - \left(\begin{array}{c}\text{Incidence in} \\ \text{nonexposed group}\end{array}\right)$$

We could instead ask, "What *proportion* of the risk in exposed persons is due to the exposure?" We could

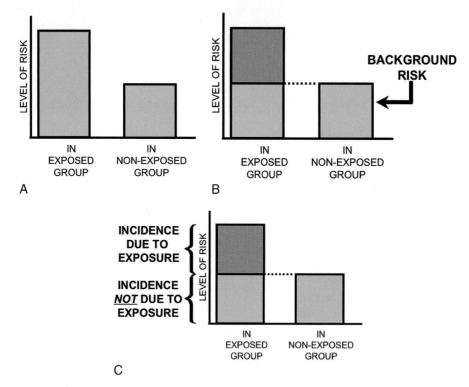

Figure 12-1. A, Total risks in exposed and nonexposed groups. **B,** Background risk. **C,** Incidence attributable to exposure and incidence not attributable to exposure.

then express the attributable risk as the *proportion* of the total incidence in the exposed group that is attributable to the exposure by simply dividing Formula 12-1 by the incidence in the exposed group, as follows:

Formula 12-2

$$\frac{\left(\begin{array}{c}\text{Incidence in}\\\text{exposed group}\end{array}\right)-\left(\begin{array}{c}\text{Incidence in}\\\text{nonexposed group}\end{array}\right)}{\text{Incidence in exposed group}}$$

The attributable risk expresses the most that we can hope to accomplish in reducing the risk of the disease if we completely eliminate the exposure. For example, if all smokers were induced to stop smoking, how much of a reduction could we anticipate in lung cancer rates? From a practical programmatic standpoint, the attributable risk may be more relevant than the relative risk. The relative risk is a measure of the strength of the association and the possibility of a causal relationship, but the attributable risk indicates the potential for prevention if the exposure could be eliminated.

The practicing clinician is mainly interested in the attributable risk *in the exposed group:* For example,

when a physician advises a patient to stop smoking, he or she is in effect telling the patient that stopping smoking will reduce the risk of coronary heart disease (CHD). Implicit in this advice is the physician's estimate that the patient's risk will be reduced by a certain proportion if he or she stops smoking; the risk reduction is motivating the physician to give that advice. Although the physician often does not have a specific value in mind for the attributable risk, he or she is in effect relying on an attributable risk for an exposed group (smokers) to which the patient belongs. The physician is implicitly addressing the question: In a population of smokers, how much of the CHD that they experience is due to smoking, and, consequently, how much of the CHD could be prevented if they did not smoke? Thus, attributable risk tells us the potential for prevention.

If all the incidence of a disease were the result of a single factor, the attributable risk for that disease would be 100%. However, this is rarely if ever the case. Both the concept and the calculation of attributable risk imply that not all of the disease incidence is due to a single specific exposure, as the disease even develops in some nonexposed individuals. Figure 12-2 recapitulates this concept.

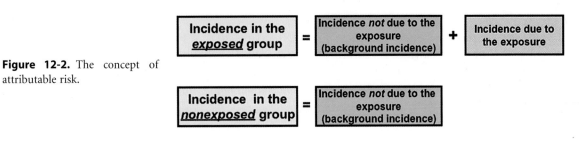

Figure 12-2. The concept of attributable risk.

Attributable Risk for the Total Population— Population Attributable Risk (PAR)

Let us turn to a somewhat different question relating to attributable risk. Assume that we know how to eliminate smoking. We tell the mayor that we have a highly effective way to eliminate smoking in the community, and we want her to provide the funds to support such a program. The mayor responds that she is delighted to hear the news, but asks, "What will the impact of your smoking cessation program be on lung cancer incidence rates in our city?" This question differs from that which was just discussed. For if we talk about lung cancer rates in the entire population of a city, and not just in exposed individuals, we are talking about a population that is composed of both smokers and nonsmokers. The mayor is not asking what impact we will have on smokers in this city, but rather what impact will we have on the entire population of the city, which includes both smokers and nonsmokers.

Let us consider this question further. In addition to the assumption that we have a terrific smoking cessation program, let us also assume that everyone in the city smokes. (Heaven forbid!) We now want to calculate the attributable risk. Clearly, because everyone in the city smokes, the attributable risk for the entire population of the city would equal the attributable risk for the exposed population. If everybody smokes, the attributable risk for the exposed group tells us what we can hope to accomplish with a smoking cessation program in the total population.

Now, let us assume that an ideal situation exists and that nobody in the city smokes. What will be the potential for preventing lung cancer through the use of the completely effective smoking cessation program that we wish to apply to the population of the city? The answer is zero; because there are no exposed people in the city, a program to eliminate the exposure would have no effect on the risk of lung cancer. Therefore, the spectrum of potential effect runs from a maximum (if everybody smokes) to zero

(if nobody smokes). Of course, in reality, the answer is generally somewhere in between, because some members of the population smoke and some do not. The latter group (all nonsmokers) clearly will not benefit from a smoking cessation program, regardless of how effective it is.

To this point, we have discussed the concept and calculation of attributable risk for *an exposed group.* For example, in a population of smokers, how much of the lung cancer that they experience is due to smoking and, consequently, how much of the lung cancer could be prevented if they did not smoke? However, to answer the mayor's question as to what effect the smoking cessation program will have on the city's population as a whole, we need to calculate the *attributable risk for the total population:* What proportion of the disease incidence in a *total population* (both exposed and nonexposed) can be attributed to a specific exposure? What would be the total impact of a prevention program on the community? If we want to calculate the attributable risk in the total population, the calculation is similar to that for exposed people, but we begin with the *incidence in the total population* and again subtract the background risk, or the incidence in the nonexposed population. The incidence in the total population that is due to the exposure* can be calculated as shown in Formula 12-3.

Formula 12-3

$$\left(\begin{array}{c} \text{Incidence in} \\ \text{total population} \end{array} \right) - \left(\begin{array}{c} \text{Incidence in} \\ \text{nonexposed group} \\ \text{(background risk)} \end{array} \right)$$

Again, if we prefer to express this as the *proportion* of the incidence in the *total population* that is attributable to the exposure, Formula 12-3 can be divided by the incidence in the total population:

---

*The incidence in the population that is due to the exposure can also be calculated as follows: Attributable risk for the exposed group × Proportion of the population exposed.

TABLE 12-1. Smoking and Coronary Heart Disease (CHD): A Hypothetical Cohort Study of 3,000 Cigarette Smokers and 5,000 Nonsmokers

	CHD Develops	CHD Does Not Develop	Total	Incidence per 1,000 per Year
Smoke cigarettes	84	2,916	3,000	28.0
Do not smoke cigarettes	87	4,913	5,000	17.4

$$\text{Incidence among smokers} = \frac{84}{3,000} = 28.0 \text{ per } 1,000$$

$$\text{Incidence among nonsmokers} = \frac{87}{5,000} = 17.4 \text{ per } 1,000$$

Formula 12-4

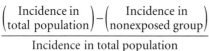

$$\frac{\left(\begin{array}{c}\text{Incidence in}\\\text{total population}\end{array}\right) - \left(\begin{array}{c}\text{Incidence in}\\\text{nonexposed group}\end{array}\right)}{\text{Incidence in total population}}$$

The attributable risk for the total population (population attributable risk) is a valuable concept for the public health worker. The question addressed is: What *proportion* of lung cancer in the *total population* can be attributed to smoking? This question could be reworded as follows: If smoking were eliminated, what *proportion* of the incidence of lung cancer in the total population (which consists of both smokers and nonsmokers) would be prevented? The answer is: the attributable risk *in the total population* also called the *population attributable risk*—or the *PAR* (as discussed earlier).*

From a public health standpoint, this is often both the critical issue and the question that is raised by policy-makers and by those responsible for funding prevention programs. They may want to know what the proposed program is going to do for the community as a whole. How is it going to change the burden on the health care system or the burden of suffering in the entire community, not just in exposed individuals? For example, if all smokers in the community stopped smoking, what would be the impact of this change on the incidence of lung cancer in the total population of the community (which includes both smokers and nonsmokers)?

An Example of an Attributable Risk Calculation for the Exposed Group

This section presents a step-by-step calculation of the attributable risk in both an exposed group and in a

total population. We will use the example previously presented of a cohort study of smoking and CHD. The data are again shown in Table 12-1.

The incidence of CHD in the exposed group (smokers) that is attributable to the exposure is calculated using Formula 12-1:

Formula 12-1

$$\left(\begin{array}{c}\text{Incidence in}\\\text{exposed group}\end{array}\right) - \left(\begin{array}{c}\text{Incidence in}\\\text{nonexposed group}\end{array}\right)$$

$$= \frac{28.0 - 17.4}{1,000} = \frac{10.6}{1,000}$$

What does this mean? It means that 10.6 of the 28/1000 incident cases in smokers are attributable to the fact that these people smoke. Stated another way, if we had an effective smoking cessation campaign, we could hope to prevent 10.6 of the $\frac{28}{1,000}$ incident cases of CHD that smokers experience.

If we prefer, we can express this as a *proportion*. The proportion of the total incidence in the exposed group that is attributable to the exposure can be calculated by dividing Formula 12-1 by the incidence in the exposed group (Formula 12-2):

Formula 12-2

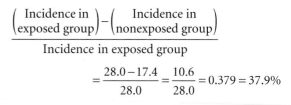

$$\frac{\left(\begin{array}{c}\text{Incidence in}\\\text{exposed group}\end{array}\right) - \left(\begin{array}{c}\text{Incidence in}\\\text{nonexposed group}\end{array}\right)}{\text{Incidence in exposed group}}$$

$$= \frac{28.0 - 17.4}{28.0} = \frac{10.6}{28.0} = 0.379 = 37.9\%$$

Thus, 37.9% of the morbidity from CHD among smokers may be attributable to smoking and could presumably be prevented by eliminating smoking.

---

*Another way to calculate the attributable risk for the total population is to use Levin's formula, which is given in the appendix to this chapter.

An Example of an Attributable Risk Calculation in the Total Population (Population Attributable Risk—PAR)

Using the same example, let us calculate the Population Attributable Risk (PAR): the attributable risk for the total population. The question we are asking is: What can we hope to accomplish with our smoking cessation program *in the total population* (i.e., the entire community, which consists of both smokers and nonsmokers)?

Remember that in the total population, the incidence that is due to smoking (the exposure) can be calculated by subtracting the background risk (i.e., the incidence in the nonsmokers, or nonexposed) from the incidence in the total population:

Formula 12-3

$$\left(\begin{array}{c}\text{Incidence in}\\\text{total population}\end{array}\right)-\left(\begin{array}{c}\text{Incidence in}\\\text{nonexposed group}\end{array}\right)$$

To calculate Formula 12-3, we must know *either* the incidence of the disease (CHD) in the total population (which we often do not know) *or* all of the following three values, from which we can then calculate the incidence in the total population:

1. The incidence among smokers
2. The incidence among nonsmokers
3. The proportion of the total population that smokes

In this example, we know that the incidence among the smokers is 28.0 per 1,000 and the incidence among the nonsmokers is 17.4 per 1,000. However, we do not know the incidence in the total population. Let us assume that, from some other source of information, we know that the proportion of smokers in the population is 44% (and therefore the proportion of nonsmokers is 56%). The incidence in the total population can then be calculated as follows:

$$\left(\begin{array}{c}\text{Incidence}\\\text{in smokers}\end{array}\right)\left(\begin{array}{c}\text{\% Smokers}\\\text{in population}\end{array}\right)$$
$$+\left(\begin{array}{c}\text{Incidence in}\\\text{nonsmokers}\end{array}\right)\left(\begin{array}{c}\text{\% Nonsmokers}\\\text{in population}\end{array}\right)$$

(We are simply weighting the calculation of the incidence in the total population, taking into account the proportion of the population that smokes and the proportion of the population that does not smoke.)

So, in this example, the incidence in the total population can be calculated as follows:

$$\left(\frac{28.0}{1,000}\right)(0.44)+\left(\frac{17.4}{1,000}\right)(0.56)=\frac{22.1}{1,000}$$

We now have the values needed for using Formula 12-3 to calculate the attributable risk in the total population:

Formula 12-3

$$\left(\begin{array}{c}\text{Incidence in}\\\text{total population}\end{array}\right)-\left(\begin{array}{c}\text{Incidence in}\\\text{nonexposed group}\end{array}\right)$$

$$=\frac{22.1}{1,000}-\frac{17.4}{1,000}=\frac{4.7}{1,000}$$

What does this tell us? How much of the total risk of CHD in this population (which consists of both smokers and nonsmokers) is attributable to smoking? If we had an effective prevention program (smoking cessation) in this population, how much of a reduction in CHD incidence could we anticipate, at best, in the total population (of both smokers and nonsmokers)?

If we prefer to calculate the *proportion* of the incidence in the *total population* that is attributable to the exposure, we can do so by dividing Formula 12-3 by the incidence in the total population as in Formula 12-4:

Formula 12-4

$$\frac{\left(\begin{array}{c}\text{Incidence in}\\\text{total population}\end{array}\right)-\left(\begin{array}{c}\text{Incidence in}\\\text{nonexposed group}\end{array}\right)}{\text{Incidence in total population}}$$

$$=\frac{22.1-17.4}{22.1}=21.3\%$$

Thus, 21.3% of the incidence of CHD in the total population can be attributed to smoking, and if an effective prevention program eliminated smoking, the best that we could hope to achieve would be a reduction of 21.3% in the incidence of CHD in the total population (consisting of both smokers and nonsmokers).

Attributable risk is a critical concept in virtually any area of public health and in clinical practice, in particular in relation to questions regarding the potential of preventive measures. For example, Mokdad and colleagues[1] estimated the actual causes of death in the United States in 2000. These estimates used published data and applied attributable risk calculations as well as other approaches. Their estimates are shown in Figure 12-3. The authors reported that tobacco and diet-activity patterns accounted for 33% of all deaths.

It is also of interest that in the legal arena, in which toxic tort litigation has become increasingly common, the concept of attributable risk has taken on great importance. One of the legal criteria used in finding a company responsible for an environmental injury, for example, is whether it is "more likely than not"

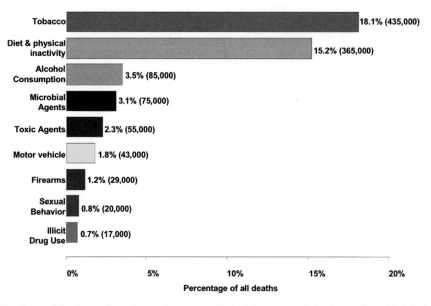

Figure 12-3. Numbers of deaths attributed to major causes, United States, 2000. (Redrawn from Mokdad AH, Marks JS, Stroup DF, Gerberding JL: Actual causes of death in the United States, 2000. JAMA 291:1238–1245, 2004, with the correction from JAMA 293:289, 2005.)

that the company caused the injury. It has been suggested that an attributable risk of greater than 50% might represent a quantitative determination of the legal definition of "more likely than not."

COMPARISON OF RELATIVE RISK AND ATTRIBUTABLE RISK

Chapters 11 and 12 have reviewed several measures of risk and of excess risk. The relative risk and the odds ratio are important as measures of the strength of the association, which is an important consideration in deriving a causal inference. The attributable risk is a measure of how much of the disease risk is attributable to a certain exposure. Consequently, the attributable risk is useful in answering the question of how much disease can be prevented if we have an effective means of eliminat-

ing the exposure in question. Thus, the relative risk is valuable in etiologic studies of disease, whereas the attributable risk has major applications in clinical practice and public health.

Table 12-2 shows an example from a study by Doll and Peto[2] that relates mortality from lung cancer and CHD in smokers and nonsmokers and provides an illuminating comparison of relative risk and attributable risk in the same set of data.

Let us first examine the data for lung cancer. (Note that in this example, we are using mortality as a surrogate for risk.) We see that the lung cancer mortality risk is 140 for smokers and 10 for nonsmokers. We can calculate the relative risk as $\frac{140}{10} = 14$.

Now, let us look at the data for CHD. The CHD mortality rate is 669 in smokers and 413 in non-

TABLE 12-2. Lung Cancer and CHD Mortality in Male British Physicians: Smokers vs. Nonsmokers

	Age-Adjusted Death Rates per 100,000		Relative Risk	Attributable Risk	% Attributable Risk
	Smokers	Nonsmokers			
Lung cancer	140	10	14.0	130	92.9
Coronary heart disease	669	413	1.6	256	38.3

From Doll R, Peto R: Mortality in relation to smoking: Twenty years' observation on male British doctors. Br Med J 2:1525–1536, 1976.

TABLE 12-3. Summary of Attributable Risk Calculations

	In Exposed Group	In Total Population
Incidence attributable to exposure	$\left(\begin{array}{c}\text{Incidence in}\\\text{exposed group}\end{array}\right) - \left(\begin{array}{c}\text{Incidence in}\\\text{nonexposed group}\end{array}\right)$	$\left(\begin{array}{c}\text{Incidence in}\\\text{total population}\end{array}\right) - \left(\begin{array}{c}\text{Incidence in}\\\text{nonexposed group}\end{array}\right)$
Proportion of incidence attributable to exposure	$\dfrac{\left(\begin{array}{c}\text{Incidence in}\\\text{exposed group}\end{array}\right) - \left(\begin{array}{c}\text{Incidence in}\\\text{nonexposed group}\end{array}\right)}{\text{Incidence in exposed group}}$	$\dfrac{\left(\begin{array}{c}\text{Incidence in}\\\text{total population}\end{array}\right) - \left(\begin{array}{c}\text{Incidence in}\\\text{nonexposed group}\end{array}\right)}{\text{Incidence in total population}}$

---

smokers. The relative risk can be calculated as $\dfrac{669}{413} = 1.6$. Thus, the relative risk is much higher for smoking and lung cancer than it is for smoking and CHD.

Now, let us turn to the attributable risks in smokers. How much of the total risk in smokers can we attribute to smoking? To calculate the attributable risk, we subtract the background risk—the risk in the nonexposed group (nonsmokers)—from the risk in the exposed group (smokers). With the data for lung cancer used, $140 - 10 = 130$.

To calculate the attributable risk for CHD and smoking, we subtract the risk in the nonexposed group (nonsmokers) from the risk in the exposed group (smokers), $669 - 413 = 256$. That is, of the total 669 deaths per 100,000 in smokers, 256 can be attributed to smoking.

If we prefer to express the attributable risk for lung cancer and smoking as a proportion (i.e., the proportion of the lung cancer risk in smokers that can be attributed to smoking), we divide the attributable risk by the risk in smokers:

$$\frac{(140-10)}{140} = 92.9\%.$$

If we prefer to express the attributable risk of CHD and smoking as a proportion (i.e., the proportion of the CHD risk in smokers that can be attributed to smoking), we divide the attributable risk by the risk in smokers:

$$\frac{(669-413)}{669} = 38.3\%.$$

What does this table tell us? First, we see a tremendous difference in the relative risks for lung cancer and for CHD in relation to smoking—14.0 for lung cancer compared with 1.6 for CHD (i.e., a much stronger association exists for smoking and lung cancer than for smoking and CHD). However, the attributable risk is almost twice as high (256) for CHD as it is for lung cancer (130). If we choose to express the attributable risk as a proportion, we find that 92.9% of lung cancer deaths in smokers can be attributed to smoking (and are potentially preventable by eliminating smoking) compared with only 38.3% of deaths from CHD in smokers that can be attributed to smoking.

Thus, the relative risk is much higher for lung cancer than for CHD, and the attributable risk expressed as a proportion is also much higher for lung cancer. However, if an effective smoking cessation program were available today and smoking were eliminated, would the preventive impact be greater on mortality from lung cancer or from CHD? If we examine the table we see that if smoking were eliminated, 256 deaths per 100,000 from CHD would be prevented in contrast to only 130 from lung cancer, despite the fact that the relative risk is higher for lung cancer and despite the fact that the proportion of deaths attributable to smoking is greater for lung cancer. Why is this so? This is a result of the fact that the mortality level in smokers is much higher for CHD than for lung cancer (669 compared to 140) and that the attributable risk (the difference between total risk in smokers and background risk) is much greater for CHD than for lung cancer.

CONCLUSION

In this chapter, we have introduced the concept of attributable risk and described how it is calculated and interpreted. Attributable risk is summarized in the four calculations shown in Table 12-3.

The concepts of relative risk and attributable risk are essential for understanding causation and the potential for prevention. Several measures of risk have now been discussed: (1) absolute risk, (2) relative risk, (3) odds ratios, and (4) attributable risk. In the next chapter, we shall briefly review study designs and concepts of risk before proceeding to a discussion of how we use estimates of excess risk to derive causal inferences.

REFERENCES

1. Mokdad AH, Marks JS, Stroup DF, Gerberding JL: Actual causes of death in the United States, 2000. JAMA 291:1238–1245, 2004. With the correction JAMA 293:298, 2005.
2. Doll R, Peto R: Mortality in relation to smoking: Twenty years' observations on male British doctors. Br Med J 2:1525–1536, 1976.
3. Levin ML: The occurrence of lung cancer in man. Acta Intern Cancer 9:531, 1953.
4. Leviton A: Definitions of attributable risk. Am J Epidemiol 98:231, 1973.

REVIEW QUESTIONS FOR CHAPTER 12

1. Several studies have found that approximately 85% of cases of lung cancer are due to cigarette smoking. This measure is an example of:
   a. An incidence rate
   b. An attributable risk
   c. A relative risk
   d. A prevalence risk
   e. A proportionate mortality ratio

Questions 2 and 3 refer to the following information:

The results of a 10-year cohort study of smoking and coronary heart disease (CHD) are shown below:

	OUTCOME AFTER 10 YRS	
At Beginning of Study	**CHD Developed**	**CHD Did Not Develop**
2,000 Healthy smokers	65	1,935
4,000 Healthy nonsmokers	20	3,980

2. The incidence of CHD in smokers that can be attributed to smoking is: _____

3. The proportion of the total incidence of CHD in smokers that is attributable to smoking is: _____

Questions 4 and 5 are based on the following information:

In a cohort study of smoking and lung cancer, the incidence of lung cancer among smokers was found to be 9/1,000 and the incidence among nonsmokers was 1/1,000. From another source we know that 45% of the total population were smokers.

4. The incidence of lung cancer attributable to smoking in the total population is: _____

5. The proportion of the risk in the total population that is attributable to smoking is: _____

APPENDIX TO CHAPTER 12: LEVIN'S FORMULA FOR THE ATTRIBUTABLE RISK FOR THE TOTAL POPULATION

Another way to calculate this proportion for the total population is to use Levin's formula[3]:

$$\frac{p(r-1)}{p(r-1)+1}$$

where p is the proportion of the population with the characteristic or exposure and r is the relative risk (or odds ratio).

Leviton[4] has shown that Levin's formula[3] and the following formula are algebraically identical:

$$\frac{\left(\begin{array}{c}\text{Incidence in}\\\text{total population}\end{array}\right)-\left(\begin{array}{c}\text{Incidence in}\\\text{nonexposed group}\end{array}\right)}{\text{Incidence in total population}}$$

Chapter 13

A Pause for Review: Comparing Cohort and Case-Control Studies

At this point in our discussion, we will pause to review some of the material that has been covered in Section II. Because the presentation proceeds in a stepwise manner, it is important to understand what has been discussed thus far.

First, let us compare the designs of cohort and case-control studies, as seen in Figure 13-1. The important point that distinguishes between the two types of study design is that, in a cohort study, exposed and nonexposed persons are compared, and in a case-control study, persons with the disease (cases) and without the disease (controls) are compared (Fig. 13-2A). In cohort studies, we compare the rates of disease in exposed and in nonexposed individuals, and in case-control studies, we compare the proportions who have the exposure of interest in people with the disease and in people without the disease (Fig. 13-2B).

Table 13-1 presents a detailed comparison of prospective cohort, retrospective (historical) cohort, and case-control study designs. If the reader has followed the discussion in Section II to this point, the entries in the table should be easy to understand.

When we begin a cohort study with exposed and nonexposed groups, we can study only the specific exposure that distinguishes one group from the other. But as shown in Figure 13-3, we can study multiple outcomes or diseases in relation to the exposure of interest. Most cohort studies start with exposed and nonexposed individuals. Less common is the situation where we start with a defined population in which the study population is selected on the basis of a factor not related to exposure, such as place of residence, and some members of the cohort become exposed and others are not exposed (Fig. 13-4). In a cohort study that starts with a defined population, it is possible to study multiple exposures. Thus, for example, in the Framingham Study, it was possible to study many exposures, including weight, blood pressure, cholesterol level, smoking, and physical activity among the participating individuals residing in Framingham, Massachusetts.

In cohort studies, incidence in both exposed and nonexposed groups *can* be calculated, and we can therefore directly calculate the relative risk. Prospective cohort studies minimize the potential for recall and other bias in assessing the exposure and have greater validity of the exposure assessments. However, in retrospective cohort studies, which require data from the past, these problems may be significant. Cohort studies are desirable when the exposure of interest is rare. In a case-control design, we are unlikely to identify a sufficient number of exposed persons when we are dealing with a rare exposure. In prospective cohort studies in particular we are likely to have better data on the temporal relationship

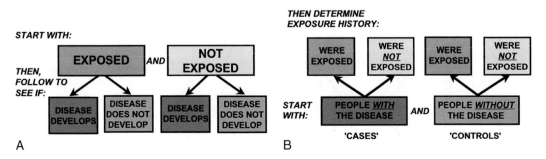

Figure 13-1. Design of cohort and case-control studies. **A,** Cohort study. **B,** Case-control study.

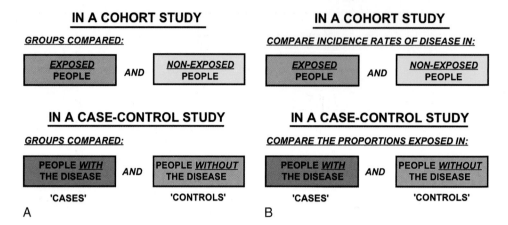

Figure 13-2. Comparison of cohort and case-control study designs. **A,** Groups compared. **B,** Outcome measurements.

between exposure and outcome; that is, did the exposure precede the outcome? Among the disadvantages of cohort studies is that they usually require large populations, and, in general, prospective cohort studies are especially expensive to carry out because follow-up of a large population over time is required. A greater potential bias for assessing the outcome is present in cohort studies. Finally, cohort studies often become impractical when the disease under study is rare.

As seen in Table 13-1, case-control studies have a number of advantages. They are relatively inexpensive and require a relatively small number of subjects for study. They are desirable when the disease occurrence is rare, because if a cohort study were performed in such a circumstance, a tremendous number of people would have to be followed to generate enough people with the disease for study. As seen in Figure 13-5, in a case-control study, because we begin with cases and controls, we are able to study more

than one possible etiologic factor and to explore interactions among the factors.

Because case-control studies often require data about past events or exposures, they are often encumbered by the difficulties encountered in using such data (including a potential for recall bias). Furthermore, as has been discussed in some detail, selection of an appropriate control group is one of the most difficult methodologic problems encountered in epidemiology. In addition, in most case-control studies, we cannot calculate disease incidence in either the total population or the exposed and nonexposed groups without some supplemental information.

The nested case-control design combines elements of both cohort and case-control studies and offers a number of advantages. The possibility of recall bias is eliminated because the data on exposure are obtained before the disease develops. Exposure data are more likely to represent the pre-illness state,

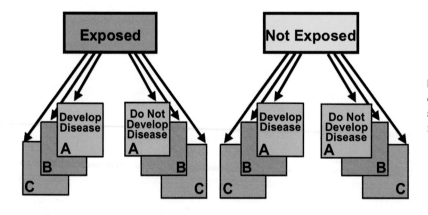

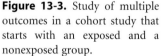

Figure 13-3. Study of multiple outcomes in a cohort study that starts with an exposed and a nonexposed group.

TABLE 13-1. Comparisons of Cohort and Case-Control Studies

	Cohort Studies		Case-Control Studies
	Prospective	*Retrospective*	
A. Study group	Exposed persons: $(a + b)$	Exposed persons: $(a + b)$	Persons with diseases (cases): $(a + c)$
B. Comparison group	Nonexposed persons: $(c + d)$	Nonexposed persons: $(c + d)$	Persons without disease (controls): $(b + d)$
C. Outcome measurements	Incidence in the exposed $\left(\dfrac{a}{a+b}\right)$ and Incidence in the nonexposed $\left(\dfrac{c}{c+d}\right)$	Incidence in the exposed $\left(\dfrac{a}{a+b}\right)$ and Incidence in the nonexposed $\left(\dfrac{c}{c+d}\right)$	Proportion of cases exposed $\left(\dfrac{a}{a+c}\right)$ and Proportion of controls exposed $\left(\dfrac{b}{b+d}\right)$
D. Measures of risk	Absolute risk Relative risk Odds ratio Attributable risk	Absolute risk Relative risk Odds ratio Attributable risk	— — Odds ratio Attributable risk†
E. Temporal relationship between exposure and disease	Easy to establish	Sometimes hard to establish	Sometimes hard to establish
F. Multiple associations	Possible to study associations of an exposure with several diseases*	Possible to study associations of an exposure with several diseases*	Possible to study associations of a disease with several exposures or factors
G. Time required for the study	Generally long because of need to follow-up the subjects	May be short	Relatively short
H. Cost of study	Expensive	Generally less expensive than a prospective study	Relatively inexpensive
I. Population size needed	Relatively large	Relatively large	Relatively small
J. Potential bias	Assessment of outcome	Susceptible to bias both in assessment of exposure and assessment of outcome	Assessment of exposure
K. Best when	Exposure is rare Disease is frequent among exposed	Exposure is rare Disease is frequent among exposed	Disease is rare Exposure is frequent among the diseased
L. Problems	Selection of nonexposed comparison group often difficult Changes over time in criteria and methods	Selection of nonexposed comparison group often difficult Changes over time in criteria and methods	Selection of appropriate controls often difficult Incomplete information on exposure

*Also possible to study multiple exposures when the study population is selected on the basis of a factor unrelated to the exposure.
†Provided additional information is available.

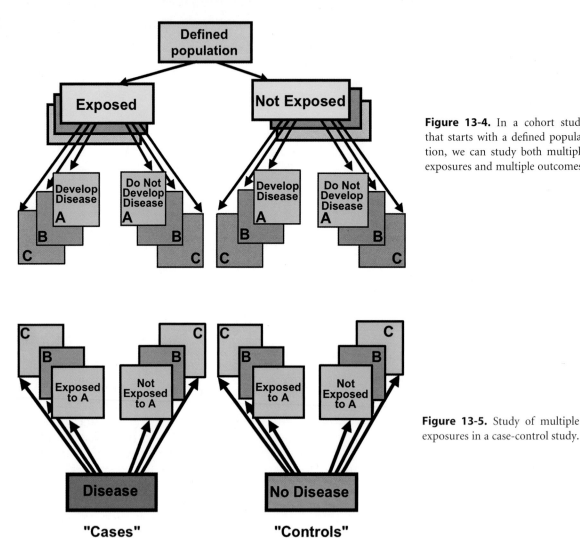

Figure 13-4. In a cohort study that starts with a defined population, we can study both multiple exposures and multiple outcomes.

Figure 13-5. Study of multiple exposures in a case-control study.

because they are obtained years before clinical illness is diagnosed. Finally, the costs are lower than with a cohort study, because laboratory tests need to be done only on specimens from subjects who are later chosen as cases or controls.

Finally, we have discussed the cross-sectional study design, in which data on both exposure and disease outcomes are collected simultaneously from each subject. The data can therefore be analyzed by comparing the prevalence of disease in exposed individuals with that in nonexposed individuals, or by comparing the prevalence of exposure in persons with the disease with that of persons without the disease. Although cross-sectional data are often obtained in surveys and can be very useful, they usually do not permit the investigator to determine the temporal relationship between exposure and the development of disease. As a result, their value for deriving causal inferences is limited. However, they can provide important directions for further research using cohort, case-control, and nested case-control designs.

Chapter 14

From Association to Causation: Deriving Inferences from Epidemiologic Studies

In the previous chapters, we discussed the designs of epidemiologic studies that are used to determine whether an association exists between an exposure and a disease (Fig. 14-1). We then addressed different types of risk measurement that are used to quantitatively express an excess in risk. If we determine that an exposure is associated with a disease, the next question is whether the observed association reflects a causal relationship (Fig. 14-2).

Although Figures 14-1 and 14-2 refer to an environmental exposure, they could just as well have specified a genetic characteristic or characteristics or a specific combination of environmental and genetic factors. As we shall see in Chapter 16, studies of disease etiology generally address the contributions of both genetic and environmental factors and their interactions.

This chapter discusses the derivation of causal inferences in epidemiology. Let us begin by asking, "What approaches are available for studying the etiology of disease?"

APPROACHES FOR STUDYING DISEASE ETIOLOGY

If we are interested in whether a certain substance is carcinogenic in human beings, a first step in the study of the substance's effect might be to expose animals to the carcinogen in a controlled laboratory environment. Although such animal studies afford us the opportunity to control the exposure dose and other environmental conditions and genetic factors precisely, and to keep loss to follow-up to a minimum, at the conclusion of the study we are left with the problem of having to extrapolate data across species, from animal to human populations. Certain diseases seen in humans have neither occurred nor been produced in animals. It is also difficult to extrapolate animal doses to human doses, and species differ in their responses. Thus, although such toxicologic studies can be very useful, they still leave a gnawing uncertainty as to whether the animal findings can be generalized to human beings.

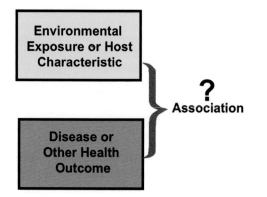

Figure 14-1. Observed association between exposure and disease.

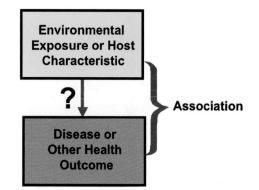

Figure 14-2. Is the association between exposure and disease causal?

We can also use in vitro systems, such as cell culture or organ culture. However, because these are artificial systems, we are again left with the difficulty of extrapolating from artificial systems to intact, whole human organisms.

In view of these limitations, if we want to be able to draw a conclusion as to whether a substance causes disease in human beings, we need to make *observations in human populations*. Because we cannot ethically or practically randomize human beings to exposure to a suspected carcinogen, we are dependent on non-randomized observations, such as those made in case-control and cohort studies.

Approaches to Etiology in Human Populations

Epidemiology capitalizes on what have been called "unplanned" or "natural" experiments. (Some think that this phrase is a contradiction in terms, in that the word "experiment" implies a planned exposure.) What we mean by *unplanned* or *natural* experiments is that we take advantage of groups of people who have been exposed for nonstudy purposes, such as occupational cohorts in specific industries, persons exposed to toxic chemicals (such as those affected by the explosion at Bhopal, India), or persons subjected to other toxic exposures (such as residents of Hiroshima and Nagasaki who were exposed to atomic bomb radiation in 1945). Each of these exposed groups can be compared to a nonexposed group to determine whether there is an increased risk of a certain adverse effect in persons who have been exposed.

In conducting human studies, the sequence shown in Figure 14-3 is frequently followed:

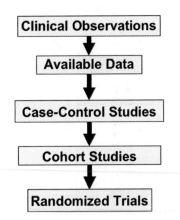

Figure 14-3. A frequent sequence of studies in human populations.

The initial step may consist of *clinical observations* at the bedside. For example, when the surgeon Alton Ochsner observed that virtually every patient on whom he operated for lung cancer gave a history of cigarette smoking, he was among the first to suggest a possible causal relationship.[1] A second step is to try to identify *routinely available data*, the analysis of which might shed light on the question. We can then carry out *new studies* such as the cohort and case-control studies discussed in Chapters 9 and 10, which are specifically designed to determine whether there is an association between an exposure and a disease, and whether a causal relationship exists.

The usual first step in carrying out new studies to explore a relationship is often a *case-control study*. For example, if Ochsner had wanted to further explore his suggestion that cigarette smoking may be associated with lung cancer, he would have compared the smoking histories of a group of his patients with lung cancer with those of a group of patients without lung cancer—a case-control study.

If a case-control study yields evidence that a certain exposure is suspect, we might next do a *cohort study* (e.g., comparing smokers and nonsmokers and determining the rate of lung cancer in each group or comparing workers exposed to an industrial toxin with workers without such an exposure). Although, in theory, a randomized trial might be the next step, as discussed earlier, randomized trials are almost never used to study the effects of putative toxins or carcinogens and are generally used only for studying potentially beneficial agents.

Conceptually, a two-step process is followed in carrying out studies and evaluating evidence. However, in practice, this process often becomes interactive and deviates from a fixed sequence:

1. We determine whether there is an association between an exposure or characteristic and the risk of a disease. To do so, we use:
   a. Studies of group characteristics: ecologic studies
   b. Studies of individual characteristics: case-control and cohort studies
2. If an association is demonstrated, we determine whether the observed association is likely to be a causal one.

Ecologic Studies

The first approach in determining whether an association exists might be to conduct studies of group characteristics, called *ecologic studies*. Figure 14-4 shows the relationship between breast cancer incidence and average dietary fat consumption in each

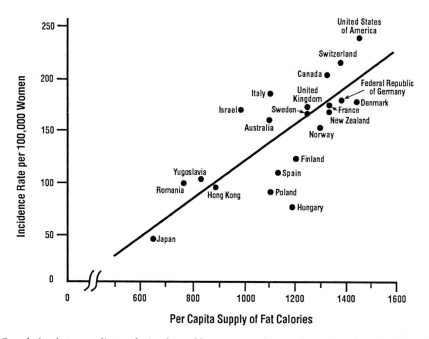

Figure 14-4. Correlation between dietary fat intake and breast cancer by country. (From Prentice RL, Kakar F, Hursting S, et al: Aspects of the rationale for the Women's Health Trial. J Natl Cancer Inst 80:802–814, 1988.)

country.[2] In this figure, each dot represents a different country.

The higher the average dietary fat consumption for a country, the higher breast cancer incidence for that country generally is. We might therefore be tempted to conclude that dietary fat may be a causal factor for breast cancer. What is the problem with drawing such a conclusion from this type of study? Consider Switzerland, for example, which has a high breast cancer incidence and a high average consumption of dietary fat. The problem is that we do not know whether the *individuals* in whom breast cancer developed in that country actually had high dietary fat intake. All we have are *average* values of dietary fat consumption for each country and the breast cancer incidence for each country. In fact, one might argue that given the same overall picture, it is conceivable that those who developed breast cancer ate very little dietary fat. Figure 14-4 alone does not reveal whether this might be true; in effect, individuals in each country are characterized by the average figure for that country. No account is taken of variability between individuals in that country in regard to dietary fat consumption. This problem is called the *ecologic fallacy*—we may be ascribing to members of a group, characteristics that they in fact do not possess as individuals. This problem arises in an ecologic study because we only have data for groups;

we do not have exposure and outcome data for each individual in the population.

Table 14-1 shows data from a study in northern California exploring a possible relation between prenatal exposure to influenza during an influenza outbreak and the later development of acute lymphocytic leukemia in a child.[3] The data presented in this table show the incidence data for children who were not in utero during a flu outbreak and for children who were in utero—in the first, second, or third trimester of the pregnancy—during the outbreak. Below these figures, the data are presented as relative risks, with the risk being set at 1.0 for those who were not in utero during the outbreak and the other rates being set relative to this. The data indicate a high relative risk for leukemia in children who were in utero during the flu outbreak in the first trimester.

What is the problem? The authors themselves wrote: "The observed association is between pregnancy during an influenza epidemic and subsequent leukemia in the offspring of that pregnancy. It is not known if the mothers of any of these children actually had influenza during their pregnancy." What we are missing are *individual data* on exposure. One might ask, why didn't the investigators obtain the necessary exposure data? The likely reason is that the investigators used birth certificates and data from a cancer registry; both types of data are relatively easy

TABLE 14-1. **Average Annual Crude Incidence Rates and Relative Risks of Acute Lymphocytic Leukemia by Cohort and Trimester of Flu Exposure for Children Younger Than 5 Years, San Francisco/Oakland (1969–1973)**

| | | Flu Exposure | | | |
| | | Trimester | | | |
	No Flu Exposure	1st	2nd	3rd	Total
Incidence rates per 100,000	3.19	10.32	8.21	2.99	6.94
Relative risks	1.0	3.2	2.6	0.9	2.2

Adapted from Austin DF, Karp S, Dworsky R, Henderson BE: Excess leukemia in cohorts of children born following influenza epidemics. Am J Epidemiol 10:77–83, 1977.

to obtain. This approach did not require follow-up and direct contact with individual subjects. If we are impressed by these ecologic data, we might want to carry out a study specifically designed to explore the possible relationship of prenatal flu and leukemia. Such a study would probably be considerably more difficult and more expensive to conduct.

In view of these problems, are ecologic studies of value? Yes, they can suggest avenues of research that may be promising in casting light on etiologic relationships. In and of themselves, however, they do not demonstrate conclusively that a causal association exists.

For many years, legitimate concerns about the ecologic fallacy gave ecologic studies a bad name and diverted attention from the importance of studying possible true ecologic relationships, such as those between the individual and the community in which the person lives. For example, Diez Roux and associates studied the relationship of characteristics of a neighborhood and the incidence of coronary heart disease (CHD).[4] They followed 13,009 people participating in the Atherosclerosis Risk in Communities Study over a 9-year period and identified 615 coronary events. They found that CHD was more likely to develop in people living in the most disadvantaged neighborhoods than in those living in the most advantaged neighborhoods, even after they controlled for personal socioeconomic indicators (income, education, and occupation) and adjusted for established individual risk factors for CHD. Thus, future studies addressing both individual risk factors and ecologic risk factors such as neighborhood characteristics and the possible interactions of both types of factors may contribute significantly to improving our understanding of the etiology and pathogenesis of many diseases and suggest new preventive interventions.

Recognizing the limitations discussed above of ecologic studies that use only group data, we turn next to studies of individual characteristics: case-control and cohort studies. It has been claimed that because epidemiologists generally show tabulated data and refer to characteristics of groups, the data in all epidemiologic studies are group data. This is not true. For what distinguishes case-control and cohort studies from studies that are exclusively ecologic is that although all of these types of studies rely on groups of individuals, in case-control or cohort studies, for each subject we have information on both exposure (whether or not and, often, how much exposure occurred) and disease outcome (whether or not the person developed the disease in question). In ecologic studies, we only have data on groups.

TYPES OF ASSOCIATIONS

Real or Spurious Associations

Let us turn next to the types of associations that we might observe in a cohort or case-control study. If we observe an association, we start by asking the question, "Is it a true (real) association or a false (spurious) one?" For example, if we designed a study to select controls in such a way that they tended to be nonexposed, we might observe an association of exposure with disease (i.e., more exposure in cases than in controls). This would not be a true association, but only a result of the study design. Recall that this issue was raised in Chapter 10 regarding a study of coffee consumption and cancer of the pancreas. The possibility was suggested that the controls selected for the study had a lower rate of

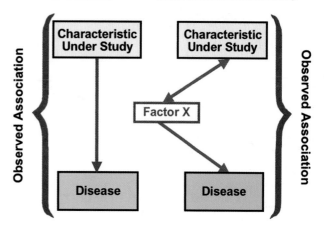

Figure 14-5. Types of associations.

coffee consumption than was found in the general population.

Interpreting Real Associations

If the observed association is real, is it causal? Figure 14-5 shows two possibilities. Figure 14-5A shows a causal association: we observe an association of exposure and disease, as indicated by the bracket, and the exposure induces development of the disease, as indicated by the arrow. Figure 14-5B shows the same observed association of exposure and disease, but they are associated only because they are both linked to a third factor, designated here as *factor X*. This association is a result of confounding and is non-causal. Confounding is discussed in greater detail in Chapter 15.

In Chapter 10 we discussed this issue in relation to McMahon's study of coffee and cancer of the pancreas. McMahon observed an association of coffee consumption with risk of pancreatic cancer. Ciga-rette smoking was known to be associated with pancreatic cancer, and coffee drinking and cigarette smoking are closely associated (few smokers do not drink coffee) (Fig. 14-6). Therefore, was the observed association of coffee drinking and cancer of the pan-creas likely to be a causal relationship, or could the association be due to the fact that coffee and cigarette smoking are associated, and that cigarette smoking is a known risk factor for cancer of the pancreas?

The same issue is exemplified by the observed association of increased serum cholesterol level and risk of coronary heart disease (CHD) (Fig. 14-7). Is increased cholesterol a causal factor for increased risk of CHD, or is the observed association due to con-founding? That is, are we observing an association of increased cholesterol and CHD because both are associated with a factor X (such as a particular genetic profile), which might cause people to have both increased levels of cholesterol and an increased risk of CHD?

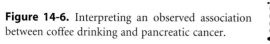

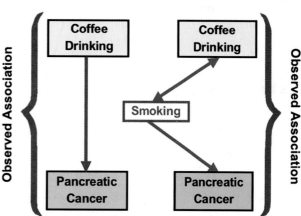

Figure 14-6. Interpreting an observed association between coffee drinking and pancreatic cancer.

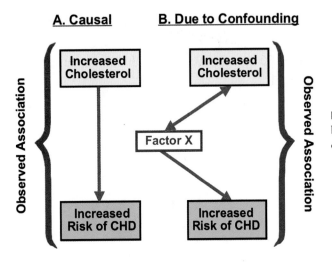

Figure 14-7. Interpreting an observed association between increased cholesterol level and increased risk of coronary heart disease (CHD).

Is this distinction really important? What difference does it make? The answer is that it makes a tremendous difference from both clinical and public health standpoints. If the relationship is causal, we will succeed in reducing the risk of CHD if we lower cholesterol levels. However, if the relationship is due to confounding, then the increased risk of CHD is caused by factor X. Therefore, changes in the level of serum cholesterol will have no effect on the risk of CHD. Thus, it is extremely important for us to be able to distinguish between an association due to a causal relationship and an association due to confounding (noncausal).

Let us look at another example. For many years it has been known that cigarette smoking by pregnant women is associated with low birth weight in their infants. As seen in Figure 14-8, the effect is not just the result of the birth of a few low-birth-weight babies in this group of women. Rather, the entire weight distribution curve is shifted to the left in the babies born to smokers. The reduction in birth weight is also not a result of shorter pregnancies. The babies of smokers are smaller than those of nonsmokers at each gestational age (Fig. 14-9). A dose-response relationship is also seen (Fig. 14-10). The more a woman smokes, the greater her risk of having a low-birth-weight baby. For many years the interpretation of this association was the subject of great controversy. Many believed the association reflected a causal relation. Others, including a leading statistician, Jacob

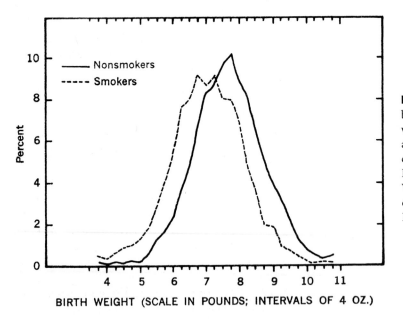

Figure 14-8. Percentage distribution by birth weight of infants of mothers who did not smoke during pregnancy and of those who smoked 1 pack of cigarettes or more per day. (From U.S. Department of Health, Education, and Welfare: The Health Consequences of Smoking. Washington, DC, Public Health Service, 1973, p 105.)

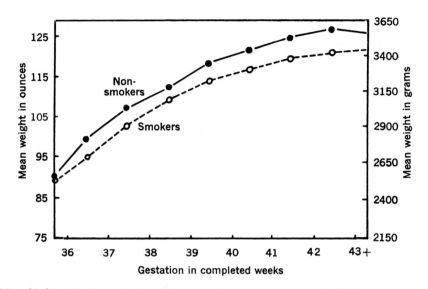

Figure 14-9. Mean birth weight for week of gestation according to maternal smoking habit. (From U.S. Department of Health, Education, and Welfare: The Health Consequences of Smoking. Washington, DC, Public Health Service, 1973, p 104.)

Yerushalmy, believed the association was due to confounding and was not causal. He wrote as follows:

A comparison of smokers and nonsmokers shows that the two differ markedly along many environmental, behavioral and biologic variables. For example, smokers are less likely to use contraceptives and to plan the pregnancy. Smokers are more likely to drink coffee, beer and whiskey and the nonsmoker,

tea, milk and wine. The smoker is more likely than the nonsmoker to indulge in these habits to excess. In general, the nonsmokers are revealed to be more moderate than the smokers who are shown to be more extreme and carefree in their mode of life. Some biologic differences are also noted between them: Thus smokers have a higher twinning rate only in whites and their age for menarche is lower than for nonsmokers.[5]

In view of these many differences between smokers and nonsmokers, Yerushalmy believed that it was not the *smoking* that caused the low birth weight, but rather that the low weight was attributable to *other characteristics of the smokers.* It is interesting to examine a study that Yerushalmy carried out to support his position at the time (Fig. 14-11).[5]

Yerushalmy examined the results of one pregnancy (the study pregnancy) in a population of women who had had several pregnancies. The rate of low-birth-weight babies in the study pregnancy was 5.3% for women who were nonsmokers in *all* of their pregnancies. However, if they were smokers in all of their pregnancies, the rate of low birth weight in the study pregnancy was almost 9%. When he examined pregnancies of women who were nonsmokers in the study pregnancy, but who later became smokers, he found that their rate of low-birth-weight babies was about equal to that of women who smoked in all pregnancies. When he examined pregnancies of women who were smokers in the study pregnancy, but who subsequently stopped smoking, he found

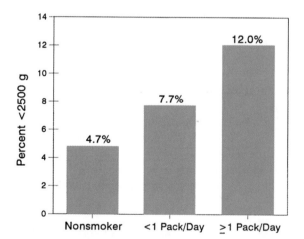

Figure 14-10. Percentage of pregnancies ($n = 50,267$) with infant weighing less than 2,500 g, by maternal cigarette smoking category. (Redrawn from Ontario Department of Health: Second Report of the Perinatal Mortality Study in Ten University Teaching Hospitals. Toronto, Ontario, Department of Health, Ontario Perinatal Mortality Study Committee, vol I, 1967, p 275.)

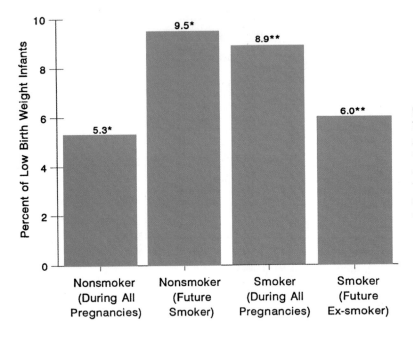

Figure 14-11. Percentage of low-birth-weight infants by smoking status of their mothers ($*P < .01$; $**P < .02$). (Redrawn from Yerushalmy J: Infants with low birth weight born before their mothers started to smoke cigarettes. Am J Obstet Gynecol 112:277–284, 1972.)

that their rate of low birth weight in the study pregnancy was similar to that of women who were nonsmokers in all of their pregnancies.

On the basis of these data, Yerushalmy came to the conclusion that it was not the smoking but rather some characteristic of the smoker that caused the low birth weight. Today, however, it is virtually universally accepted that smoking is a cause of low birth weight. The causal nature of this relation has also been demonstrated in randomized trials that have reduced the frequency of low birth weight by initiating programs for smoking cessation in pregnant women. Although this issue has now largely been resolved, it is illuminating to review both the controversy and the study, as they exemplify the reasoning that is necessary in trying to distinguish causal from noncausal interpretations of observed associations.

TYPES OF CAUSAL RELATIONSHIPS

A causal pathway can be either *direct* or *indirect* (Fig. 14-12). In direct causation, a factor directly causes a disease without any intermediate step. In indirect causation, a factor causes a disease, but only through an intermediate step or steps. In human biology, intermediate steps are virtually always present in any causal process.

If a relationship is causal, four types of causal relationships are possible: (1) necessary and sufficient; (2) necessary, but not sufficient; (3) sufficient, but not necessary; and (4) neither sufficient nor necessary.

Necessary and Sufficient

In the first type of causal relationship, a factor is both necessary and sufficient for producing the disease. Without that factor, the disease never develops (the factor is necessary), and in the presence of that factor, the disease always develops (the factor is sufficient) (Fig. 14-13). This situation rarely if ever occurs. For example, in most infectious diseases, a number of people are exposed, some of whom will manifest the disease and others who will not. Members of households of a person with tuberculosis do not uni-

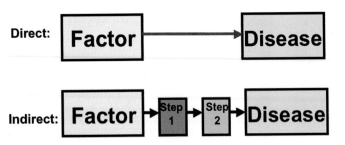

Figure 14-12. Direct versus indirect causes of disease.

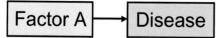

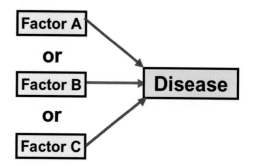

Figure 14-13. Types of causal relationships: I. A factor is both necessary and sufficient.

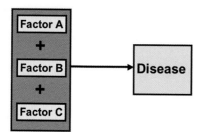

Figure 14-15. Types of causal relationships: III. Each factor is sufficient, but not necessary.

Figure 14-14. Types of causal relationships: II. Each factor is necessary, but not sufficient.

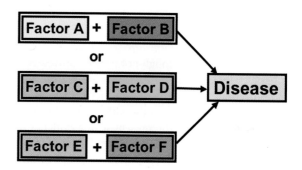

Figure 14-16. Types of causal relationships: IV. Each factor is neither sufficient nor necessary.

formly acquire the disease from the index case. If the exposure dose is assumed to be the same, there are likely differences in immune status, genetic susceptibility, or other characteristics that determine who develops the disease and who does not. A one-to-one relationship of exposure to disease, which is a consequence of a necessary and sufficient relationship, rarely if ever occurs.

Necessary, But Not Sufficient
In another model, each factor is necessary, but not, in itself, sufficient to cause the disease (Fig. 14-14). Thus, multiple factors are required, often in a specific temporal sequence. For example, carcinogenesis is considered to be a multistage process involving both initiation and promotion. For cancer to result, a promoter must act after an initiator has acted. Action of an initiator or a promoter alone will not produce a cancer.

Again, in tuberculosis, the tubercle bacillus is clearly a necessary factor, even though its presence may not be sufficient to produce the disease in every infected individual.

Sufficient But Not Necessary
In this model, the factor alone can produce the disease, but so can other factors that are acting alone (Fig. 14-15). Thus, either radiation exposure or benzene exposure can each produce leukemia without the presence of the other. Even in this situation, however, cancer does not develop in everyone who has experienced radiation or benzene exposure, so although both factors are not needed, other cofactors probably are. Thus, the criterion of *sufficient* is rarely met by a single factor.

Neither Sufficient Nor Necessary
In the fourth model, a factor, by itself, is neither sufficient nor necessary to produce disease (Fig. 14-16). This is a more complex model, which probably most accurately represents the causal relationships that operate in most chronic diseases.

EVIDENCE FOR A CAUSAL RELATIONSHIP

Many years ago, when the major disease problems faced by man were infectious in origin, the question arose as to what evidence would be necessary to prove that an organism causes a disease. In 1840, Henle proposed postulates for causation that were expanded by Koch in the 1880s.[6] The postulates for causation were as follows:

1. The organism is *always* found with the disease.
2. The organism is *not* found with any other disease.
3. The organism, isolated from one who has the disease, and cultured through several generations, produces the disease (in experimental animals).

Koch added that "Even when an infectious disease cannot be transmitted to animals, the 'regular' and

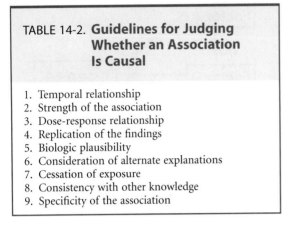

TABLE 14-2. **Guidelines for Judging Whether an Association Is Causal**

1. Temporal relationship
2. Strength of the association
3. Dose-response relationship
4. Replication of the findings
5. Biologic plausibility
6. Consideration of alternate explanations
7. Cessation of exposure
8. Consistency with other knowledge
9. Specificity of the association

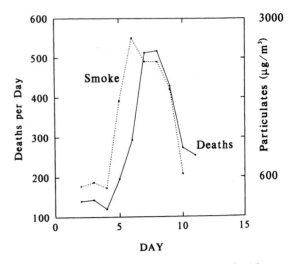

Figure 14-17. The mean concentration of airborne particles ($\mu g/m^3$) from the four inner monitoring stations in London and the count of daily deaths in the London Administrative County during the beginning of December 1952. (From Schwartz J: Air pollution and daily mortality: A review and meta analysis. Environ Res 64: 36–52, 1994.)

'exclusive' presence of the organism [postulates 1 and 2] proves a causal relationship."[6]

These postulates, though not perfect, proved very useful for infectious diseases. However, as apparently noninfectious diseases assumed increasing importance toward the middle of the 20th century, the issue arose as to what would represent strong evidence of causation in diseases that were generally not of infectious origin. In such disease there was no organism that could be cultured and grown in animals. Specifically, as attention was directed to a possible relationship between smoking and lung cancer, the U.S. Surgeon General appointed an expert committee to review the evidence. The committee developed a set of guidelines,[7] which have been revised over the years. The next few pages present a modified list of these guidelines (Table 14-2) with some brief comments.

GUIDELINES FOR JUDGING WHETHER AN ASSOCIATION IS CAUSAL

1. Temporal Relationship. It is clear that if a factor is believed to be the cause of a disease, exposure to the factor must have occurred before the disease developed. Figure 14-17 shows the number of deaths per day and the mean concentration of airborne particles in London in early December 1952.[8] The pattern of a rise in particle concentration followed by a rise in mortality and a subsequent decline in particle concentration followed by a decline in mortality strongly supported the increase in mortality being due to the increase in air pollution. This example demonstrates the use of ecologic data for exploring a temporal relationship. Further investigation revealed that the increased mortality consisted almost entirely of respiratory and cardiovascular deaths and was highest in the elderly.

It is often easier to establish a temporal relationship in a prospective cohort study than in a case-control study or a retrospective cohort study. In the last two types of studies, exposure information may need to be obtained or re-created from past records and the timing may therefore be imprecise.

The temporal relationship of exposure and disease is important not only for clarifying the order in which the two occur but also in regard to the length of the interval between exposure and disease. For example, asbestos has been clearly linked to increased risk of lung cancer, but the latent period between the exposure and the appearance of lung cancer is at least 15 to 20 years. Therefore, if, for example, lung cancer develops after only 3 years since the asbestos exposure, it is safe to conclude that the lung cancer was not a result of this exposure.

2. Strength of the Association. The strength of the association is measured by the relative risk (or odds ratio). The stronger the association, the more likely it is that the relation is causal.

3. Dose-Response Relationship. As the dose of exposure increases, the risk of disease also increases. Figure 14-18 shows an example of the dose-response relationship for cigarette smoking and lung cancer. If a dose-response relationship is present, it is strong evidence for a causal relationship. However, the absence of a dose-response relationship does not necessarily rule out a causal relationship. In some

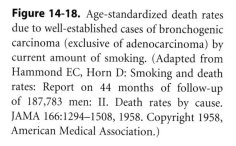

Figure 14-18. Age-standardized death rates due to well-established cases of bronchogenic carcinoma (exclusive of adenocarcinoma) by current amount of smoking. (Adapted from Hammond EC, Horn D: Smoking and death rates: Report on 44 months of follow-up of 187,783 men: II. Death rates by cause. JAMA 166:1294–1508, 1958. Copyright 1958, American Medical Association.)

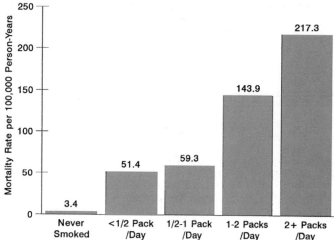

cases in which a threshold may exist, no disease may develop up to a certain level of exposure (a threshold); above this level, disease may develop.

*4. **Replication of the Findings.*** If the relationship is causal, we would expect to find it consistently in different studies and in different populations. Replication of findings is particularly important in epidemiology. If an association is observed, we would also expect it to be seen consistently within subgroups of the population and in different populations, unless there is a clear reason to expect different results.

*5. **Biologic   Plausibility.*** Biologic plausibility refers to coherence with the current body of biologic knowledge. Examples may be cited to demonstrate that epidemiologic observations have sometimes preceded biologic knowledge. Thus, as discussed in an earlier chapter, Gregg's observations on rubella and congenital cataracts preceded any knowledge of teratogenic viruses. Similarly, the implication of high oxygen concentration in the causation of retrolental fibroplasia, a form of blindness that occurs in premature infants, preceded any biologic knowledge supporting such a relationship. Nevertheless, we seek consistency of the epidemiologic findings with existing biologic knowledge, and when this is not the case, interpreting the meaning of the observed association may be difficult. We may then be more demanding in our requirements about the size and significance of any differences observed and in having the study replicated by other investigators in other populations.

*6. **Consideration of Alternate Explanations.*** We have discussed the problem in interpreting an observed association in regard to whether a relationship is causal or is the result of confounding. In judging whether a reported association is causal, the extent to which the investigators have taken other possible explanations into account and the extent to which they have ruled out such explanations are important considerations.

*7. **Cessation of Exposure.*** If a factor is a cause of a disease, we would expect the risk of the disease to decline when exposure to the factor is reduced or eliminated. Figure 14-19 shows such data for cigarette smoking and lung cancer.

Eosinophilia myalgia syndrome (EMS) reached epidemic proportions in 1989. Characterized by severe muscle pain and a high blood eosinophil count, the syndrome was found to be associated with manufactured preparations of L-tryptophan. In November 1989, a nationwide recall by the Food and Drug Administration of over-the-counter preparations of L-tryptophan was followed by dramatic reductions in numbers of cases of EMS reported each month (Fig. 14-20). This is another example of a reduction in incidence being related to cessation of exposure, which adds to the strength of the causal inference regarding the exposure.

When cessation data are available, they provide helpful supporting evidence for a causal association. However, in certain cases, the pathogenic process may have been irreversibly initiated, and the disease occurrence may have been determined by the time the exposure is removed. Emphysema is not reversed with cessation of smoking, but its progression is reduced.

*8. **Consistency with Other Knowledge.*** If a relationship is causal, we would expect the findings to be consistent with other data. For example, Figure 14-21 shows data regarding lung cancer rates in

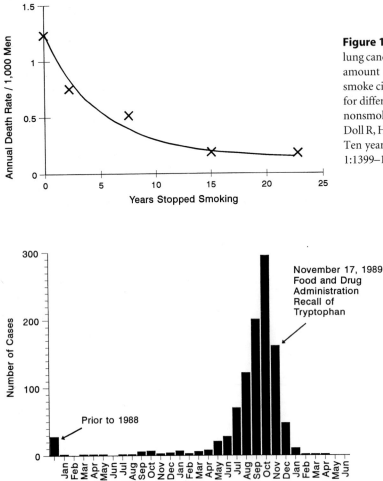

Figure 14-19. Effects of terminating exposure: lung cancer death rates, standardized for age and amount smoked, among men continuing to smoke cigarettes and men who gave up smoking for different periods. The corresponding rate for nonsmokers was 0.07 per 1,000. (Adapted from Doll R, Hill AB: Mortality in relation to smoking: Ten years' observations of British doctors. BMJ 1:1399–1410, 1964.)

Figure 14-20. Reported dates of illness onset by month and year for cases of eosinophilia-myalgia syndrome, as reported to the Centers for Disease Control and Prevention, Atlanta, as of July 10, 1990. (Adapted from Swygert LA, Maes EF, Sewell LE, et al: Eosinophilia-myalgia syndrome: Results of national surveillance. JAMA 264:1698–1703, 1990. Copyright 1990, American Medical Association.)

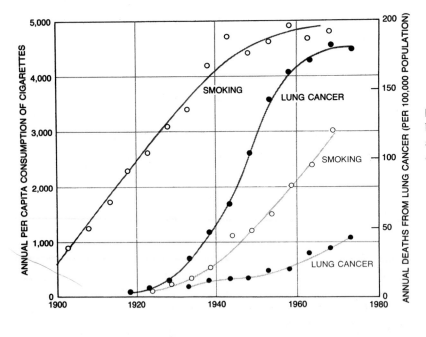

Figure 14-21. Parallel trends between cigarette consumption and lung cancer in men (two curves on left) and in women (two curves on right), in England and Wales. (From Cairns J: The cancer problem. Sci Am 235: 64–72, 77–78, 1975.)

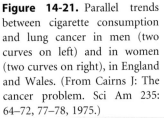

men and women and cigarette smoking in men and women.

We see a consistent direction in the curves, with the increase in lung cancer rates following the increase in cigarette sales in both men and women. These data are consistent with what we would expect if the relationship between smoking and lung cancer is established as a causal one. Although the absence of such consistency would not completely rule out this hypothesis, if we observed rising lung cancer rates after a period of declining cigarette sales, for example, we would need to explain how this observation could be consistent with a causal hypothesis.

9. Specificity of the Association. An association is specific when a certain exposure is associated with only one disease; this is the weakest of all the guidelines and should probably be deleted from the list. Cigarette manufacturers have pointed out that the diseases attributed to cigarette smoking do not meet the requirements of this guideline, because cigarette smoking has been linked to lung cancer, pancreatic cancer, bladder cancer, heart disease, emphysema, and other conditions.

The possibility of such multiple effects from a single factor is not, in fact, surprising: regardless of the tissue that comprises them, all cells have common characteristics, including DNA, RNA, and various subcellular structures, so a single agent could have effects in multiple tissues. Furthermore, cigarettes are not a single factor but constitute a mixture of a large number of compounds; consequently, a large number of effects might be anticipated.

When specificity of an association is found, it provides additional support for a causal inference. However, as with a dose-response relationship, absence of specificity in no way negates a causal relationship.

Any conclusion that an observed association is causal is greatly strengthened when different types of evidence from multiple sources support such reasoning. Thus, it is not so much a count of the number of guidelines present that is relevant to causal inference but rather an *assessment of the total pattern of evidence observed* that may be consistent with one or more of the guidelines.

DERIVING CAUSAL INFERENCES: TWO EXAMPLES

Peptic Ulcers and Gastric Cancer in Relation to Infection with *Helicobacter pylori*

Although the preceding guidelines do not permit a quantitative estimation of whether or not an asso-

ciation is causal, they can nevertheless be very helpful, as seen in the following examples:

Until the 1980s, the major causes of peptic ulcer disease were considered to be stress and lifestyle factors, including smoking. Peptic ulcer disease had long been attributed to the effects of gastric acid. Susceptibility to gastric acid had been linked to cigarette smoking, alcohol consumption, and use of nonsteroidal anti-inflammatory agents. Therapy was primarily directed at inhibiting acid secretion and protecting mucosal surfaces from acid. Although these therapies helped healing, relapses were common.

In 1984, Australian physicians Drs. Barry J. Marshall and J. Robin Warren reported that they had observed small curved bacteria colonizing the lower part of the stomach in patients with gastritis and peptic ulcers.[9] After several attempts, Marshall succeeded in cultivating a hitherto unknown bacterial species (later named *Helicobacter pylori*) from several of these biopsies (Fig. 14-22). Together they found that the organism was present in almost all patients with gastric inflammation or peptic ulcer. Many of these patients had biopsies performed which showed evidence of inflammation present in the gastric mucosa close to where the bacteria were seen. Based on these results, they proposed that *Helicobacter pylori* is involved in the etiology of these diseases. It

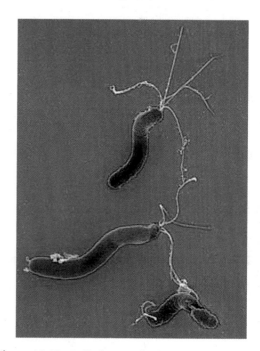

Figure 14-22. *Helicobacter pylori* [Photograph]. Encyclopædia Britannica Online. 12 June 2007; http://www.britannica.com/eb/art-94921.

was subsequently shown that the ulcer was often not cured until *Helicobacter pylori* had been eliminated.

It is now firmly established that *Helicobacter pylori* causes more than 90% of duodenal ulcers and up to 80% of gastric ulcers. The link between *Helicobacter pylori* infection and subsequent gastritis and peptic ulcer disease has been established through studies of human volunteers, antibiotic treatment studies, and epidemiological studies. Thus, many of the study designs discussed in previous chapters and many of the guidelines for causal inferences discussed earlier

in this chapter, were involved in elucidating the role of *Helicobacter pylori* in peptic ulcer and gastritis. In 2005, the Nobel Prize for Physiology or Medicine was shared by Drs. Marshall and Warren, "for their discovery of the bacterium *Helicobacter pylori* and its role in gastritis and peptic ulcer disease."

Table 14-3 categorizes this evidence according to several of the guidelines for causation just discussed. Thus, as seen here, the guidelines can be extremely helpful in characterizing the evidence supporting a causal relationship.

TABLE 14-3. Assessment of the Evidence Suggesting *Helicobacter pylori* as a Causative Agent of Duodenal Ulcers

1. Temporal relationship.
   - *Helicobacter pylori* is clearly linked to chronic gastritis. About 11% of chronic gastritis patients will go on to have duodenal ulcers over a 10-year period.
   - In one study of 454 patients who underwent endoscopy 10 years earlier, 34 of 321 patients who had been positive for *Helicobacter pylori* (11%) had duodenal ulcer compared with 1 of 133 *Helicobacter pylori*-negative patients (0.8%).
2. Strength of the relationship.
   - *Helicobacter pylori* is found in at least 90% of patients with duodenal ulcer. In at least one population reported to lack duodenal ulcers, a northern Australian aboriginal tribe that is isolated from other people, it has never been found.
3. Dose-response relationship.
   - Density of *Helicobacter pylori* per square millimeter of gastric mucosa is higher in patients with duodenal ulcer than in patients without duodenal ulcer. Also see item 2 above.
4. Replication of the findings.
   - Many of the observations regarding *Helicobacter pylori* have been replicated repeatedly.
5. Biologic plausibility.
   - Although originally it was difficult to envision a bacterium that infects the stomach antrum causing ulcers in the duodenum, it is now recognized that *Helicobacter pylori* has binding sites on antral cells and can follow these cells into the duodenum.
   - *Helicobacter pylori* also induces mediators of inflammation.
   - *Helicobacter pylori*-infected mucosa is weakened and is susceptible to the damaging effects of acid.
6. Consideration of alternate explanations.
   - Data suggest that smoking can increase the risk of duodenal ulcer in *Helicobacter pylori*-infected patients but is not a risk factor in patients in whom *Helicobacter pylori* has been eradicated.
7. Cessation of exposure.
   - Eradication of *Helicobacter pylori* heals duodenal ulcers at the same rate as histamine receptor antagonists.
   - Long-term ulcer recurrence rates were zero after *Helicobacter pylori* was eradicated using triple-antimicrobial therapy, compared with a 60% to 80% relapse rate often found in patients with duodenal ulcers treated with histamine receptor antagonists.
8. Specificity of the association.
   - Prevalence of *Helicobacter pylori* in patients with duodenal ulcers in 90% to 100%. However, it is found in some patients with gastric ulcer and even in asymptomatic individuals.
9. Consistency with other knowledge.
   - Prevalence of *Helicobacter pylori* infection is the same in men as in women. The incidence of duodenal ulcer, which in earlier years was believed to be higher in men than in women, has been equal in recent years.
   - The prevalence of ulcer disease is believed to have peaked in the latter part of the 19th century, and the prevalence of *Helicobacter pylori* may have been much higher at that time because of poor living conditions. This reasoning is also based on observations today that the prevalence of *Helicobacter pylori* is much higher in developing countries.

Data from Megraud F, Lamouliatte H: *Helicobacter pylori* and duodenal ulcer: Evidence suggesting causation. Dig Dis Sci 37:769–772, 1992; and DeCross AJ, Marshall BJ: The role of *Helicobacter pylori* in acid-peptic disease. Am J Med Sci 306:381–391, 1993.

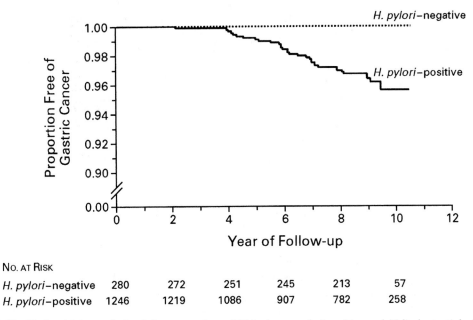

Figure 14-23. Kaplan-Meier analysis of the proportion of *Helicobacter pylori*-positive and *Helicobacter pylori*-negative patients who remained free of gastric cancer. During follow-up, gastric cancer developed in 36 of the 1,246 *H. pylori*-infected patients (2.9%), but in none of the 280 uninfected patients (*P* < .001). (From Uemura N, Okamoto S, Yamomoto S, et al: *Helicobacter pylori* infection and the development of gastric cancer. N Engl J Med 345:784–789, 2001.)

Increasing evidence now also supports the association of *Helicobacter pylori* infection and the development of gastric cancer. Uemura and coworkers[10] prospectively studied 1,526 Japanese patients who had duodenal or gastric ulcers, gastric hyperplasia, or non-ulcer hyperplasia. Of this group, 1,246 had *Helicobacter pylori* infection and 280 did not. The mean follow-up period was 7.8 years. Gastric cancers developed in 36 (2.9%) of the infected patients, but in none of the noninfected patients. Individuals who carry antibodies to *Helicobacter pylori* may have a 2 to 3 times higher risk of stomach cancer than those who do not (Fig. 14-23). The risk of stomach cancer also appears to be related to the type of strain of *Helicobacter pylori* which is infecting a person. Evidence is accumulating to support the idea that therapy against *Helicobacter pylori* may prevent gastric cancer. In the future, gastric cancer may come to be viewed as a largely preventable cancer of infectious origin.

Age of Onset of Alcohol Use and Lifetime Alcohol Abuse

In 1997, Grant and Dawson[11] reported data on the relationship of age at first use of alcohol and prevalence of lifetime alcohol dependence and abuse. They analyzed data from 27,616 current and former drinkers who were interviewed as part of the 1992 National

Longitudinal Alcohol Epidemiologic Survey. The rates of lifetime *dependence* decreased from more than 40% among individuals who began drinking at age 14 years or younger to about 10% among those who started drinking at age 20 years or older (Fig. 14-24). The configuration of the curve in Figure 14-24 suggests a dose-response relationship as has been observed for longer duration of smoking associated with increased risk of lung cancer. However, the data may also point to a period of particularly high susceptibility, namely, that the period of pre-adolescence and early adolescence is a period of increased risk for developing a disorder of alcohol use. Therefore, interventions should be targeted to this group in the hope of delaying drinking onset. However, adopting such an approach assumes that the relationship between early onset of drinking and subsequent lifetime abuse is a causal one, so that delaying age at onset of drinking would reduce the risk of lifetime alcohol dependence. Another possible explanation is that those who are destined for lifetime alcohol dependence tend to begin drinking earlier, but that the earlier age at drinking onset is not necessarily a cause of the later dependence. Further research is therefore needed to explain the intriguing association that has been observed. We shall return to this example in Chapter 16.

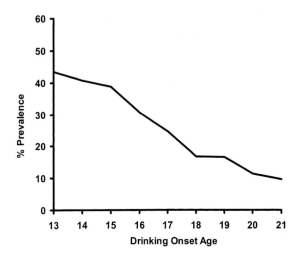

Figure 14-24. Relation of age of onset of alcohol use to prevalence of lifetime alcohol abuse. (Adapted from Grant BF, Dawson DA: Age at onset of alcohol use and its association with DSM-IV alcohol abuse and dependence: Results from the National Longitudinal Alcohol Epidemiologic Survey. J Subst Abuse 9:103–110, 1997.)

MODIFICATIONS OF THE GUIDELINES FOR CAUSAL INFERENCES

In 1986, the U.S. Public Health Service brought together a group of 19 experts to examine the scientific basis of the content of prenatal care and to answer the question: Which measures implemented during prenatal care have actually been demonstrated to be associated with improved outcome? The panel's report was issued in 1989 and served as the basis of a comprehensive report.[12] As the panel began its deliberations, it became clear that questions of causation were at the heart of the panel's task, and that guidelines were needed for assessing the relationship of prenatal measures to health outcomes. A subcommittee reviewed the current guidelines (just enumerated in the preceding text) and defined a process for using evidence that includes (1) categorization of the evidence by the quality of its sources, and (2) evaluation of the evidence of a causal relationship using standardized guidelines.[13] These recommendations are excerpted in Table 14-4. Although these modified guidelines clearly use the original components, they establish reasonable priorities in weighting them. They thus define an approach for looking at causation that may have applicability far beyond questions of the effectiveness of prenatal measures.

A similar approach, ranking studies by the quality of the study and its evidence, is used by the U.S.

Preventive Services Task Force, which is responsible for developing clinical practice guidelines for prevention and screening (Table 14-5).[14] The Task Force is an independent committee of experts supported by the U.S. Government. Members include experts in primary care, prevention, evidence-based medicine, and research methods. Various clinical areas and experience in preventive medicine, public health, and health policy are also represented.

For each topic the Task Force considers, it defines the questions that need to be addressed and identifies and retrieves the relevant evidence. The quality of each individual study is assessed after which the strength of the totality of available evidence is judged. Estimates are made of the balance of benefits and harms. This balance is expressed as the net benefit (the difference between benefits and harms). The Task Force prepares recommendations for preventive interventions based on these considerations.

Figure 14-25 shows a generic example of the analytic plan which is prepared by the Task Force as a framework for evaluating the evidence for a screening program. The straight arrows show possible pathways of benefit, and the blue curved arrows show possible adverse effects relating to different stages. The primary question (question 1 in the figure) is generally one of whether screening is effective in reducing the risk of an adverse outcome such as mortality and if so, to what extent.

Generally, few if any studies have examined this overarching question so that the deliberations of the Task Force often deal with the different steps or linkages that comprise this overall pathway. The purple arrow in the figure (step 5) shows the relation of treatment to outcome. Red arrows in the figure, steps 3, 4, and 6, show individual components of question 1. These assessments generally depend on a review of relevant randomized trials in order to prepare a chain of supporting evidence on which to base an answer to question 1. The evidence for each linkage is summarized in the evidence review and then summarized across the different linkages to provide an overall assessment of the supporting evidence for the preventive service being evaluated.

The quality of the overall evidence is graded on a 3-point scale: good, fair, or poor (see Table 14-5). The recommendations of the Task Force are based on a combined consideration of the quality of the evidence and the magnitude of the net benefit as shown in the matrix in Figure 14-26, in which a grading system of A, B, C, D, and I, is used. The meaning of each letter grade is explained in Table 14-6.

TABLE 14-4. The Process for Using the Evidence in Developing Recommendations on the Effectiveness of Prenatal Interventions

Stage I: Categorizing the Evidence by the Quality of Its Source. (*In each category, studies are listed in descending order of quality.*)
1. Trials (planned interventions with contemporaneous assignment of treatment and nontreatment)
   a. Randomized, double-blind, placebo-controlled with sufficient power appropriately analyzed.
   b. Randomized, but blindness not achieved.
   c. Nonrandomized trials with good control of confounding, that are well conducted in other respects.
   d. Randomized, but with deficiencies in execution or analysis (insufficient power, major losses to follow-up, suspect randomization, analysis with exclusions).
   e. Nonrandomized trials with deficiencies in execution or analysis.
2. Cohort or case-control studies
   a. Hypothesis specified before analysis, good data, confounders accounted for.
   b. As above, but hypothesis not specified before analysis.
   c. Post hoc, with problem(s) in the data or the analysis.
3. Time-series studies
   a. Analyses that take confounding into account.
   b. Analyses that do not consider confounding.
4. Case-series studies: Series of case reports without any specific comparison group
   Among other issues that must be considered in reviewing the evidence are the precision of definition of the outcome being measured, the degree to which the study methodology has been described, adequacy of the sample size, and the degree to which characteristics of the population studied and of the intervention being evaluated have been described.
   A study can be well designed and carried out in an exemplary fashion (internal validity), but if the population studied is an unusual or highly selected one, the results may not be generalizable (external validity).

Stage II: Guidelines for Evaluating the Evidence of a Causal Relationship. (*In each category, studies are listed in descending priority order.*)
1. Major criteria
   a. Temporal relationship: An intervention can be considered evidence of a reduction in risk of disease or abnormality only if the intervention was applied before the time the disease or abnormality would have developed.
   b. Biological plausibility: A biologically plausible mechanism should be able to explain why such a relationship would be expected to occur.
   c. Consistency: Single studies are rarely definitive. Study findings that are replicated in different populations and by different investigators carry more weight than those that are not. If the findings of studies are inconsistent, the inconsistency must be explained.
   d. Alternative explanations (confounding): The extent to which alternative explanations have been explored is an important criterion in judging causality.
2. Other considerations
   a. Dose-response relationship: If a factor is indeed the cause of a disease, usually (but not invariably) the greater the exposure to the factor, the greater the risk of the disease. Such a dose-response relationship may not always be seen because many important biologic relationships are dichotomous, and reach a threshold level for observed effects.
   b. Strength of the association: The strength of the association is usually measured by the extent to which the relative risk or odds depart from unity, either above 1 (in the case of disease-causing exposures) or below 1 (in the case of preventive interventions).
   c. Cessation effects: If an intervention has a beneficial effect, then the benefit should cease when it is removed from a population (unless carryover effect is operant).

Adapted from Gordis L, Kleinman JC, Klerman LV, et al: Criteria for evaluating evidence regarding the effectiveness of prenatal interventions. In Merkatz IR, Thompson JE (eds): New Perspectives on Prenatal Care. New York, Elsevier, 1990, pp 31–38.

The work of the Task Force has dealt with screening for many diseases and conditions. Some examples will illustrate the breadth of the Task Force's activities. It has reviewed the evidence for screening for different cancers, for cardiovascular diseases including hyper-tension, coronary heart disease, and abdominal aortic aneurysm, for infectious diseases, such as gonorrhea, Chlamydia, and hepatitis B and C, and for mental conditions such as dementia, depression, and suicide risk, and screening for glaucoma and for type 2 diabe-

TABLE 14-5. Criteria Used by the U.S. Preventive Services Task Force for Grading the Quality of the Overall Evidence

GOOD	Evidence includes consistent results from well-designed, well-conducted studies of representative populations that directly assess effects on health outcomes.
FAIR	Evidence is sufficient to determine effects on health outcomes, but the strength of the evidence is limited by the number, quality, or consistency of the individual studies, generalizability to routine practice, or indirect nature of the evidence on health outcomes.
POOR	Evidence is insufficient to assess the effects on health outcomes because of limited number or power of studies, important flaws in their design or conduct, gaps in the chain of evidence, or lack of information on important health outcomes.

From the Guide to Clinical Preventive Services: Recommendations of the U.S. Preventive Services Task Force, 2006, Agency for Health Care Research and Quality, AHRQ Publication No. 06-0588, June 2006.

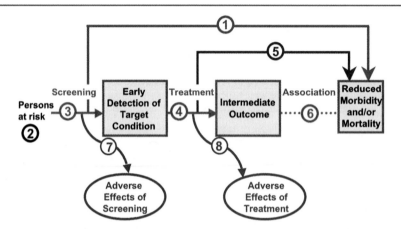

Figure 14-25. Generic analytic framework for screening topics used by the U.S. Preventive Services Task Force. Numbers refer to key questions in the figure. (1) Is there direct evidence that screening reduces morbidity and/or mortality? (2) What is the prevalence of disease in the target population? (3) Can screening accurately detect the target condition? (4) Does treatment reduce the incidence of the intermediate outcome? (5) Does treatment improve health outcomes for people diagnosed clinically? (6) Is reduced incidence of the intermediate outcome reliably associated with reduced morbidity and/or mortality? (7) Does screening result in adverse effects? (8) Does treatment result in adverse effects? (Adapted from Harris RP, Helfand M, Woolf SH, et al: Current methods of the U.S. Preventive Services Task Force: A review of the process. Am J Prev Med 20[Suppl 3]:21–35, 2001. A more detailed discussion of the methodology used by the Task Force can be found in this paper.)

tes. The Task Force has also reviewed the evidence for the effectiveness of counseling for many conditions such as counseling to prevent tobacco use and tobacco-related diseases, counseling to prevent alcohol misuse, counseling to promote a healthy diet, and counseling to promote physical activity. The above issues have been addressed in adults, but childhood conditions have also been reviewed by the Task Force including prevention of dental caries in preschool children, screening for scoliosis in adolescents, newborn hearing screening, and screening for visual impairment in children younger than 5 years of age. These and many more evidence reviews and recommendations of the Task Force can be found on the website of the Agency for Health Care Research and Quality (www.ahrq.gov). The deliberations and recommendations of the

Strength of Overall Evidence of Effectiveness	Estimates of Net Benefit (Benefits Minus Harms)			
	Substantial	Moderate	Small	Zero/Negative
Good	A	B	C	D
Fair	B	B	C	D
Poor	I = Insufficient Evidence			

Figure 14-26. Grid used by the U.S Preventive Services Task Force for combining the certainty of benefit and the magnitude of net benefit in determining the grade of its recommendations. (Adapted from the Guide to Clinical Preventive Services: Recommendations of the U.S. Preventive Services Task Force, 2006, Agency for Health Care Research and Quality, AHRQ Publication No. 06-0588, June 2006.)

TABLE 14-6. How the U.S. Preventive Services Task Force Grades Its Recommendations*

A   The USPSTF **strongly recommends** that clinicians provide [the service] to eligible patients. *The USPSTF found good evidence that [the service] improves important health outcomes and concludes that benefits substantially outweigh harms.*

B   The USPSTF **recommends** that clinicians provide [the service] to eligible patients. *The USPSTF found at least fair evidence that [the service] improves important health outcomes and concludes that benefits outweigh harms.*

C   The USPSTF **makes no recommendation** for or against routine provision of [the service]. *The USPSTF found at least fair evidence that [the service] can improve health outcomes but concludes that the balance of benefits and harms is too close to justify a general recommendation.*

D   The USPSTF recommends against routinely providing [the service] to asymptomatic patients. *The USPSTF found at least fair evidence that [the service] is ineffective or that the harms outweigh the benefits.*

I   The USPSTF concludes that **the evidence is insufficient** to recommend for or against routinely providing [the service]. *Evidence that [the service] is effective is lacking, or poor quality, or conflicting, and the balance of benefits and harms cannot be determined.*

---

*The U.S. Preventive Services Task Force (USPSTF) grades its recommendations based on the strength of evidence and magnitude of net benefit (benefits minus harms).

From the Guide to Clinical Preventive Services: Recommendations of the U.S Preventive Services Task Force, 2006, Agency for Health Care Research and Quality, AHRQ Publication No. 06-0588, June 2006.

Task Force provide a highly useful model of assessing the strength of the evidence and moving from causal inferences to policy recommendations.

CONCLUSION

Although causal guidelines discussed in this chapter are often referred to as *criteria*, this term does not seem entirely appropriate. Although it may be a desirable goal to place causal inferences on a firm quantitative and structural foundation, at present we generally do not have all the information needed for doing so. The preceding list should therefore be considered to be only guidelines that can be of most value when coupled with reasoned judgment about the entire body of available evidence, in making decisions about causation.

In the next chapter, we address several additional issues that need to be considered in deriving causal inferences from epidemiologic studies.

REFERENCES

1. DeBakey M, Ochsner A: Primary pulmonary malignancy. Surg Gynecol Obstet 68:562, 1939.
2. Prentice RL, Kakar F, Hursting S, et al: Aspects of the rationale for the Women's Health Trial. J Natl Cancer Inst 80:802–814, 1988.
3. Austin DF, Karp S, Dworsky R, Henderson BE: Excess leukemia in cohorts of children born following influenza epidemics. Am J Epidemiol 101:77–83, 1977.
4. Diez Roux AV, Merkin SS, Arnett D, et al: Neighborhood of residence and incidence of coronary heart disease. N Engl J Med 345:99–106, 2001.
5. Yerushalmy J: Infants with low birth weight born before their mothers started to smoke cigarettes. Am J Obstet Gynecol 112:277–284, 1972.
6. Evans AS: Causation and Disease: A Chronological Journey. New York, Plenum, 1993, pp 13–39.
7. United States Department of Health, Education and Welfare: Smoking and Health: Report of the Advisory Committee to the Surgeon General. Washington, DC, Public Health Service, 1964.
8. Schwartz J: Air pollution and daily mortality: A review and meta analysis. Environ Res 64:36–52, 1994.
9. Marshall BJ, Warren JR: Unidentified curved bacilli in the stomachs of patients with gastritis and peptic ulceration. Lancet 1(8390):1311–1315, 1984.
10. Uemura N, Okamoto S, Yamomoto S, et al: *Helicobacter pylori* infection and the development of gastric cancer. N Engl J Med 345:784–789, 2001.
11. Grant BF, Dawson DA: Age at onset of alcohol use and its association with DSM-IV alcohol use and dependence: Results from the National Longitudinal Alcohol Epidemiologic Survey. J Subst Abuse 9:103–110, 1997.
12. Merkatz IR, Thompson JE (eds): New Perspectives on Prenatal Care. New York, Elsevier, 1990.
13. Gordis L, Kleinman JC, Klerman LV, et al: Criteria for evaluating evidence regarding the effectiveness of prenatal interventions. In Merkatz IR, Thompson JE (eds): New Perspectives on Prenatal Care. New York, Elsevier, 1990, pp 31–38.
14. Harris RP, Helfand M, Woolf SH, et al: Current methods of the U.S. Preventive Services Task Force: A review of the process. Am J Prev Med 20(Suppl 3):21–35, 2001.

REVIEW QUESTIONS FOR CHAPTER 14

1. In a large case-control study of patients with pancreatic cancer, 17% of the patients were found to be diabetic at the time of diagnosis, compared to 4% of a well-matched control group (matched by age, sex, ethnic group, and several other characteristics) that was examined for diabetes at the same time as the cases were diagnosed. It was concluded that the diabetes played a causal role in the pancreatic cancer. This conclusion:
   a. Is correct
   b. May be incorrect because there is no control or comparison group
   c. May be incorrect because of failure to establish the time sequence between onset of the diabetes and diagnosis of pancreatic cancer
   d. May be incorrect because of less complete ascertainment of diabetes in the pancreatic cancer cases
   e. May be incorrect because of more complete ascertainment of pancreatic cancer in nondiabetic persons

2. An investigator examined cases of fetal death in 27,000 pregnancies and classified mothers according to whether they had experienced sexual intercourse within 1 month before delivery. It was found that 11% of the mothers of fetuses that died and 2.5% of the mothers of fetuses that survived had had sexual intercourse during the period. It was concluded that intercourse during the month preceding delivery caused the fetal deaths. This conclusion:
   a. May be incorrect because mothers who had intercourse during the month before childbirth may differ in other important characteristics from those who did not
   b. May be incorrect because there is no comparison group
   c. May be incorrect because prevalence rates are used where incidence rates are needed
   d. May be incorrect because of failure to achieve a high level of statistical significance
   e. Both *b* and *c*

3. All of the following are important criteria when making causal inferences *except:*
   a. Consistency with existing knowledge
   b. Dose-response relationship
   c. Consistency of association in several studies
   d. Strength of association
   e. Predictive value

4. Ecologic fallacy refers to:
   a. Assessing exposure in large groups rather than in many small groups
   b. Assessing outcome in large groups rather than in many small groups
   c. Ascribing the characteristics of a group to every individual in that group
   d. Examining correlations of exposure and outcomes rather than time trends
   e. Failure to examine temporal relationships between exposures and outcomes

Questions 5 and 6 are based on the following information.

Factor A, B, or C can each individually cause a certain disease without the other two factors, but only when followed by exposure to factor X. Exposure to factor X alone is not followed by the disease, but the disease never occurs in the absence of exposure to factor X.

5. Factor X is:
   a. A necessary and sufficient cause
   b. A necessary, but not sufficient, cause
   c. A sufficient, but not necessary, cause
   d. Neither necessary nor sufficient
   e. None of the above

6. Factor A is:
   a. A necessary and sufficient cause
   b. A necessary, but not sufficient, cause
   c. A sufficient, but not necessary, cause
   d. Neither necessary nor sufficient
   e. None of the above

Chapter 15

More on Causal Inferences: Bias, Confounding, and Interaction

In this chapter, we continue the discussion of causation that was begun in Chapter 14. Our discussion here focuses on three important issues in deriving causal inferences: (1) bias, (2) confounding, and (3) interaction.

BIAS

Bias has been addressed in many of the previous chapters because it is a major issue in virtually any type of epidemiologic study design. Therefore, only a few additional comments are made here.

What do we mean by *bias?* Bias has been defined as "any systematic error in the design, conduct or analysis of a study that results in a mistaken estimate of an exposure's effect on the risk of disease."[1]

Selection Bias

What types of bias do we encounter in epidemiologic studies? The first is *selection bias.* If the way in which cases and controls, or exposed and nonexposed individuals, were selected is such that an apparent association is observed—even if, in reality, exposure and disease are not associated—the apparent association is the result of selection bias.

One form that selection bias can take results from nonresponse of potential study subjects. For example, if we are studying the possible relationship of an exposure and a disease and the response rate of potential subjects is higher in people with the disease who were exposed than in people with the disease who were not exposed, an apparent association could be observed even if in reality there is no association.

In general, people who do not respond in a study often differ from those who do in regard to many demographic, socioeconomic, cultural, lifestyle, and medical characteristics. One study that attempted to characterize nonresponders was reported by Ronmark et al. in 1999.[2] In the course of carrying out a prevalence study of asthma, chronic bronchitis, and respi-

ratory symptoms, they studied the characteristics of nonresponders and the reasons for nonresponse. In this study, 9,132 people living in Sweden were invited to participate. Data were obtained by a mailed questionnaire, and the response rate was 85%. A sample of nonresponders was contacted by telephone and interviewed using the same questionnaire. The authors found a significantly higher proportion of current smokers and manual laborers among the nonresponders than among the responders. In addition, the prevalence rates of wheezing, chronic cough, sputum production, attacks of breathlessness, and asthma and use of asthma medications were significantly higher among the nonresponders than among the responders.

Since in many studies no information is obtained from the nonresponders, nonresponse may introduce a serious bias that may be difficult to assess. It is therefore important to keep nonresponse to a minimum. In addition, any nonresponders should be characterized as much as possible by using whatever information is available to determine ways in which they differ from responders and to gauge the likely impact of their nonresponse on the results of the study.

It is important to keep in mind the distinction between *selecting subjects for a study* and *selection bias.* Virtually every study conducted in human populations selects study subjects from a larger population. The nature of this selection potentially affects the *generalizability* or *external validity* of the study but does not necessarily affect the validity of the comparisons made within the study or the study's *internal validity.* On the other hand, when a systematic error is made in selecting one or more of the study groups that will be compared, *selection bias* may result. Such a bias can result in odds ratios or relative risks that may not be correct estimates and consequently lead to nonvalid inferences regarding associations of exposure and disease. Selection bias is therefore an error in selecting a study group or groups within the study and can have a major impact on the internal validity of the study and the legitimacy of the conclusion. But the virtually universal need that arises in designing and implementing any study, to select a study population from a larger referent population, should not be confused with selection bias, which results from a systematic error in selecting subjects in one or more of the study groups, such as exposed or nonexposed, or cases or controls.

An interesting example of selection bias was demonstrated in 1974 with publication of data that appeared to suggest a relationship between use of reserpine (a commonly used antihypertensive agent) and increased risk of breast cancer. Three articles supporting such an association were published in the same issue of the *Lancet* in September 1974.[3–5] The three papers reported three studies conducted in Boston, Great Britain, and Helsinki, respectively.

Let us consider one of these articles, which exemplifies the problem we are discussing. Heinonen et al.[5] reported a matched-pair case-control study carried out in surgical patients at a hospital in Helsinki. Women with breast cancer were compared to women without breast cancer in terms of use of reserpine. Women with newly diagnosed breast cancer were identified from a hospital discharge register and from records that logged operations at the hospital. They served as "cases," and each was pair-matched by age and year of her operation to a control who was a woman admitted for elective surgery for some benign condition. A total of 438 case-control pairs were available for analysis. As seen in Table 15-1, there were 45 pairs in which the case used reserpine and the control did not and 23 pairs in which the control used reserpine and the case did not. The resulting matched pair odds ratio was 45/23 or 1.96.

A problem was recognized, however, in the method used for selecting controls. In selecting the controls, the authors excluded women with the following operations: cholecystectomy, thyroidectomy for thyrotoxicosis, surgery for renal disease, and any cardiac operation, sympathectomy, or vascular graft. They were excluded because at the time the study was conducted, reserpine was one of the agents often used in treating these conditions. The authors were concerned that if patients with these conditions were included in this case-control study, the prevalence of reserpine use in the controls would be artificially

high, so that even if reserpine use was increased in breast cancer cases, the increase might not be detected.

Unfortunately, in trying to address this concern, the authors created a different problem because these exclusions were not applied to the cases. By excluding patients with these conditions from the controls, they created a control group in which the prevalence of reserpine use was artificially lower because a large group of potential reserpine users were excluded. Thus, even if in reality reserpine use was not increased in women who developed breast cancer, this study could show a difference in reserpine use between the cases and the controls only because of the way the controls were selected.

This type of selection bias has been called *exclusion bias*.[6] It results from the investigators' applying different eligibility criteria to the cases and to the controls in regard to which clinical conditions in the past would permit eligibility in the study and which would serve as the basis for exclusion. Horwitz and Feinstein[6] tried to replicate the reserpine study in 257 women with breast cancer and 257 controls, calculating odds ratios in two ways: first, including all the women and second after excluding from the controls women with a history of cardiovascular disease. The odds ratio including all women was 1.1, but when women with cardiovascular disease were excluded, the odds ratio rose to 2.5. The findings support the suggestion that the apparent

---

TABLE 15-1. Results of a Matched-Pairs Analysis of a Case-Control Study of Reserpine Use and Breast Cancer

Breast Cancer Cases	Controls	
	Used Reserpine	*Did Not Use Reserpine*
Used Reserpine	8	45
Did Not Use Reserpine	23	362

Matched-pairs odds ratio $= \dfrac{45}{23} = 1.96$

Adapted from Heinonen OP, Shapiro S, Tuominen L, Turunen MI: Reserpine use in relation to breast cancer. Lancet 2:675–677, 1974.

relation of reserpine use and breast cancer in the Helsinki study resulted from selection bias due to the different criteria for selecting controls in the study. Another study that dealt with coffee and pancreatic cancer had a similar problem and was discussed in Chapter 10.

Information Bias

Information bias can occur when the means for obtaining information about the subjects in the study are inadequate so that as a result some of the information gathered regarding exposures and/or disease outcome is incorrect.

Given inaccuracies in methods of data acquisition, we may at times misclassify subjects and thereby introduce a *misclassification bias.* For example, in a case-control study, some people who have the disease (cases) may be misclassified as controls, and some without the disease (controls) may be misclassified as cases. This may result, for example, from limited sensitivity and specificity of the diagnostic tests involved or from inadequacy of information derived from medical or other records. Another possibility is that we may misclassify a person's exposure status: we may believe the person was exposed when this was not the case, or we may believe that the person was not exposed when, in fact, exposure did occur. If exposure data are based on interviews, for example, subjects may either not be aware of their exposure or may erroneously think that it did not occur. If ascertainment of exposure is based on old records, data may be incomplete or inaccurate.

Misclassification may occur in two forms: differential and nondifferential. In *differential misclassification*, the rate of misclassification differs in different study groups. For example, misclassification of exposure may occur such that cases are misclassified as being exposed more often than controls are. This was seen in the hypothetical example of recall bias presented in the discussion of case-control studies (see Chapter 10). Women who had a baby with a malformation tended to remember more mild infections that occurred during their pregnancies than did mothers of normal infants. Thus, there was a tendency for differential misclassification in regard to prenatal infection, in that more unexposed cases were misclassified as exposed than were unexposed controls. The result was an apparent association of malformations with infections, even though none existed. So a differential misclassification bias can lead either to an apparent association even if one

does not really exist or to an apparent lack of association when one does in fact exist.

In contrast, *nondifferential misclassification* results from the degree of inaccuracy that characterizes how information is obtained from any study group—either cases and controls or exposed and nonexposed persons. Such misclassification is not related to exposure status or to case or control status; it is just a problem inherent in the *data collection methods.* The usual effect of nondifferential misclassification is that the relative risk or odds ratio tends to be diluted, and it is shifted toward 1.0. In other words, we are less likely to detect an association even if one really exists.

This can be seen intuitively. Let us say that in reality there is a strong association of an exposure and a disease—that is, people without the disease have much less exposure than do people with the disease. By mistake, we have included some diseased persons in our control group and some nondiseased persons in our case group. We have, in other words, misclassified some of the subjects in regard to diagnosis. In this situation, our controls will not have such a low rate of exposure because some diseased people have been mistakenly included in this group, and our cases will not have such a high rate of exposure because some nondiseased people have been mistakenly included in the case group. As a result, a smaller difference in exposure will be found between our cases and our controls than actually exists between diseased and nondiseased people.

Some of the types and sources of information bias in epidemiologic studies are shown in Table 15-2.

Bias may be introduced in the way that information is abstracted from medical, employment, or other records or from the manner in which interviewers ask questions. Bias may also result from *surrogate interviews.* What does this mean? Suppose that we are carrying out a case-control study of pan-

---

TABLE 15-2. Some Types and Sources of Information Bias

Bias in abstracting records
Bias in interviewing
Bias from surrogate interviews
Surveillance bias
Recall bias
Reporting bias

creatic cancer. The case-fatality from this disease is very high, and the survival time is very short. When we prepare to interview cases, we find that many of them have died and that many of those who have survived are too ill to be interviewed. We may then approach a family member to obtain information about the case's employment history, diet, and other exposures and characteristics. The person interviewed is most often a spouse or a child. Several problems arise in obtaining information from such surrogates. First, they may not have accurate information about the case's history. A spouse may not know the work-related exposures of the case. Children often know even less than do spouses. Second, there is evidence that when a wife reports on her husband's work and lifestyle after he dies, she tends to elevate his occupational level and lifestyle. She may ascribe to him a higher occupation category than that in which he was actually engaged. She may also convert him posthumously to a nondrinker or nonsmoker or both.

If a population is monitored over a period of time, disease ascertainment may be better in the monitored population than in the general population, and may introduce a *surveillance bias*, which leads to an erroneous estimate of the relative risk or odds ratio. For example, some years ago a great deal of interest centered on the possible relationship of oral contraceptive use to thrombophlebitis. It was suggested that physicians monitored patients who had been prescribed oral contraceptives much more closely than they monitored their other patients. As a result, they were more apt to identify cases of thrombophlebitis that developed in those patients who were taking oral contraceptives (and who were therefore being more closely monitored) than among other patients who were not as well monitored. As a result, just through better ascertainment of thrombophlebitis in women receiving oral contraceptives, an apparent association of thrombophlebitis with oral contraceptive use may be observed, even if no true association exists.

In Chapter 10, we discussed *recall bias* in case-control studies. This bias operates to enhance recall in cases compared with controls. Thus a certain piece of information, such as a potentially relevant exposure, may be recalled by a case but forgotten by a control. A related type of bias is *reporting bias*, in which a subject may be reluctant to report an exposure he is aware of because of attitudes, beliefs, and perceptions. If such underreporting is more frequent either among the cases or among the controls, a bias may result. One example is presented below.

The term *wish bias* was coined by Wynder and coworkers[7] to denote the bias introduced by subjects who have developed a disease and who in attempting to answer the question "Why me?" seek to show, often unintentionally, that the disease is not their fault. Thus, they may deny certain exposures related to lifestyle (such as smoking or drinking); if they are contemplating litigation, they may overemphasize workplace-related exposures. Wish bias can be considered one type of reporting bias.

A point to remember is that *bias is a result of an error in the design or conduct of a study.* Efforts should therefore be made to reduce or eliminate bias or, at the very least, to recognize it and take it into account when interpreting the findings of a study. However, the data needed to document and assess the type and extent of bias may not always be available.

Let us consider an example. The relationship of induced abortion to risk of breast cancer has been a subject of considerable interest in recent years. Although in general no association has been reported for *spontaneous* abortion and risk of breast cancer, the data have been mixed in regard to the possible relationship of *induced* abortion and breast cancer. It was suggested that reporting bias might have played a role in those case-control studies that reported a positive association: healthy controls may have been more reluctant than women with breast cancer to report that they had had an induced abortion.

A study of induced abortion and risk of breast cancer provided an opportunity for the investigators to assess the extent and possible role of such reporting bias which is one type of information bias. Rookus and van Leeuwen[8] reported a case-control study in The Netherlands in which an overall estimated adjusted relative risk was 1.9 for induced abortion and breast cancer in parous women. (No association was found in nulliparous women.) They then compared the findings in two regions of the country—the southeastern region, which has a greater Roman Catholic, more conservative population, and the western region including Amsterdam, which has more liberal attitudes toward abortion. This difference in attitudes is reflected in the fact that the rates of induced abortions in the southeast have always been lower than in the west. As seen in Table 15-3, the authors found the association of induced abortion and breast cancer to be much stronger in the conservative southeast (estimated adjusted relative risk = 14.6) than in the more liberal west (estimated adjusted relative risk = 1.3), suggesting

TABLE 15-3. **Relative Risks* (RR) and 95% Confidence Intervals (CI) of the Development of Breast Cancer at Ages 20–45 Years in Relation to Previous Induced Abortions Reported by Parous Women in All Regions and in Western and Southeastern Regions of The Netherlands**

	Unadjusted RR	Adjusted RR[†]	95% CI
All regions	1.8	1.9	1.1–3.2
Western region	1.2	1.3	0.7–2.6
Southeastern region	12.3	14.6	1.8–120

*Relative risks estimated using conditional logistic regression methods for matched pairs.
[†]Adjusted for spontaneous or induced abortion, age at first full-term pregnancy, number of full-term pregnancies, weeks of breast-feeding, family history of breast cancer, and use of injectable contraceptives.
Adapted from Rookus MA, van Leeuwen FE: Induced abortion and risk for breast cancer: Reporting (recall) bias in a Dutch case-control study. J Natl Cancer Inst 88:1759–1764, 1996.

that the overall finding of an association of breast cancer and induced abortion in this study was largely attributable to underreporting of abortions by the controls in the southeast. Furthermore, since this study was part of a population-based case-control study of oral contraceptive use and breast cancer risk, it was possible to seek support for the possibility of such an underreporting bias as an explanation for regional differences. In the oral contraceptive study, when women's responses were compared with their physicians' prescriptions, controls in the southeastern region were found to have underreported the duration of their oral contraceptive use by more than 6 months more than did controls in the western region.

CONFOUNDING

A problem posed in many epidemiologic studies is that we observe a true association and are tempted to derive a causal inference when, in fact, the relationship may not be causal. This brings us to the subject of *confounding*, one of the most important problems in observational epidemiologic studies.

What do we mean by *confounding?* In a study of whether factor A is a cause of disease B, we say that a third factor, factor X, is a confounder if the following are true:

1. Factor X is a known risk factor for disease B.
2. Factor X is associated with factor A, but is not a result of factor A.

Recall the example we discussed in Chapter 10 of the relationship between coffee and cancer of the pancreas. Smoking was a confounder, because although we were interested in a possible relationship between coffee consumption (factor A) and pancreatic cancer (disease B), the following are true of smoking (factor X):

1. Smoking is a known risk factor for pancreatic cancer.
2. Smoking is associated with coffee drinking, but is not a result of coffee drinking.

So if an association is observed between coffee drinking and cancer of the pancreas, it may be (1) that coffee actually causes cancer of the pancreas, or (2) that the observed association of coffee drinking and cancer of the pancreas may be a result of confounding by cigarette smoking (i.e., we observe the association of coffee drinking and pancreatic cancer because cigarette smoking is a risk factor for pancreatic cancer and cigarette smoking is associated with coffee drinking) (Fig. 15-1).

When we observe an association we ask whether it is causal (see Fig. 15-1A) or whether it is a result

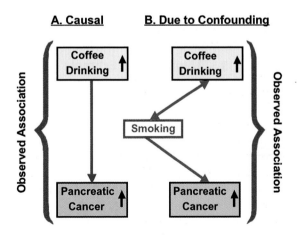

Figure 15-1. The association between coffee drinking and pancreatic cancer.

TABLE 15-4. Hypothetical Example of Confounding in an Unmatched Case-Control Study: I. Numbers of Exposed and Nonexposed Cases and Controls

Exposed	Cases	Controls
Yes	30	18
No	70	82
Total	100	100

$$\text{Odds ratio} = \frac{30 \times 82}{70 \times 18} = 1.95$$

TABLE 15-6. Hypothetical Example of Confounding in an Unmatched Case-Control Study: III. Relationship of Exposure to Age

Age (yr)	Total	Exposed	Not Exposed	% Exposed
<40	130	13	117	10
≥40	70	35	35	50

of confounding by a third factor that is both a risk factor for the disease and is associated with the exposure in question (see Fig. 15-1B).

Let us look at a hypothetical example: Table 15-4 shows data from an unmatched case-control study of an exposure and a disease, in which 100 cases and 100 controls were studied.

We calculate an unmatched odds ratio of 1.95. The question arises "Is this association of the exposure with the disease a causal one, or could it have resulted from differences in age distributions?" In other words, is the observed relationship confounded by age? The first question to ask in addressing this issue is whether age is related to being a case or a control. This question is answered by the analysis in Table 15-5.

We see that 80% of the controls are younger than 40 years of age, compared with only 50% of the cases. Thus, older age is associated with being a case (having the disease), and younger age is associated with being a control (not having the disease).

The next question is whether age is related to whether or not a person has been exposed.

Table 15-6 looks at the relationship of age to exposure for all 200 subjects studied, regardless of their case-control status. We see that 130 people were younger than 40 years (the 50 + 80 in the top row of Table 15-5), and of these, 13 (10%) were exposed. Among the 70 subjects who were older than 40 years, 35 (50%) were exposed. Thus, age is clearly related to exposure. So at this point we know that age is related to being a case (the cases were older than the controls); we also know that being exposed is related to older age.

As shown in Figure 15-2, the question is: Is the association of exposure and disease causal (Fig. 15-2A), or could we be seeing an association of exposure with disease only because there is an age difference between cases and controls, and older age is also related to being exposed (Fig. 15-2B)? Does exposure cause the disease (i.e., whether a person is a case or a control), or is the observation a result of confounding by a third factor (in this case, age)?

How can we clarify this issue? One approach is seen in Table 15-7. We can carry out a stratified analysis with subjects in two age groups: younger than 40 years and older than 40 years. Within each stratum a 2 × 2 table is created, and an odds ratio is calculated for each. When we calculate the odds ratio separately for the younger and the older subjects, we find the

TABLE 15-5. Hypothetical Example of Confounding in an Unmatched Case-Control Study: II. Distribution of Cases and Controls by Age

Age (yr)	Cases	Controls
<40	50	80
≥40	50	20
Total	100	100

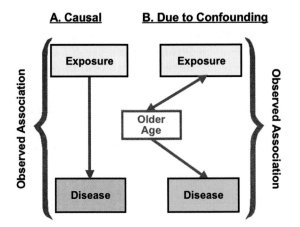

Figure 15-2. Schematic representation of the issue of potential confounding.

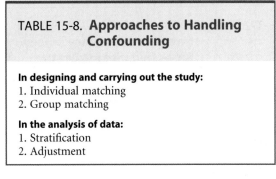

TABLE 15-8. **Approaches to Handling Confounding**

In designing and carrying out the study:
1. Individual matching
2. Group matching

In the analysis of data:
1. Stratification
2. Adjustment

TABLE 15-7. **Hypothetical Example of Confounding in an Unmatched Case-Control Study: IV. Calculations of Odds Ratios after Stratifying by Age**

Age (yr)	Exposed	Cases	Controls	Odds Ratio
<40	Yes	5	8	$\dfrac{5\times72}{45\times8}=\dfrac{360}{360}=1.0$
	No	45	72	
	Total	**50**	**80**	
≥40	Yes	25	10	$\dfrac{25\times10}{25\times10}=\dfrac{250}{250}=1.0$
	No	25	10	
	Total	**50**	**20**	

odds ratio to be 1.0 in each stratum. Thus, the only reason we originally had an odds ratio of 1.95 in Table 15-4 was because there was a difference in age distributions between the cases and the controls. Thus, in this example age is a confounder.

How can we address the problem of confounding? As seen in Table 15-8, the issue of confounding can be addressed either in designing and carrying out a study or in analysis of the data. In *designing and carrying out a study*, we can match the cases to the controls, as discussed in Chapter 10 (by either group matching or individual matching), for the factor that

we suspect could be a possible confounder. In this example, we could match by age to eliminate any age difference between the cases and the controls. If, after matching in this way, we then observe an association of exposure and disease, we would know that we could not attribute the association to an age difference.

Alternatively, we can handle the problem of confounding in the *data analysis* in one of two ways: stratification or adjustment. Let us briefly discuss stratification, which was just demonstrated in the hypothetical example. Let us say we are interested in the relationship of smoking and lung cancer. We want to know whether the observed higher risks of lung cancer in smokers could be a result of confounding by air pollution and/or urbanization. Perhaps we are observing a relationship of smoking and lung cancer not because smoking causes lung cancer, but because air pollution causes lung cancer and smoking is more frequent in polluted areas (i.e., in urban areas). Perhaps smokers just happen to live in the cities.

How can we address this question? One approach would be to stratify the data by degree of urbanization—rural, town, or major city. We then calculate the lung cancer rates in smokers and nonsmokers in each urbanization stratum (Table 15-9).

If the relationship of lung cancer to smoking is due to smoking, and not to the confounding effect of pollution and/or urbanization, then *in each stratum of urbanization* the incidence of lung cancer should be higher in smokers than in nonsmokers. It would then be clear that the observed association of smoking and lung cancer could not be due to degree of urbanization.

We may prefer not just to dichotomize smoking groups into smokers and nonsmokers, but to

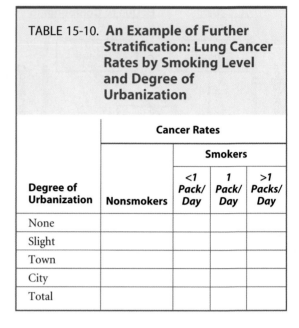

TABLE 15-9. **An Example of Stratification: Lung Cancer Rates by Smoking Status and Degree of Urbanization**

Degree of Urbanization	Cancer Rates	
	Nonsmokers	Smokers
None		
Slight		
Town		
City		
Total		

TABLE 15-10. **An Example of Further Stratification: Lung Cancer Rates by Smoking Level and Degree of Urbanization**

Degree of Urbanization	Cancer Rates			
		Smokers		
	Nonsmokers	<1 Pack/ Day	1 Pack/ Day	>1 Packs/ Day
None				
Slight				
Town				
City				
Total				

include in the analysis the number of cigarettes smoked.

In Table 15-10, we have expanded cigarette smoking into categories of amount smoked. Again, we can calculate the incidence in each cell of the table. If the observed association of cigarette smoking and lung cancer is not due to confounding by urbanization or pollution or both, we would expect to see a dose-response pattern *in each stratum of urbanization.*

Figure 15-3 shows actual age-adjusted lung cancer mortality rates per 100,000 man-years by urban-rural classification and smoking category. For each degree of urbanization, lung cancer mortality rates in smokers are shown by the blue bars, and non-smoker mortality rates are indicated by light green bars. From these data we see that in every level (or stratum) of urbanization, lung cancer mortality is higher in smokers than in nonsmokers. Therefore, the observed association of smoking and lung cancer cannot be attributed to level of urbanization. By examining each stratum separately, we are, in effect, holding urbanization constant, and we still find much higher lung cancer mortality in smokers than in nonsmokers.

At the same time, it is interesting to examine the data for nonsmokers (shown by the green bars). If we draw a line connecting the tops of these bars, we see that the higher the urbanization level, the higher the incidence of lung cancer in nonsmokers (Fig. 15-4). Thus, there is a dose-response relationship of lung cancer and urbanization in nonsmokers.

However, as we have seen, this relationship cannot explain the association of lung cancer with smoking as the latter relationship holds within each level of urbanization.

Figure 15-5 shows the relationship among smoking, drinking, and cancer of the esophagus. Four strata (levels) of amount smoked are shown. Within each smoking stratum, the risk of esophageal cancer is plotted in relation to the amount of alcohol consumed.

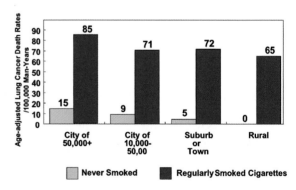

Figure 15-3. Age-adjusted lung cancer death rates per 100,000 man-years by urban-rural classification and by smoking category. (Adapted from Hammond EC, Horn D: Smoking and death rates: Report on 44 months of follow-up of 187,783 men: II. Death rates by cause. JAMA 166:1294–1308, 1958. Copyright 1958, American Medical Association.)

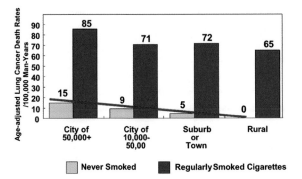

Figure 15-4. Relationship of degree of urbanization to lung cancer death rates in nonsmokers. The *sloping line* connects the age-adjusted lung cancer death rates per 100,000 man-years by urban-rural classification in nonsmokers. (Adapted from Hammond EC, Horn D: Smoking and death rates: Report on 44 months of follow-up of 187,783 men: II. Death rates by cause. JAMA 166:1294–1308, 1958. Copyright 1958, American Medical Association.)

It is interesting to note that in this presentation of data, we cannot compare smokers with nonsmokers or drinkers with nondrinkers because the authors have pooled the group that smokes 0 to 9 g of tobacco per day, and they have also pooled nondrinkers with minimal drinkers. Thus we have no rates for persons who are *nonexposed* to alcohol or tobacco. It would have been preferable to have kept the data for non-exposed persons separate so that relative risks could have been calculated based on rates in nonexposed persons.

Two final points on confounding: First, when we identify a confounder, we generally consider it a problem and want to find ways to address the issue of confounding. But sometimes finding a con-founded relationship can also be very useful. For even if the apparent association between factor A (the factor in which we are primarily interested) and disease B is actually due to some third confounding factor X so that factor A is not causally related to disease B, screening for factor A can nevertheless be useful because it permits us to identify people who are at high risk for the disease and direct appropri-ate preventive and therapeutic interventions to them. Thus, a confounded relationship may still be a helpful guide in screening populations even when we do not identify the specific etiologic agent involved.

What do we observe? The more a person smokes, the higher the levels of esophageal cancer. However, within each stratum of smoking, there is a dose-response relationship of esophageal cancer and the amount of alcohol consumed. Therefore, we cannot attribute to smoking the effects of alcohol con-sumption on esophageal cancer. Both smoking and alcohol have separate effects on the risk of esophageal cancer.

Second, confounding is not an error in the study, but rather is a true phenomenon that is identified in a study and must be understood. Bias is a result of an error in the way that the study has been

Figure 15-5. Relative risk of developing cancer of the esophagus in relation to smoking and drinking habits. (Adapted from Tuyns AJ, Pequignot G, Jensen OM: Esophageal cancer in Ille-et-Vilaine in relation to levels of alcohol and tobacco consumption: Risks are multiplying. Bull Cancer 64:45–60, 1977.)

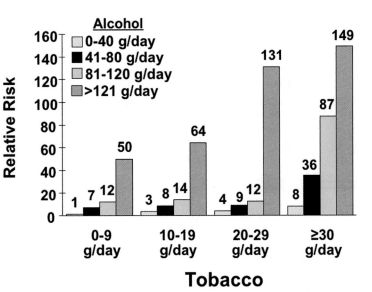

carried out, but confounding is a valid finding that describes the nature of the relationship among several factors and the risk of disease. However, *failure to take confounding into account in interpreting the results of a study* is indeed an error in the conduct of the study and can bias the conclusions of the study.

INTERACTION

To this point, our discussion has generally assumed the presence of a single causal factor in the etiology of a disease. Although this approach is useful for discussion purposes, in real life, we rarely deal with single causes. In the previous examples of the relationship of lung cancer to smoking and urbanization and the relationship of esophageal cancer to drinking and smoking, we have already seen more than one factor involved in disease etiology. In this section, we ask the question, "How do multiple factors interact in causing a disease?"

What do we mean by *interaction?* MacMahon[9] defined interaction as follows: "When the incidence rate of disease in the presence of two or more risk factors differs from the incidence rate expected to result from their individual effects." The effect can be greater than what we would expect (positive interaction, synergism) or less than what we would expect (negative interaction, antagonism). The problem is to determine what we would *expect* to result from the individual effects of the exposures.

Figure 15-6 shows an algorithm for exploring the possibility of interaction.

In examining our data, the first question is whether an association has been observed between an exposure and a disease. If so, is it due to confounding? If we decide that it is *not* due to confounding—that is, it is causal—then we ask whether the association is equally strong in each of the strata that are formed on the basis of some third variable. For example, is the association of smoking and lung cancer equally strong in strata formed on the basis of degree of urbanization? If the association is equally strong in all strata, there is no interaction. But if the association is of different strengths in different strata formed on the basis of age, for example (if the association is stronger in older people than in younger people), an interaction has been observed between age and exposure in producing the disease. If there were no interaction, we would expect the association to be of the same strength in each stratum.

Let us look more closely at interaction. Table 15-11 shows the incidence in persons exposed to either one of two risk factors (A or B), to both factors, or to neither factor, in a hypothetical example.

In persons with neither exposure, the incidence is 3.0. In persons exposed to factor A only and not to factor B, the incidence is 9.0. In persons exposed to factor B only and not to factor A, the incidence is 15.0. These are the individual effects of each factor considered separately.

What would we expect the incidence to be in persons who are exposed to both factors A and B (the lower right-hand cell in the table) if those people experienced the risk resulting from the independent contributions of both factors? The answer depends on the type of model that we propose. Let us assume that when there are two exposures, the effect of one exposure is *added* to the effect of the second expo-

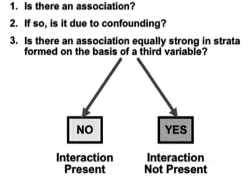

1. **Is there an association?**

2. **If so, is it due to confounding?**

3. **Is there an association equally strong in strata formed on the basis of a third variable?**

NO	YES
Interaction Present	Interaction Not Present

Figure 15-6. Questions to ask regarding possible interaction.

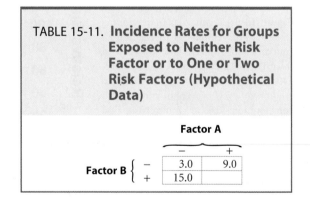

TABLE 15-11. **Incidence Rates for Groups Exposed to Neither Risk Factor or to One or Two Risk Factors (Hypothetical Data)**

		Factor A	
		−	+
Factor B	−	3.0	9.0
	+	15.0	

sure—that is, the model is *additive*. What, then, would we expect to see in the lower right-hand cell of the table? Let us use as an example the people who have neither exposure, whose risk in the absence of both exposures is 3.0. How does exposure to factor A affect their risk? It adds 6.0 to the 3.0 to produce a risk of 9.0. If factor A adds a risk of 6.0 to the risk that exists without factor A, it should have the same effect both in people exposed to factor B and in those not exposed to factor B. Because factor A adds 6.0 to the 3.0, it would also be expected to add 6.0 to the 15.0 rate of people exposed to factor B when they have exposure to A added as well. Thus, we would expect the effects of exposures to both factors to yield an incidence of 21.0.

We can also view this as follows: If factor B adds 12.0 to the 3.0 incidence of people with neither exposure, we would expect it to add 12.0 to any group, including the group exposed only to factor A, whose incidence is 9.0. Therefore, the effect of exposure to both A and B would be expected to equal 9.0 added to 12.0, or 21.0. (Remember that the 3.0 is a background risk that is present in the absence of both A and B. When we calculate the combined effect of factors A and B, we cannot just add 9.0 and 15.0—we must be sure that we do not count the background risk [3.0] twice.) The left-hand side of Table 15-12 shows the completed table from the partial data presented in Table 15-11.

Recall that when we discuss differences in risks, we are talking about *attributable risks*. This is shown on the right side of Table 15-12. If we examine

persons who have neither exposure, they have a background risk, but the attributable risk—that is, the risk attributable to exposure to factor A or B—is 0. As stated earlier, exposure only to factor A adds 6, and exposure only to factor B adds 12. What will the attributable risk be for both exposures? The answer is 18, that is, 18 more than the background risk. The additive model is summarized in Table 15-13.

What if an additive model does not describe correctly the effect of exposure to two independent factors? Perhaps a second exposure does not *add* to the effect of the first exposure but instead *multiplies* the effect of the first exposure. If having a certain exposure doubles a person's risk, we might expect it to double that risk regardless of whether or not that person had another exposure. For example, if the effect of alcohol is to double a person's risk for a certain cancer, we might expect it to double that risk for both smokers and nonsmokers. The appropriate model for the effects of two independent factors might therefore be a *multiplicative* rather than an additive model.

Let us return to our original data on risk resulting from neither exposure, or from exposure to factor A or B. These data are shown again in Table 15-14.

We see that exposure to factor A triples the risk, compared with that seen when factor A is absent (9.0 compared with 3.0). What would we therefore expect to find in the lower right-hand cell of the table when both exposures are present? Since in the absence of factor B, factor A has tripled the risk of 3.0, we would

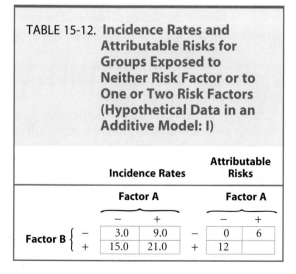

TABLE 15-12. **Incidence Rates and Attributable Risks for Groups Exposed to Neither Risk Factor or to One or Two Risk Factors (Hypothetical Data in an Additive Model: I)**

		Incidence Rates			Attributable Risks	
		Factor A			Factor A	
		−	+		−	+
Factor B	−	3.0	9.0	−	0	6
	+	15.0	21.0	+	12	

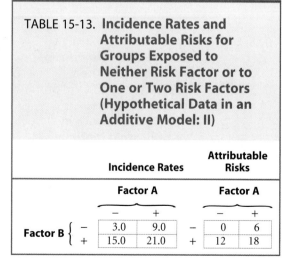

TABLE 15-13. **Incidence Rates and Attributable Risks for Groups Exposed to Neither Risk Factor or to One or Two Risk Factors (Hypothetical Data in an Additive Model: II)**

		Incidence Rates			Attributable Risks	
		Factor A			Factor A	
		−	+		−	+
Factor B	−	3.0	9.0	−	0	6
	+	15.0	21.0	+	12	18

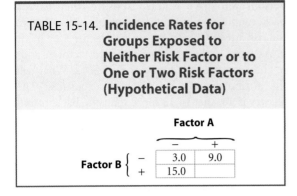

TABLE 15-14. **Incidence Rates for Groups Exposed to Neither Risk Factor or to One or Two Risk Factors (Hypothetical Data)**

		Factor A	
		−	+
Factor B	−	3.0	9.0
	+	15.0	

also expect it to triple the risk of 15.0 observed when exposure to factor B is present. If so, the effect from exposure to both factors would be 45.0. Again, we can calculate this in a different fashion. Factor B multiplies the risk by 5 (15.0 compared to 3.0) when factor A is absent. We would therefore expect it to have the same effect when factor A is present. Because the risk when factor A is present is 9.0, we would expect the presence of factor B to yield a risk of 45.0 (9.0 × 5) (Table 15-15).

The left-hand side of Table 15-15 shows the completed incidence rate table. Our discussion of a multiplicative model is of a *relative risk model*. This is shown on the right-hand side of the table. What value would we expect to find in the blank cell?

If we now assign the background risk (3.0) a value of 1, against which to compare the other values in the table, exposure to factor A triples the risk, yielding a

TABLE 15-16. **Incidence Rates and Relative Risks for Groups Exposed to Neither Risk Factor or to One or Two Risk Factors (Hypothetical Data in a Multiplicative Model: II)**

		Incidence Rates		Relative Risks	
		Factor A		Factor A	
		−	+	−	+
Factor B	−	3.0	9.0	1	3
	+	15.0	45.0	5	15

relative risk of 3 for factor A in the absence of factor B. Factor B multiplies the risk by 5, yielding a relative risk of 5 for exposure to factor B in the absence of factor A. When both factors A and B are operating, we would expect to see a relative risk of 15—(45.0/3.0) as seen on the left or 3 × 5 as seen on the right in Table 15-16.

We have considered two models: additive and multiplicative. The questions remain, "What would we expect to see as a result of the independent effects of two risk factors? Do we expect an additive model or a multiplicative model?"

The answers may not be obvious. If two factors are operating and the incidence is 21.0, the result is consistent with an additive model. If the incidence is 45.0, the result is consistent with a multiplicative model. However, if the incidence resulting from two factors is 60.0, for example, even the value for a multiplicative model is clearly exceeded, and an interaction is present—that is, an effect greater than would be expected from the independent effects of the two separate factors.

However, if the incidence is 30.0, it is less than expected from a multiplicative model and more than expected from an additive model. The question again is, "Is this more than we would expect from the independent effects of the two factors?" It is difficult to know the answer without more information about the biology of the disease, the mechanisms involved in the pathogenesis of the disease, and how such factors operate at cellular and molecular levels. Most experts accept any effect greater than additive as evidence of positive interaction, which is also called

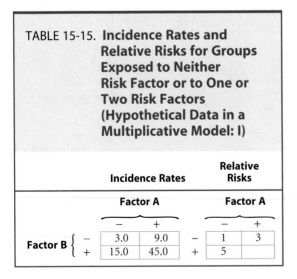

TABLE 15-15. **Incidence Rates and Relative Risks for Groups Exposed to Neither Risk Factor or to One or Two Risk Factors (Hypothetical Data in a Multiplicative Model: I)**

		Incidence Rates		Relative Risks	
		Factor A		Factor A	
		−	+	−	+
Factor B	−	3.0	9.0	1	3
	+	15.0	45.0	5	

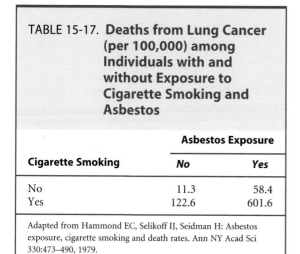

TABLE 15-17. Deaths from Lung Cancer (per 100,000) among Individuals with and without Exposure to Cigarette Smoking and Asbestos

	Asbestos Exposure	
Cigarette Smoking	*No*	*Yes*
No	11.3	58.4
Yes	122.6	601.6

Adapted from Hammond EC, Selikoff IJ, Seidman H: Asbestos exposure, cigarette smoking and death rates. Ann NY Acad Sci 330:473–490, 1979.

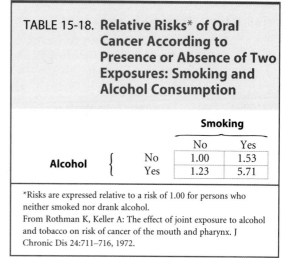

TABLE 15-18. Relative Risks* of Oral Cancer According to Presence or Absence of Two Exposures: Smoking and Alcohol Consumption

		Smoking	
		No	Yes
Alcohol {	No	1.00	1.53
	Yes	1.23	5.71

*Risks are expressed relative to a risk of 1.00 for persons who neither smoked nor drank alcohol.
From Rothman K, Keller A: The effect of joint exposure to alcohol and tobacco on risk of cancer of the mouth and pharynx. J Chronic Dis 24:711–716, 1972.

synergism. However, this opinion is often based on statistical considerations, whereas the validity of the model should ideally be based on biologic knowledge. The model may differ from one disease to another and from one exposure to another.

Let us consider a few examples. In a cohort study of smoking and lung cancer, Hammond and colleagues[10] studied the risk of lung cancer in 17,800 asbestos workers in the United States and in 73,763 men who were not exposed to asbestos in relation to their smoking habits. Table 15-17 shows the findings for deaths from lung cancer in relation to exposure. If the relationship between smoking and asbestos exposure were additive, we would expect the risk in those exposed to both smoking and asbestos (the lower right-hand cell) to be 58.4 + 122.6 − 11.3, or 169.7. (The 11.3 background risk is subtracted to avoid counting it twice.) Clearly, the observed value of 601.6 is much greater than the expected additive value. In fact, the data in this table closely approximate a multiplicative model and strongly suggest synergism between asbestos exposure and smoking.

A second example is seen in Table 15-18, which shows the relative risk of oral cancer by presence or absence of two exposures: smoking and alcohol consumption. The risk is set at 1.00 for persons with neither exposure. Is there evidence of an interaction? What would we expect the risk to be if the effect were multiplicative? We would expect 1.53 × 1.23, or 1.88. Clearly, the observed effect of 5.71 is higher than a multiplicative effect and indicates the presence of interaction.

Let us look at more detailed data for these relationships using dose data for alcohol consumption and for smoking (Table 15-19).

Again, the risk in those who do not drink and do not smoke is set at 1.0. In those with the highest level of alcohol consumption and the highest level of smoking, the risk is 15.50. Is an interaction evident? The data appear to support this. The highest values in smokers who are nondrinkers and in drinkers who are nonsmokers are 2.43 and 2.33, respectively; the value of 15.5 clearly exceeds the resulting product of

TABLE 15-19. Risk Ratios* for Oral Cancer According to Level of Exposure to Alcohol and Smoking—I

Alcohol Consumption (oz/day)	Cigarette Equivalents per Day			
	0	*<20*	*20–39*	*≥40*
0	1.00	1.52	1.43	2.43
<0.4	0.40	1.67	3.18	3.25
0.4–1.5	1.60	4.36	4.46	8.21
>1.5	2.33	4.13	9.59	15.50

*Risks are expressed relative to a risk of 1.00 for persons who neither smoked nor drank.
From Rothman K, Keller A: The effect of joint exposure to alcohol and tobacco on risk of cancer of the mouth and pharynx. J Chronic Dis 25:711–716, 1972.

TABLE 15-20. Risk Ratios* for Oral Cancer According to Level of Exposure to Alcohol and Smoking—II

Alcohol Consumption (oz/Day)	Cigarette Equivalents per Day			
	0	**<20**	**20–39**	**≥40**
None	1.00	1.52	1.43	2.43
<0.4	0.40	1.67	3.18	3.25
0.4–1.5	1.60	4.36	4.46	8.21
>1.5	2.33	4.13	9.59	15.50

*Risks are expressed relative to a risk of 1.00 for persons who neither smoked nor drank.
From Rothman K, Keller A: The effect of joint exposure to alcohol and tobacco on risk of cancer of the mouth and pharynx. J Chronic Dis 25:711–716, 1972.

TABLE 15-21. Relative Risks of Lung Cancer According to Smoking and Radiation Exposure in Two Populations

Radiation Level	Uranium Workers (Smoking Level)		A-bomb Survivors (Smoking Level)	
	Low	**High**	**Low**	**High**
Low	1.0	7.7	1.0	9.7
High	18.2	146.8	6.2	14.2

From Blot WJ, Akiba S, Kato H: Ionizing radiation and lung cancer: A review including preliminary results from a case-control study among A-bomb survivors. In Prentice RL, Thompson DJ (eds): Atomic Bomb Survivor Data: Utilization and Analysis. Philadelphia, Society for Industrial and Applied Mathematics, 1984, pp 235–248.

5.66 that would be expected with a multiplicative effect.

However, a problem with these data should be mentioned. Note that each category of smoking or drinking has upper and lower boundaries except for the highest categories, which have no upper boundaries. Therefore, the high risk of 15.50 could result from the presence of one or a few extreme outliers—either extraordinarily heavy smokers or extraordinarily heavy drinkers.

Is there a way to avoid this problem and still use the data shown here? We could ignore the right-hand column and the bottom row and look only at the resulting 3 × 3 table (Table 15-20). Now all of the categories have both upper and lower boundaries. If the model was multiplicative we would expect to see 1.43 × 1.60, or 2.29, rather than the 4.46 actually observed. Thus, we still see evidence of interaction, but much weaker evidence than we had seen in the full table, with its indefinite high-exposure categories. This suggests that the problem of the lack of upper boundaries of categories was indeed a contributor to the high value of 15.50 seen in the 4 × 4 table.

As we have said, the decision as to whether an additive model or a multiplicative model is most relevant in a given situation should depend on the biology of the disease. Table 15-21 shows interesting data regarding the risks of cancer from radiation and smoking in two different populations: uranium workers (left) and survivors of the atomic bomb

(right). Each table shows low and high levels of smoking and low and high levels of radiation.

What kind of model is suggested by the table on the left? Clearly, a multiplicative relationship is suggested; 146.8 is close to the product of 7.7 × 18.2. The table on the right suggests an additive model; 14.2 is close to the sum of 9.7 + 6.2 − 1.0. Therefore, although the data address radiation and smoking in two populations, in one setting, the exposures relate in an additive way, and in the other, they relate in a multiplicative way. It is not known whether this is a result of differences in radiation exposure in uranium mines compared with that from atomic bombs. Such a hypothesis is not unreasonable; we know that there was even a difference in the radiation emitted by the atomic bombs at Hiroshima and Nagasaki and that the dose-response curves for cancer were different in the two cities. In any case, the fact that two exposures that are ostensibly the same (or, at least, similar) may have different interrelationships in different settings is an intriguing observation that requires further exploration.

Finally, a dramatic example of interaction is seen in the relationship of aflatoxin and chronic hepatitis B infection to the risk of liver cancer (Table 15-22). In this study, hepatitis B infection alone multiplied the risk of liver cancer by 7.3; aflatoxin exposure alone multiplied the risk by 3.4. However, when both exposures were present, the relative risk rose to

TABLE 15-22. Risks* of Liver Cancer for Persons Exposed to Aflatoxin or Chronic Hepatitis B Infection: An Example of Interaction

	Aflatoxin-Negative	Aflatoxin-Positive
HBsAg[†] negative	1.0	3.4
HBsAg positive	7.3	59.4

*Adjusted for cigarette smoking.
[†]HBsAg, hepatitis B surface antigen.
Adapted from Qian GS, Ross RK, Yu MC, et al: A follow-up study of urinary markers of aflatoxin exposure and liver cancer risk in Shanghai, People's Republic of China. Cancer Epidemiol Biomarkers Prev 3:3–10, 1994.

59.4, far in excess of what we might expect in an additive model. Such an observation of synergy is of major clinical and public health interest, but also suggests important directions for further laboratory research into the etiology and pathogenesis of liver cancer.

The finding of interaction or synergism may also have practical policy implications involving issues such as who is responsible for a disease and who should pay compensation to the victims. For example, earlier in this chapter we discussed the relationship of smoking and asbestos exposure in producing cancer, a relationship that clearly is strongly interactive or synergistic. Litigation against asbestos manufacturers dates back at least to the 1970s and large awards were made by the courts. In 1998, at a time of increasing legal actions against the tobacco companies, a coalition of some of the victims of asbestos exposure joined forces with asbestos manufacturers to demand that Congress set aside a large amount of money from any national tobacco settlement bill to compensate people whose cancer was caused by the combined exposure to both asbestos and tobacco, a claim they justified by pointing to the synergistic relationship of these exposures. Those who objected to this demand claimed that those making the demand were in effect freeing the asbestos manufacturers from paying their obligation and were doing so only because they believed that it might be easier to obtain significant compensation from tobacco companies than from asbestos manufacturers. In so doing, they were willing to forge an alliance with asbestos manufacturers who had previously been found responsible for their disease. The basis for this approach was the well-documented synergism of asbestos and tobacco smoking in causing cancer.

CONCLUSION

This chapter has reviewed the concepts of bias, confounding, and interaction in relation to the derivation of causal inferences. Biases reflect inadequacies in the design or conduct of a study and clearly affect the validity of the findings. Biases therefore need to be assessed and, if possible, eliminated. Confounding and interaction, on the other hand, describe the reality of the interrelationships between certain factors and a certain outcome. Confounding and interaction characterize virtually every situation in which etiology is addressed, because most causal questions involve the relationships of multiple exposures and multiple, possibly etiologic, factors. Such relationships are particularly important in investigating the roles of genetic and environmental factors in disease causation and in assigning responsibility for adverse health outcomes from environmental exposures. Assessing the relative contributions of genetic and environmental factors is discussed in Chapter 16.

REFERENCES

1. Schlesselman JJ: Case-Control Studies: Design, Conduct, and Analysis. New York, Oxford University Press, 1982.
2. Ronmark E, Lundqvist A, Lundback B, Nystrom L: Non-responders to a postal questionnaire on respiratory symptoms and diseases. Eur J Epidemiol 15:292–299, 1999.
3. Boston Collaborative Drug Surveillance Program: Reserpine and breast cancer. Lancet 2:669–671, 1974.
4. Armstrong B, Stevens B, Doll R: Retrospective study of the association between use of *Rauwolfia* derivatives and breast cancer in English women. Lancet 2:672–675, 1974.
5. Heinonen OP, Shapiro S, Tuominen L, Turunen MI: Reserpine use in relation to breast cancer. Lancet 2:675–677, 1974.
6. Horwitz RI, Feinstein AR: Exclusion bias and the false relationship of reserpine and breast cancer. Arch Intern Med 145:1873–1875, 1985.
7. Wynder EL, Higgins IT, Harris RE: The wish bias. J Clin Epidemiol 43:619–621, 1991.

8. Rookus MA, van Leeuwen FE: Induced abortion and risk for breast cancer: Reporting (recall) bias in a Dutch case-control study. J Natl Cancer Inst 88:1759–1764, 1996.

9. MacMahon B: Concepts of multiple factors. In Lee DH, Kotin P (eds): Multiple Factors in the Causation of Envi-

ronmentally Induced Disease. New York, Academic Press, 1972.

10. Hammond EC, Selikoff IJ, Seidman H: Asbestos exposure, cigarette smoking and death rates. Ann NY Acad Sci 330: 473–490, 1979.

REVIEW QUESTIONS FOR CHAPTER 15

1. Which of the following is an approach to handling confounding?
   a. Individual matching
   b. Stratification
   c. Group matching
   d. Adjustment
   e. All of the above

2. It has been suggested that physicians may examine women who use oral contraceptives more often or more thoroughly than women who do not. If so, and if an association is observed between phlebitis and oral contraceptive use, the association may be due to:
   a. Selection bias
   b. Interviewer bias
   c. Surveillance bias
   d. Nonresponse bias
   e. Recall bias

Questions 3 through 6 are based on the information given below:

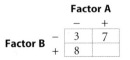

Factor A

		−	+
Factor B	−	3	7
	+	8	

3. Fill in the blank cell in the first table using the additive model of interaction: _____

4. Fill in the blank cell in the first table using the multiplicative model of interaction: _____

Convert the numbers in the above table to attributable risks for the additive model (below, left) and relative risks for the multiplicative model (below, right).

5. Fill in the bottom right cell of the table at the bottom of the left column for the attributable risk of having both factors A and B (additive model): _____

6. Fill in the bottom right cell of the table at the bottom of the left column for the relative risk of having both factors A and B (multiplicative model): _____

Question 7 is based on the information given below:

In a case-control study of the relationship of radiation exposure and thyroid cancer, 50 cases admitted for thyroid cancer and 100 "controls" admitted during the same period for treatment of hernias were studied. Only the cases were interviewed, and 20 of the cases were found to have been exposed to x-ray therapy in the past, based on the interviews and medical records. The controls were not interviewed, but a review of their hospital records when they were admitted for hernia surgery revealed that only 2 controls had been exposed to x-ray therapy in the past.

7. Based on the description given above, what source of bias is *least likely* to be present in this study?
   a. Recall bias
   b. Bias due to controls being nonrepresentative of the nondiseased population
   c. Bias due to use of different methods of ascertainment of exposure in the cases and controls
   d. Bias due to loss of subjects from the control group over time
   e. Selection bias for exposure to x-ray therapy in the past

8. In 1990, a case-control study was conducted to investigate the positive association between artificial sweetener use and bladder cancer. Controls were selected from a hospital sample of patients diagnosed with obesity-related conditions. Obesity-related conditions have been positively

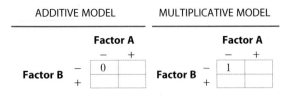

ADDITIVE MODEL		MULTIPLICATIVE MODEL	
Factor A		**Factor A**	

		−	+			−	+
Factor B	−	0		**Factor B**	−	1	
	+				+		

associated with artificial sweetener use. How would the use of these patients as controls affect the estimate of the association between artificial sweetener use and bladder cancer?

a. The estimate of association would accurately reflect the true association regardless of the association between artificial sweetener use and obesity-related conditions

b. The estimate of association would tend to underestimate the true association

c. More information is needed on the strength of association between artificial sweetener use and obesity-related conditions before any judgment can be made

d. The estimate of association would tend to overestimate the true association

e. More information is needed on the strength of association between artificial sweetener use and bladder cancer before any judgment can be made

Chapter 16

Identifying the Roles of Genetic and Environmental Factors in Disease Causation

To produce another Wolfgang Amadeus Mozart, we would need not only Wolfgang's genome but his mother's uterus, his father's music lessons, his parents' friends and his own, the state of music in 18th century Austria, Haydn's patronage, and on and on, in ever-widening circles. Without Mozart's set of genes, the rest would not suffice; there was, after all, only one Wolfgang Amadeus Mozart. But we have no right to the converse assumption: that his genome, cultivated in another world at another time, would result in the same musical genius. If a particular strain of wheat yields different harvests under different conditions of climate, soil and cultivation, how can we assume that so much more complex a genome as that of a human being would yield its desired crop of operas, symphonies and chamber music under different circumstances of nurture?[1]
—Leon Eisenberg, MD

In previous chapters we discussed study designs for identifying the causes of disease and focused primarily on the possible etiologic role of environmental factors. However, in order to prevent disease, we must take into account the major part played by genetic factors and look at the interaction of genetic susceptibility and exposure to environmental factors. Human beings clearly differ from one another in physical characteristics, personality, and other factors. They also differ in genetically determined susceptibility to disease. When we investigate the etiology of a disease, we are explicitly or implicitly asking the question: How much of the incidence of the disease is due to genetic factors, how much is due to environmental factors, and how do these types of factors interact with each other in increasing or decreasing the risk of disease?

Clearly, disease does not necessarily develop in everyone exposed to an environmental risk factor. Even if the relative risk for a specific factor and a disease is very high, the notion of attributable risk conveys the message that not all occurrence of a disease is due only to the specific exposure in question. For example, the relationship of cigarette smoking and lung cancer has been clearly demonstrated. However, lung cancer does not develop in everyone who smokes, and it does develop in some nonsmokers. Either another environment cofactor is needed in addition to cigarette smoking or individuals differ in genetic susceptibility or both.

People often adopt a fatalistic approach if a disease is primarily genetic in origin. But even in diseases that are primarily of genetic origin, a tremendous amount of environmental interaction often occurs. For example, phenylketonuria is characterized by a genetically determined deficiency of phenylalanine hydroxylase; the affected child cannot metabolize the essential amino acid phenylalanine, and the result of the phenylalanine accumulation is irreversible mental retardation. Can we prevent the genetic abnormality? No, we cannot. Can we reduce the likelihood that a child afflicted with this genetic abnormality will manifest mental retardation? Yes, we can do so by reducing or eliminating the child's exposure to phenylalanine by providing a diet that is low in phenylalanine. In this example, the adverse effects of a genetic disease can be prevented by controlling the affected person's environment so that the manifestations are not expressed. Thus, from standpoints of both clinical and public health, it is important to keep in mind the interrelationships between genetic and environmental factors in disease causation and expression.

Another example is Down syndrome, in which a trisomy of chromosome 21 occurs in one of two forms: either a nondisjunction occurs—that is, the chromosomes fail to separate during cell division, or a translocation of chromosome 21 is passed on together with a normal chromosome 21 from a balanced carrier. Nondisjunction is more common in older women. Thus nondisjunction Down syndrome is more common in babies born to women who are older than 35 years at the time of pregnancy. Why is there a greater likelihood of nondisjunction in babies of women who are in their late 30s than in those of women who are in their late 20s? Something must happen to cause the increased risk—possibly an accumulation of environmental insults or some other manifestation of biologic aging. To say that Down syndrome is genetic does not account for the age-related change in risk, which may well reflect the interrelation of genetic and environmental factors.

The interaction of genetic and environmental factors was succinctly described many years ago by Lancelot Hogben, who wrote:

> Our genes cannot make bricks without straw. The individual differences which men and women display are partly due to the fact that they receive different genes from their parents and partly due to the fact that the same genes live in different houses.[2]

In this chapter, we discuss some of the approaches used by epidemiologists to distinguish the relative contributions of genetic and environmental factors to disease causation. The discussion covers the use of classical epidemiologic methods and also introduces some of the newer approaches that have been made possible by advances in laboratory genetics and molecular biology.

ASSOCIATION WITH KNOWN GENETIC DISEASES

If we are interested in whether a certain disease has a strong genetic component, one question we can ask is whether the disease is associated with other diseases or conditions that are known to have strong genetic components. Several examples are seen in Table 16-1. Children with Down syndrome are known to be at high risk for leukemia. Down syndrome has also shown to be associated with Alzheimer's disease. Breast cancer is known to have a high incidence in males with Klinefelter's syndrome (XXY syndrome). Familial adenomatous polyposis is associated with colon cancer, and homocystinuria is linked to throm-

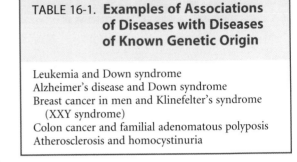

TABLE 16-1. Examples of Associations of Diseases with Diseases of Known Genetic Origin

Leukemia and Down syndrome
Alzheimer's disease and Down syndrome
Breast cancer in men and Klinefelter's syndrome (XXY syndrome)
Colon cancer and familial adenomatous polyposis
Atherosclerosis and homocystinuria

bosis and atherosclerosis. If we identify such associations between the condition of interest and a disease that has a known genetic etiology, it does not prove that the disease is genetically determined, but it does indicate that at least some components of the causation of the disease or some cases of this disease are likely to be due to genetic factors.

A related approach when a disease occurs in both hereditary and nonhereditary forms is to try to identify genes responsible for the hereditary form in the hope that such identification will provide a clue to the role of genetic factors in nonhereditary cases. In 1994, Miki and coworkers identified a gene designated *BRCA1 (Breast Cancer 1)* that when mutated appeared to be responsible for most hereditary breast cancer cases as well as ovarian cancer cases.[3]

Studies of breast cancer pedigrees not linked to *BRCA1* subsequently led to the discovery of the *BRCA2* gene. While the relative risk of early onset breast cancer is increased in women with *BRCA2* mutations, it is lower than in women with *BRCA1* mutations. Although the risk for ovarian cancer is also increased, it appears to be lower in women with *BRCA2* than in women with *BRCA1* mutations. Small increases in prostate and pancreatic cancers have also been seen in *BRCA2* pedigrees. About half of all inherited cases of breast cancer (5% of all breast cancer cases) seem to result from mutations in *BRCA1* or *BRCA2*. In Ashkenazi Jewish women, two mutations in *BRCA1* and one in *BRCA2* appear to account for about 25% of early onset breast cancer.

With the isolation of these candidate genes, the prospects for improved understanding of the role of genetic factors in nonhereditary cases of breast cancer seemed greatly enhanced. However, in contrast to mutations in other tumor-suppressor genes, *BRCA1* and *BRCA2* mutations are rarely seen in noninherited forms of breast cancer, suggesting that the genetic pathways or mechanisms operating in inherited breast cancers may differ from those operating in noninherited cases.

It has been estimated that the lifetime risk of breast cancer in women with a *BRCA1* or *BRCA2* mutation ranges from about 50% to 85%, compared to 12% in the general population. Up to 40% of women with a *BRCA1* mutation and 20% of women with a *BRCA2* mutation will develop ovarian cancer, compared to 1.5% in the general population. The findings regarding *BRCA1* and *BRCA2* have suggested the possibility that genetic testing might be recommended for certain high-risk population subgroups such as Ashkenazi Jews. However, many ethical and policy issues arise relating to possible genetic testing in such groups, and these have been further complicated by the fact that over time, the risk estimates reported for these mutations have tended to be lower than those originally reported, probably because the original estimates were generated in high-risk families with strong family histories. Multiple family members were affected, often with an early age at onset. The more recent lower estimates were derived from studies in less selected populations and from a population-based study in Washington, DC.[4] Thus, definitive recommendations regarding screening for these mutations in Ashkenazi Jewish women not selected for family history of breast cancer must await better data regarding the level of risk associated with these mutations in populations not selected on the basis of family history.

In 1995, Savitsky and associates, working with others on a team led by Shiloh, discovered a gene that when mutated causes the serious and rare autosomal recessive disorder, ataxia telangiectasia (AT).[5] The gene called *ATM* (for AT, mutated) may also be the most important cause of hereditary breast cancer. This possibility is based on epidemiologic evidence from studies of relatives of AT patients that suggest that the risk of breast cancer is increased fivefold in female carriers of the *ATM* gene. Identification of the *ATM* gene permits study of its role in cases of hereditary breast cancer that have not been linked to other breast cancer genes such as *BRCA1*. Although AT is a rare disease, about 0.5% to 1.4% of the population carries one defective gene, so that the gene could account for up to 8% of all breast cancers.[6]

USE OF GENETIC MARKERS

Genetic markers are genes or gene products that can be evaluated by laboratory methods. Transmission of markers from parent to offspring is observable, and the chromosomal location of genetic markers is often known. Several types of genetic markers can now be tested for in the laboratory as the direct result of revolutionary advances in molecular biology. The new methods which have been developed have helped clarify the process of protein synthesis, in which DNA codes for the production of amino acids and proteins.

Protein synthesis comprises two steps: (1) transcription and (2) translation. In step 1, *transcription,* one strand of a DNA double helix serves as a template for the synthesis of a messenger RNA (mRNA) by mRNA polymerase. In step 2, *translation,* the mRNA guides synthesis of the protein by adding amino acids one by one, as originally determined by the DNA sequences and represented by the messenger RNA.[7] Increased understanding of this process has provided a framework for the two approaches to studying genetic markers in the laboratory listed in Table 16-2: A, Analysis of DNA markers, and B, Analysis of gene products, namely, proteins.

It has also been recognized that virtually every cell in the body has a full set of chromosomes and identical genes, but in any specific type of cell only a small subset of these genes is turned on. These "expressed" genes confer unique properties on each cell type. Gene expression is regulated by an "on and off" switch and by a "volume control" that increases or decreases the level of expression of various genes as needed. By studying the kinds and amounts of mRNA produced by a cell, we can determine which genes are

---

TABLE 16-2. Types and Examples of Genetic Markers Used in Studies of Associations of an Allele and a Disease

A. Analysis of DNA markers
1. Allelic variants of genes
2. Restriction fragment length polymorphisms (RFLP)
3. Variable tandem repeats (VTRs)
4. Single nucleotide polymorphisms (SNPs)

B. Analysis of gene products or their phenotypic expression
1. Blood groups
2. Human leukocyte antigens (HLA)
3. Protein polymorphisms (apoliprotein E)

Modified from Khoury MJ, Beaty TH, Cohen BH: Fundamentals of Genetic Epidemiology. New York, Oxford University Press, 1993.

expressed and to what extent each is expressed. In this way we can gain insight into how the cell responds to changing demands including those resulting from environmental challenges.[8]

A major methodologic advance has been DNA microarray technology which capitalizes on the ability of a given mRNA molecule to bind specifically (hybridize) to the DNA template from which it originated. By using an array containing many DNA samples, we can determine in a single experiment the levels of expression of hundreds or thousands of genes in a cell by measuring the amount of mRNA bound to each site on the array and thus generate a profile of gene expression in that cell. The Human Genome Project has produced vast amounts of information about the DNA sequence of the human genome. In the future, use of microarrays will likely clarify the interactions of different genes with each other and contribute to determining how variations in genetic profiles resulting from differences in gene expression contribute to differences in risk of disease in human populations.[8]

Evidence of the potential importance of this method is already available. For example, in a study reported in 2002, van de Vijver and colleagues[9] used microarray analysis to classify 295 patients younger than 53 years who had primary breast carcinomas into those with a gene expression "signature" associated with a poor prognosis and those with a "signature" associated with a good prognosis. The probability of remaining free of distant metastases after 10 years was 85.2% in patients classified as having a good prognosis compared to 50.6% in those classified as having a poor prognosis. The prognosis profile based on microarrays was a strong independent predictor of disease outcome and in young patients was a much more powerful predictor of outcome than were standard systems based on clinical and histologic criteria.

Considerable interest has focused on HLA (human leukocyte antigen) types, which are genetically determined. Certain diseases have been shown to be associated with certain HLA antigens as seen in Table 16-3. For example, ankylosing spondylitis has a strong association with HLA type B27. Interest in such associations is strong, both because such an association may cast light on the pathogenetic mechanisms involved, and because the possibility arises of using HLA as a marker to identify population subsets at increased risk. Furthermore, if ankylosing spondylitis is associated with a certain HLA antigen that is known to be genetically determined, is it because ankylosing spondylitis itself is also genetically determined?

Some of the problems in methodology and interpretation of results that were addressed in earlier chapters apply to identifying associations between diseases and particular gene products. For example, cancer of the pancreas has been reported to be associated with blood group A. How would we design a study to determine whether cancer of the pancreas is in fact associated with blood group A? We could determine the blood group distribution in a group of patients with cancer of the pancreas (cases), but how do we obtain an "expected rate" of the prevalence of blood group A in the general population from which these cases were drawn? This is again the difficult problem of control selection, as was discussed earlier. Investigators have used blood donors at blood banks for comparison, but even 20 years ago there were major selection biases in groups who donated blood and those who did not; the group of persons who donated blood was not representative of the general population. Today, with human immunodeficiency virus (HIV) and acquired immunodeficiency syndrome (AIDS) presenting such a major problem, there is even a greater selection bias in those who donate blood, so that it is even more difficult to interpret the results when such a group is used as a control group.

Another approach for studying the possible association of a certain blood group with cancer of the pancreas is to conduct a case-control study of pancreatic cancer, in which blood group is one of the "exposures" studied. In such a study, the problem of selecting appropriate controls is an important one. When presented with a list of associations with blood groups, we should ask how were the conclusions regarding such associations arrived at and what comparison groups were used for generating the expected rates?

AGE AT ONSET

Epidemiologic observations can be useful in elucidating or confirming biologic or genetic mechanisms. An example is age at onset of a disease. Consider retinoblastoma, a tumor of the eye in children. This tumor occurs in two forms: unilateral and bilateral. The unilateral form (about 60% of cases) generally has a low rate of heritability with little familial pattern, whereas the bilateral form (40% of cases) has a strong familial predisposition and is often transmitted from parents to children.

TABLE 16-3. **HLA Disease Associations**

Disease and HLA Type	Race	Patients (% Positive)	Controls (%)	Odds Ratio*
Ankylosing spondylitis				
B27	White	89	9	69.1
B27	Asian	85	15	207.9
B27	Black	58	4	54.4
Idiopathic hemochromatosis				
A3	White	72	28	6.7
B7	White	48	26	2.9
B14	White	19	6	2.7
Insulin-dependent diabetes mellitus				
B8	White	40	21	2.5
B15	White	22	14	2.1
DR3	White	52	22	3.8
DR4	White	74	24	9.0
DR2	White	4	29	0.1
Rheumatoid arthritis				
DR4	White	68	25	3.8
Celiac disease				
B8	White	68	22	7.6
DR3	White	79	22	11.6
DR7	White	60	15	7.7
Multiple sclerosis				
B7	White	37	24	1.8
DR2	White	51	27	2.7
Narcolepsy				
DR2	White	100	22	129.8
DR2	Asian	100	34	358.1

*Odds ratio values are combined estimates from a number of studies and cannot be directly calculated from the table.
Data from Tiwari JL, Terasaki PI: HLA and Disease Associations. New York, Springer-Verlag, 1985; and from Thomson G, Robinson WP, Kuhner MK, et al: Genetic heterogeneity, modes of inheritance and risk estimates from a joint study of Caucasians with insulin dependent diabetes mellitus. Am J Hum Genet 43:799–816, 1988 (as cited in Thomson G: HLA disease associations: Models for insulin-dependent diabetes mellitus and the study of complex human genetic disorders. Ann Rev Genet 22:31–50, 1988).

Children who survive retinoblastoma have an increased risk of developing a second primary tumor at another site, usually osteogenic sarcoma (a bone tumor). In a large series of patients who survived hereditary retinoblastoma, more than 50% developed a second primary tumor during the subsequent 30 years, and most of these tumors were osteogenic sarcomas. Although it was initially suggested that these tumors might be a result of the radiation therapy that had been given, it was subsequently shown that these tumors may occur at sites distant from the field of radiation, which suggests an underlying susceptibility to the development of osteogenic sarcoma. Moreover, some families of retinoblastoma patients include relatives who have osteogenic sarcoma and who have never had retinoblastoma. These observations suggest the presence of a genetically determined pattern of tumor susceptibility that is specific to the type of tumor. Clearly, such issues become very important considerations when we design studies to investigate the etiology of such conditions.

When we look at the age at onset of familial and nonfamilial retinoblastomas, we see that nonfamilial tumors are distributed throughout childhood, with most occurring in early childhood, whereas almost all familial tumors tend to occur only in very early childhood (Fig. 16-1).

This is commonly observed in other diseases: When a disease occurs in both genetic and nongenetic forms, the genetic form develops in patients at much earlier ages than does the nongenetic form. This observation seems reasonable, for a disease that is not primarily genetic in origin requires an accumulation of environmental insults or exposures that can only build up over time. Consequently, it takes

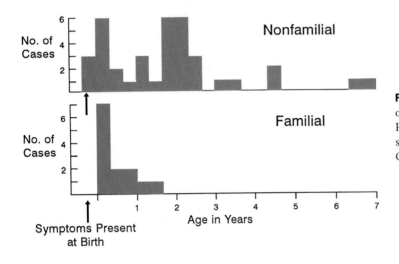

Figure 16-1. Retinoblastoma: age at onset of symptoms. (From Aherne GE, Roberts DF: Retinoblastoma: A clinical survey and its genetic implications. Clin Genet 8:275–290, 1975.)

longer for such diseases to develop than for those that are primarily genetic in origin.

Retinoblastoma has been studied extensively. In 1971, Knudson reviewed the clinical and epidemiologic information regarding retinoblastoma—specifically, the age distribution of the tumor—and on the basis of a statistical study proposed what has become known as the "two-hit" hypothesis for the development of retinoblastoma[10] (Fig. 16-2).

According to this model, two mutations in the same cell of the retina are required for the development of cancer. In the genetically determined form

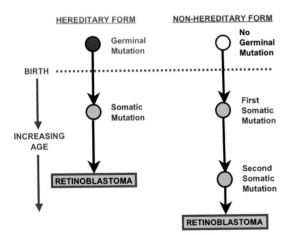

Figure 16-2. Two-hit model for the development of retinoblastoma. (Adapted from Knudson AG Jr: The genetics of childhood cancer. Cancer 35 [Suppl 3]: 1022–1026, 1975. Copyright © 1975 American Cancer Society. Adapted by permission of Wiley-Liss, Inc., a subsidiary of John Wiley & Sons, Inc.)

of retinoblastoma, a child is born with one mutation in the germ cells. Therefore, only one more (somatic) mutation is needed for cancer to develop. However, in the nonfamilial form, a child is born without any germ cell mutation. Consequently, for a retinoblastoma to develop, two mutations in a somatic retinal cell are needed. Because these events are very rare, cases of genetically determined retinoblastoma occur at earlier ages than do nongenetic cases. Thus, epidemiologic observations about age at onset can be linked to current hypotheses about biologic mechanisms in the development of cancer.

Retinoblastoma has been shown to be associated with a deletion from a single band on the long arm of chromosome 13 (13q14). In 1983 Cavenee and coworkers suggested that homozygosity for a mutant allele in this band is probably needed for development of retinoblastoma; this would in effect constitute a loss of the normal tumor suppressor activity at this locus.[11] A gene responsible for the development of both retinoblastoma and osteogenic sarcoma was identified and isolated in 1988.[12]

Figure 16-3 shows another example of different age distributions in genetic and nongenetic forms of a disease. Cumulative age distributions are shown for patients with basal or squamous cell skin cancer in the U.S. population and in 84 persons with basal cell cancer who also have a genetically determined condition—xeroderma pigmentosum—in which a defect in DNA repair predisposes them to cancer. Age at onset is clearly earlier in patients with the genetically determined form of the disease.

Another example relates to age of onset. Evidence has confirmed a role for the APO lipoprotein E

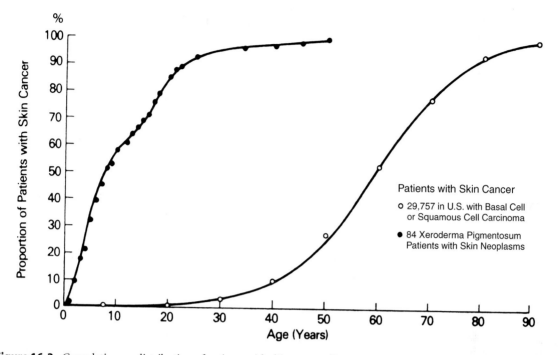

Figure 16-3. Cumulative age distribution of patients with skin cancer. (From Kraemer KH, Lee MM, Scotto J: Early onset of skin and oral cavity neoplasms in xeroderma pigmentosum [letter]. Lancet 1:56–57, 1982.)

(APOE) locus on chromosome 19 in late onset Alzheimer's disease. APOE has three alleles: APOE-ε2, APOE-ε3, and APOE-ε4. APOE-ε4 has been implicated in the etiology of at least half of all Alzheimer's disease cases. In a study of 42 families with late onset Alzheimer's disease, Corder and colleagues[13] found that the risk for Alzheimer's disease increased with the number of APO-ε4 alleles, from 20% for individuals with no APO-ε4 alleles, to 47% of individuals with one such allele, and to 91% of individuals with two such alleles (the 4/4 genotype). Figure 16-4 shows the age at onset for subjects with 0, 1, and 2 APO-ε4 alleles. The more alleles that are present the younger the age at onset. For example, at age 75, about 24% of individuals with no APO-ε4 alleles were diagnosed with Alzheimer's disease, compared to 61% of those with one APO-ε4 allele and 86% of those with 2 APO-ε4 alleles.

Childs and Scriver analyzed the age at onset of many genetic and nongenetic diseases and also found a pattern of earlier age at onset of genetic diseases.[14] Presumably, disease develops relatively rapidly in genetically susceptible persons; hence, the early age at onset. An accumulation of environmental insults over time is required for development of the remaining diseases.

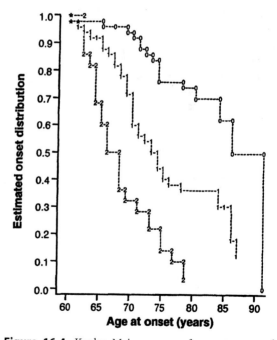

Figure 16-4. Kaplan-Meier curves of age at onset of Alzheimer's disease for subjects with 0, 1, and 2 APO-ε4 alleles. Each curve is labeled with the number 0, 1, or 2 to indicate the number of alleles. (From Corder EH, Saunders AM, Strittmatter WJ, et al: Gene dose of apolipoprotein E type 4 allele and the risk of Alzheimer's disease in late onset families. Science 261:921–923, 1993.)

FAMILY STUDIES

When a disease aggregates in families, what does it tell us about the relative contributions of genetic and environmental factors to its causation? Such aggregation could be a result of genetic determination. But could familial aggregation be observed if the disease were environmentally determined? Yes, because certain environmental exposures are also shared by families. Let us examine the methods used to study familial aggregation and the approaches used to interpret the data from such studies.

Risk of the Disease in First-Degree Relatives

When a person with a certain disease is identified, it is valuable to examine his or her first-degree relatives for evidence of a greater-than-expected prevalence of disease. Such an excess in first-degree relatives would suggest, though not prove, a genetic component. It is also possible to examine family pedigrees such as the one shown in Figure 16-5, which shows a family with retinoblastoma in four successive generations. Such pedigrees not only give a visual picture of the familial impact of the disease, but can also be used to estimate the genetic component in the causation of the disease. This pedigree also demonstrates that the disease or susceptibility to it may skip generations and may be transmitted by individuals who are not affected themselves because other factors may influence expression.

When a person has a disease and there is spousal concordance—that is, husbands and wives of the persons with the disease tend also to have the disease—environmental factors are implicated, as spouses are generally not genetically linked (except in unusually inbred populations).

Applying Molecular Biologic Methods to Family Studies

If familial aggregation of disease is observed, the techniques of epidemiology can be coupled with those of molecular biology to determine whether there is a major identifiable gene transmitted from parent to child that is associated with an increased risk of disease. The techniques involve exploring the observed familial aggregation by using segregation analyses and linkage analyses.

Segregation analyses test whether the observed pattern of a disease in families is compatible with a Mendelian model of inheritance (e.g., autosomal dominant inheritance). This is done by statistically testing competing models.[15]

Linkage analyses seek to determine whether alleles from two loci segregate together in a family and are passed as a unit from parent to child. Genes that are physically near each other on the same chromosome tend to be transmitted together. Linkage can only be identified through family studies. However, even when linkage is demonstrated, it does not necessarily imply a causal relationship.

The ultimate purpose of these analyses is to identify and isolate the genes associated with susceptibility to the disease in order to enhance our understanding of disease pathogenesis and to facilitate the development of appropriate preventive strategies. The search for disease susceptibility genes uses two approaches:

1. Search for an *association* between an allele and a disease using the methods for studying genetic markers listed in Table 16-2:
   a. Analysis of DNA polymorphisms
   b. Analysis of gene products or their phenotypic expression

   These two steps (**a** and **b**) should be viewed in the context of the progression from genotype to phenotype shown schematically in Figure 16-6. Often, DNA probes may be used, even before the specific gene products underlying the disease are known.

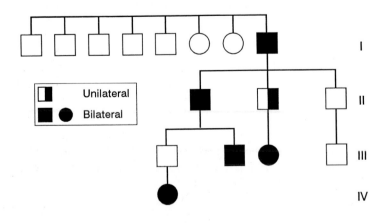

Figure 16-5. Pedigree of family reported with retinoblastoma occurring in four successive generations. Squares, men; circles, women. (From Migdal C: Retinoblastoma occurring in four successive generations. Br J Ophthalmol 60:151–152, 1976.)

Unilateral
Bilateral

I

II

III

IV

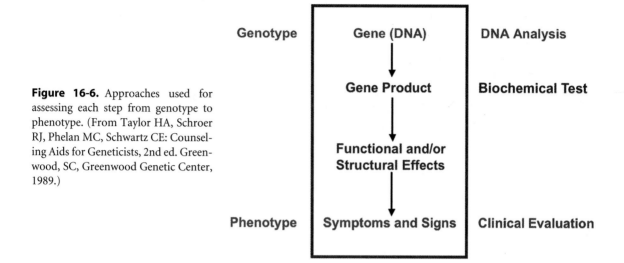

Figure 16-6. Approaches used for assessing each step from genotype to phenotype. (From Taylor HA, Schroer RJ, Phelan MC, Schwartz CE: Counseling Aids for Geneticists, 2nd ed. Greenwood, SC, Greenwood Genetic Center, 1989.)

2. Use of family studies to identify a *linkage* or cosegregation between a certain locus and a possible disease locus.[15] The coinheritance of genetic markers and disease is used to localize defective genes to a specific chromosome location.

Linkage often casts light on the biologic mechanisms underlying the transmission and pathogenesis of disease. Linkage can be demonstrated using the statistical methods of linkage analysis or various laboratory techniques.

For example, the gene for polycystic kidney disorder, an autosomal dominant disease, has been characterized. As seen in the family shown in Figure 16-7, the 1-allele has been demonstrated to be linked with the appearance of the condition and is seen in the father and two of the offspring, all of whom were affected. In the case of cystic fibrosis (Fig. 16-8), an autosomal recessive condition, the 1/4 combination is needed for expression of the disease and must be inherited from both the father and the mother. Thus, the disease is not seen in either parent, but only in the child who has both alleles.

Twin Studies

Studies of twins have been of great value in enriching our understanding of the relative contributions of genetic and environmental factors to the causation of human disease. There are two types of twins: monozygotic (identical) and dizygotic (fraternal). Monozygotic twins arise from the same fertilized ovum and share 100% of their genetic material. However, dizygotic twins are like ordinary siblings who just happened to develop in the uterus at the same time. Like ordinary siblings, they share, on the average, 50% of their genetic material.

If we look at the occurrence of a disease in identical twins—who, in effect, have identical genetic material—what are the possible findings? Both twins (twin A and twin B) may have the disease, or both twins may not have the disease—that is, the members of the pair may be *concordant* for the disease. It is also possible that we find that twin A has the disease and twin B does not or that twin B has the disease and twin A does not; in this case, the twin pairs are *discordant* for the disease.

If monozygotic twins are concordant for a disease, what does that tell us about the role of genetic factors? Could the disease be genetic? Yes, because the twins have identical genetic material. Could it be environmental? Yes, because it is well recognized that parents often raise identical twins in a similar fashion, so that they are exposed to many of the same environmental factors. So an observed concordance in monozygotic twins does not clearly indicate whether a disease is genetic or environmental in origin.

What if monozygotic twins are discordant for a certain disease; that is, one has the disease and the other does not? Is this observation consistent with a genetic hypothesis? No. Because the discordant twins share the same genetic material but have a different disease experience, the disease would have to be mainly environmental in origin.

In dizygotic twins, both environmental and genetic factors are operant. If a disease is genetic, we would expect less concordance in dizygotic twins than in monozygotic twins.

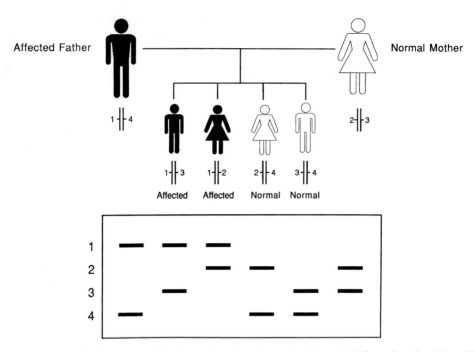

Figure 16-7. DNA analysis of autosomal dominant disorders. Example: Polycystic kidney disorder. (From Taylor HA, Schroer RJ, Phelan MC, Schwartz CE: Counseling Aids for Geneticists, 2nd ed. Greenwood, SC, Greenwood Genetic Center, 1989.)

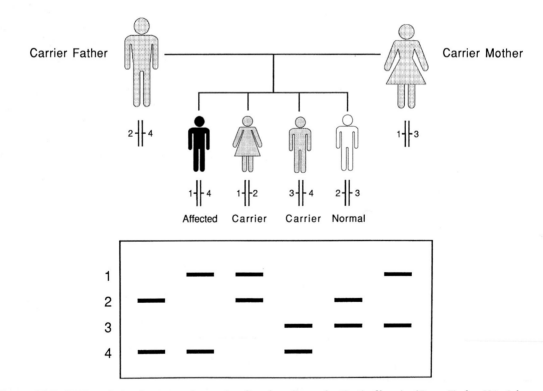

Figure 16-8. DNA analysis of autosomal recessive disorders. Example: Cystic fibrosis. (From Taylor HA, Schroer RJ, Phelan MC, Schwartz CE: Counseling Aids for Geneticists, 2nd ed. Greenwood, SC, Greenwood Genetic Center, 1989.)

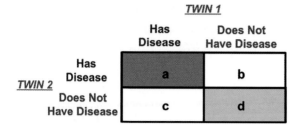

Figure 16-9. Concordance in twins for a dichotomous variable, such as leukemia.

How do we calculate the rates of concordance and of discordance in twins? Figure 16-9 shows a cross-tabulation of twins 1 and 2. The numbers in each cell are therefore numbers of *twin pairs:* thus, there are *a* pairs (in which both twin 1 and 2 have the disease); *d* pairs (in which neither twin 1 nor 2 has the disease); *b* pairs (in which twin 1 does not have the disease but twin 2 does); and *c* pairs (in which twin 1 has the disease but twin 2 does not).

If we want to calculate the concordance rate in twins, most twins will fall into the *d* category—that is, neither will have the disease. We therefore usually look at the other three cells—those twin pairs in which at least one of the twins has the disease. We can calculate the concordance rate in twin pairs in which at least one twin has the disease as follows:

$$\text{Concordance rate} = \frac{a}{a+b+c}$$

We can also calculate the discordance rate in all twin pairs in which at least one twin has the disease as:

$$\text{Discordance rate} = \frac{b+c}{a+b+c}$$

Table 16-4 shows concordance data for leukemia in monozygotic and dizygotic twin pairs. We see that the percentage of concordant pairs is notably high for congenital leukemia, which strongly suggests a major genetic component in causation when the disease occurs near the time of birth.

How are concordance data used? Let us look at a few examples. Table 16-5 shows reported concordance rates for alcoholism in monozygotic and dizygotic twins reported in several studies.[16–19] Almost all of the reported studies show higher concordance rates for monozygotic than for dizygotic twins; the findings from only one study of a relatively small number of twins were not consistent with the findings of the other studies. Thus, in general, the data reported in the literature strongly suggest a genetic component in the etiology of alcoholism.

Table 16-6 shows concordance rates in New York State for neural tube defects (anencephaly and spina bifida). Notice that the table refers only to co-twins and does not distinguish between monozygotic and dizygotic twins. The reason for this is that the data were obtained from birth certificates in which zygosity data are generally not available. No contacts were made with individuals and families. As seen in this study, routinely available data may be useful for certain studies, but because they are not gathered for study purposes, such data often are limited in the detail needed to answer specific questions. It should be pointed out that good evidence of zygosity is often not obtained in many twin studies, and when examining data such as those shown in Tables 16-3 and 16-4, we must ask on what basis were the twin pairs labeled monozygotic or dizygotic? (Remember the caveat discussed earlier: If you are shown differences between groups or changes over time, the first ques-

TABLE 16-4. Age Distribution in Published Clinical Reports of Childhood Leukemia in Twins, 1928–1974

	MONOZYGOTIC PAIRS		DIZYGOTIC PAIRS	
	Concordant	Discordant	Concordant	Discordant
Perinatal-congenital	14	1	1	1
Age 2–7 yr	6	13	3	5
Age 7–12 yr	1	8	–	1
Age 12 yr and older	5	14	0	3
Total	26	36	4	10

From Keith L, Brown ER, Ames B, et al: Leukemia in twins: Antenatal and postnatal factors. Acta Genet Med Gemellol 25:336–341, 1976.

TABLE 16-5. Concordance for Alcoholism in Monozygotic (MZ) and Dizygotic (DZ) Twin Pairs Identified Through an Alcoholic Member

	CONCORDANCE			
Author (Year)	**Number of Twin Pairs**	**MZ (%)**	**DZ (%)**	**Ratio of MZ:DZ Concordance**
Kaij (1960)	174	71	32	2.2
Hrubec et al. (1981)	15,924	26	13	2.0
Murray et al. (1983)	56	21	25	0.8
Pickens et al. (1991)	86 (M)	59	36	1.6
	44 (F)	25	5	5.0

Adapted from Lumeng L, Crabb DW: Genetic aspects and risk factors in alcoholism and alcoholic liver disease. Gastroenterology 107:572–578, 1994.

TABLE 16-6. Concordance Rates of Anencephaly and Spina Bifida (ASB) in New York State, 1955–1974

Incidence of ASB	1.3/1,000
Concordance rates	
Among co-twins	4/59 (6.8%)
Among full siblings	19/1,037 (1.8%)
Among half siblings	1/133 (0.8%)

From Janerich DT, Piper J: Shifting genetic patterns in anencephaly and spina bifida. J Med Genet 15:101–105, 1978.

tion to ask is, Are they real? If you are convinced that a difference or change is real and not artifactual, then and only then should you proceed to interpret the findings.)

One problem in interpreting concordance data is *publication bias*—that is, a selection bias related to which cases are reported and which are ultimately accepted for publication by a journal. An observation of an infrequent or unusual disease in both members of a pair of twins is often clinically striking. A clinician is therefore much more likely to report such a concordant pair than to report a discordant pair. Journals may also be more likely to accept reports of concordant twin pairs for publication than they are to accept reports of discordant twin pairs. Therefore, many discordant pairs that are never reported are probably missing in tables that summarize data from the literature.

So far, we have discussed concordance for a discrete variable, such as leukemia or schizophrenia,

that is either present or absent. However, we are often interested in determining concordance for a continuous variable, such as blood pressure. In this case, we would plot the data for twin 1 against the data for twin 2 for all twin pairs and calculate the correlation coefficient *(r)*, as seen in Figure 16-10. The correlation coefficient can range from −1 to +1.

A correlation coefficient of +1 indicates a full positive correlation, 0 indicates no correlation, and −1 indicates a full inverse correlation. If we plot such data for monozygotic twin pairs and for dizygotic twin pairs, as shown in Figure 16-11, we would expect to find a stronger correlation for monozygotic twins than for dizygotic twins if the disease or characteristic is genetically determined.

Table 16-7 shows correlation coefficients for systolic blood pressure among relatives. The highest

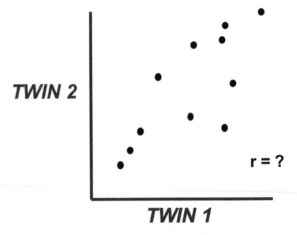

Figure 16-10. Concordance in twins for a continuous variable, such as systolic blood pressure.

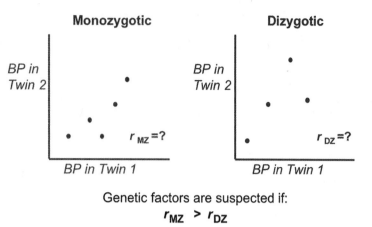

Figure 16-11. Use of concordance rates for continuous variables, such as blood pressure (BP), to explore the etiologic role of genetic factors.

TABLE 16-7. **Correlation among Relatives for Systolic Blood Pressure**

Relatives Compared	Correlation Coefficients
Monozygotic twins	0.55
Dizygotic twins	0.25
Siblings	0.18
Parents and offspring	0.34
Spouses	0.07

Adapted from Feinleib M, Garrison MS, Borhani N, et al: Studies of hypertension in twins. In Paul O (ed): Epidemiology and Control of Hypertension. New York, Grune & Stratton, 1975, pp 3–20.

---

coefficient is seen in monozygotic twins; the values for dizygotic twins and ordinary siblings are close. Also of interest is that virtually no correlation exists between spouses. A strong correlation between spouses (who are not biologically related) would suggest a role for environmental factors. (An alternate suggestion, however, could be that people seek out individuals like themselves for marriage. Thus, individuals with type A personalities, for example, may seek out other individuals with type A personalities for marriage. In such a situation we might arrive at a high spousal correlation even for conditions that are not environmentally determined.)

Another example of the value of family studies and twin studies in assessing the relative contributions of genetic and environmental factors to disease causation is seen in the case of Hodgkin's disease. Years ago the incidence of Hodgkin's disease was shown to be bimodal when plotted against age: one peak occurred in the 20s and a second occurred at about age 70 years[20] (Fig. 16-12). Data suggest that the histologic type of disease varies by age: the young adult form of the disease is mainly the nodular sclerosing form, and the mixed-cell type increases with increasing age.[21]

Over the years a large number of studies have implicated both environmental and genetic factors. Environmentally, small number of siblings and higher socioeconomic status have been associated with increased risk of Hodgkin's disease, suggesting that Hodgkin's disease may be a rare sequel to a common childhood infection.[22] Epstein-Barr virus infection has been implicated. At the same time, familial clusters and increased risk of the disease among siblings of Hodgkin's disease patients have suggested a strong genetic component. In 1995, Mack and coworkers reported a study of concordance for Hodgkin's disease in monozygotic and dizygotic twin pairs that had been identified by Hodgkin's disease in one of its members.[23] As indicated in Table 16-8, 6% of the monozygotic twin pairs were concordant for Hodgkin's disease compared with 0% of the dizygotic pairs.

The median age at diagnosis of the concordant twins was 25.5 years, and most of the cases in the concordant pairs for whom information was available were of the nodular sclerosing histologic subtype. Most of the previously reported sibships with multiple cases were also of this subtype. Although these data suggest a genetic susceptibility to Hodgkin's disease, such a susceptibility does not itself appear to account fully for all cases of the disease. The findings are therefore also consistent with a role for, and possibly an interaction with, environmental factors such as infection.

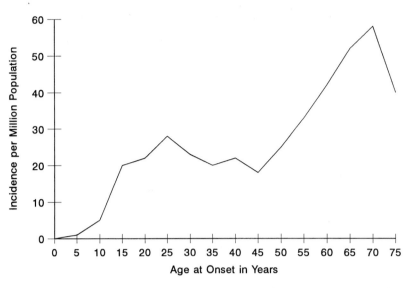

Figure 16-12. Incidence of Hodgkin's disease in the white population of Brooklyn, 1943–1957. (From MacMahon B: Epidemiologic evidence of the nature of Hodgkin's disease. Cancer 10:1045–1054, 1957. Copyright © 1957 American Cancer Society. Reprinted by permission of Wiley-Liss, Inc., a subsidiary of John Wiley & Sons, Inc.)

TABLE 16-8. **Concordance Rates for Hodgkin's Disease in Twin Pairs with an Affected Member**

Types of Pairs	Number of Pairs	CONCORDANT PAIRS	
		Number	%
Monozygotic	179	10	6
Dizygotic	187	0	0

Adapted from Mack TM, Cozen W, Shibata DK, et al: Concordance for Hodgkin's disease in identical twins suggesting genetic susceptibility to the young-adult form of the disease. N Engl J Med 332:413–418, 1995.

Another example is from research on Parkinson's disease (PD), a neurodegenerative disease that affects a half million to a million adults in the United States. About 90% of cases develop after age 50. The etiology is not known, nor are the relative contributions of genetic and environmental factors. An intriguing study was published in 1999 by Tanner and coworkers who investigated concordance and discordance rates for PD in both monozygotic and dizygotic twins.[24] Almost 20,000 white male twins enrolled in the National Academy of Science/National Research Council World War II Veteran Twins Registry were screened for PD by physical examination and questionnaires. Zygosity was established by polymerase chain reaction or questionnaire. Since all twins listed in the registry were studied, the possibility of selection bias was reduced or eliminated.

In 161 twin pairs at least one twin had PD; 71 of these pairs were monozygotic and 90 were dizygotic. As seen in Table 16-9 (*top*), the concordance rate was 15.5% for monozygotic twins and 11.1% for dizygotic twins. However, when the twin pairs were stratified according to age of onset of the first case of PD, an interesting difference was found: When the first twin developed PD before age 50, 100% of the monozygotic twin pairs were concordant compared with only 16.7% of the dizygotic pairs (see Table 16-9, *middle*). In contrast, when the first twin developed PD after age 50, there was no difference in concordance rates between monozygotic and dizygotic twins (see Table 16-9, *bottom*). The numbers of affected twin pairs were small, and the study remains to be replicated and its findings confirmed. Nevertheless, the results suggest that genetic factors may

TABLE 16-9. Concordance Rates for Parkinson's Disease (PD) in Twin Pairs with at Least One Affected Member

Types of Pairs	Number of Pairs	CONCORDANT PAIRS	
		Number	%
All twin pairs			
Monozygotic	71	11	15.5
Dizygotic	90	10	11.1
Onset before age 50 yr			
Monozygotic	4	4	100.0
Dizygotic	12	2	16.7
Onset after age 50 yr			
Monozygotic	65	7	10.8
Dizygotic	76	8	10.5

From Tanner CH, Ottman R, Goldman SM, et al: Parkinson disease in twins: An etiologic study. JAMA 281:341–346, 1999.

TABLE 16-10. Types of Subjects Compared in Studies of Schizophrenia in Adopted Offspring

1. Offspring of normal biologic parents reared by schizophrenic adopting parents
2. Offspring of normal biologic parents reared by normal adopting parents
3. Offspring of schizophrenic biologic parents reared by normal adopting parents

play a significant role in PD that develops before age 50, but that in cases developing after age 50, genetic factors may be less important and the role of environmental factors should be explored.

A large twin study was reported by Lichtenstein and colleagues in 2000.[25] This study was conducted to estimate the relative contributions of environmental and heritable factors in the causation of cancer. Data from 44,788 twin pairs listed in the Swedish, Danish, and Finnish twin registries were used to assess cancer risks at 28 anatomic sites in twins of people with cancer. Twins of persons with stomach, colorectal, lung, breast, and prostate cancer had an increased risk of developing the same type of cancer. The large effect of heritability at those sites (for example, heritable factors accounted for 42% of the risk of prostate cancer) contrasted with the picture for most cancers in which genetic factors made a relatively minor contribution to susceptibility. The findings of this and other studies emphasize the need to consider the effects of both genetic and environmental factors and their interactions in addressing the etiology of different cancers.

Adoption Studies

We have said that one problem in interpreting the findings from twin studies is that even monozygotic twins who share the same genetic constitution also share much of the same environment. In such studies,

it is therefore difficult to tease out the relative contributions of genetic and environmental factors to the cause of disease. One approach to addressing this problem would be to identify twin pairs in which one twin was adopted by another family and the other was not, so that they do not share a common environment. This is the basis for *adoption studies*. However, because such twins are difficult to find, a frequently used approach is to compare different groups of adopted children as follows:

Suppose we are interested in whether schizophrenia is primarily genetic or environmental in origin, and we are considering conducting a study using adopted children (Table 16-10). We can examine offspring of normal biologic parents who are adopted and reared by schizophrenic parents. If the disease is genetic in origin, what would we expect the risk of schizophrenia to be in these children? It should approximate what is seen in the rest of the population because the environment would not have an effect in increasing the risk. If the disease is largely environmental, we would expect that being reared in an environment with schizophrenic adoptive parents would increase the risk of schizophrenia in these children. We could also examine offspring of normal biologic parents reared by normal adoptive parents and we would expect them to have the usual rate of schizophrenia.

We could also examine the offspring of biologic parents with schizophrenia who have been adopted and reared by normal parents. In this case, if the disease is genetic, we would expect the children to be at increased risk for schizophrenia. If the disease is environmental, we would expect them to have the usual rate of schizophrenia.

When interpreting data from adoption studies, certain factors need to be kept in mind. The first is the age at which the adoption took place. For example, if the adoption occurred in late childhood, part of

TABLE 16-11. **Schizophrenia in Biologic and Adoptive Relatives of Adoptees Who Became Schizophrenic (National Study of Adoptees in Denmark)**

| | BIOLOGIC RELATIVES | | | ADOPTIVE RELATIVES | | |
| | | Schizophrenic | | | Schizophrenic | |
	Total Number	Number	%	Total Number	Number	%
Adoptees who became schizophrenic (N = 34)	275	14	5.0	111	0	0
Control adoptees (no serious mental disease) (N = 34)	253	1	0.4	124	0	0

From Kety SS, Ingraham LJ: Genetic transmission and improved diagnosis of schizophrenia from pedigrees of adoptees. J Psychiatr Res 26:247–255, 1992.

the child's environment may have been that of the biologic parents. Ideally, we would like to study children who are adopted at birth. Another complicating issue is that, after adoption, some children maintain relationships with their biologic parents, including visits and other exposures to the environment of the biologic parents, so that the separation between the environment of the biologic parents and that of the adoptive parents is not complete.

Many fine adoption studies have been conducted in Scandinavian countries, which have excellent disease registries and record linkage systems. They also have adoption registries and psychiatric registries. As an example, Table 16-11 shows data from a study of schizophrenia carried out by Kety and Ingraham in which they studied rates of schizophrenia in biologic and in adoptive relatives of adopted children.[26] Using the adoption registry and the psychiatric registry, they identified 34 adoptees who later became schizophrenic and also identified 34 adoptees without serious mental disease. They then examined the rates of schizophrenia in the biologic and in the adoptive relatives of the schizophrenic adoptees and in the control adoptees. The rate of schizophrenia in the biologic relatives of the schizophrenic adoptees was 5.0%, compared with 0.4% in the biologic relatives of control adoptees without serious mental disease. The findings strongly suggest that there is a significant genetic component in the cause of schizophrenia.

Table 16-12 shows correlation coefficients for parent-child aggregation of blood pressure, comparing biologic children with adopted children. Clearly, the correlations are much weaker (and approach 0) for correlations between parents and adopted children than between parents and biologic children.

TABLE 16-12. **Correlation Coefficients for Parent-Child Aggregation of Blood Pressure**

| | BETWEEN PARENTS AND | |
	Biologic Child	Adopted Child
Systolic	0.32 (P < .001)	0.09 (NS)
Diastolic	0.37 (P < .001)	0.10 (NS)

NS, not significant.
Adapted from Biron P, Mongeau JG, Bertrand D: Familial aggregation of blood pressure in 558 adopted children. Can Med Assoc J 115:773–774, 1976.

The findings strongly suggest a genetic component in the determination of blood pressure.

TIME TRENDS IN DISEASE INCIDENCE

If we observe time trends in disease, with incidence either increasing or decreasing over a period of time, and if we are convinced that the trend is real, the observation implicates environmental factors in the causation of the disease. Clearly, genetic characteristics of human populations generally do not change over relatively short periods. Thus the change in mortality from coronary heart disease in men from 1979 to 2004 seen in Figure 16-13 is primarily due to changes in exposure to environmental factors.

INTERNATIONAL STUDIES

Figure 16-14 shows age-adjusted death rates for stomach cancer in men in several countries. The

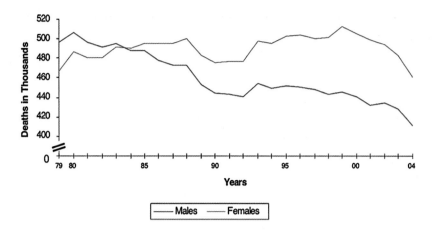

Figure 16-13. Cardiovascular disease mortality trends for men and women, United States: 1979–2000. (From CDC and NCHS. Cited by the American Heart Association: Heart Disease and Stroke Statistics, 2003 Update. Dallas, American Heart Association, 2002.)

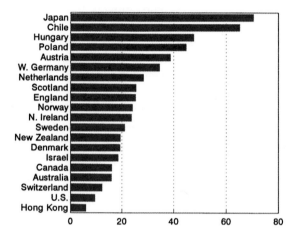

Figure 16-14. Age-adjusted death rates per 100,000 for stomach cancer in 20 countries, men, 1976–1977. (Data from Page HS, Asire AJ: Cancer Rates and Risks, 3rd ed. Washington, DC, NIH publication no. 85–691, 1985.)

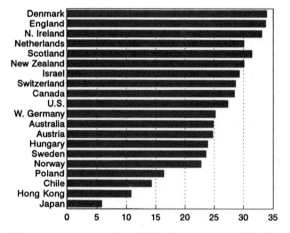

Figure 16-15. Age-adjusted death rates per 100,000 for breast cancer in 20 countries, women, 1976–1977. (Data from Page HS, Asire AJ: Cancer Rates and Risks, 3rd ed. Washington, DC, NIH publication no. 85–691, 1985.)

highest rate is seen in Japan, and the rates in the United States are quite low. Are these differences real? Could they be due to differences in quality of medical care or in access to medical care in different countries? Could they be due to international differences in how death certificates are completed? Results of other studies suggest that these differences are real.

Figure 16-15 shows comparable data for breast cancer in women. Here we see that one of the lowest rates in the world is in Japan. Are differences between countries due to environmental or to genetic factors? The answer is probably both. How can we tease apart the relative contributions of genetic and environmental factors to international differences in risk of

disease? We can do so by studying migrants in a manner analogous to that just described for studying adoptees.

Migrant Studies

Let us assume that a Japanese individual living in Japan, a country with a high risk for stomach cancer, moves to the United States, a country with a low risk of stomach cancer. What would we expect to happen to this person's risk of stomach cancer? If the disease is primarily genetic in origin, we would expect the high risk of stomach cancer to be retained even when people move from a high-risk to a low-risk area.

TABLE 16-13. **Standardized Mortality Ratios for Cancer of the Stomach in Japanese Men, Issei, Nisei, and U.S. White Men**

Group	Standardized Mortality Ratio
Japanese men	100
Issei*	72
Nisei*	38
U.S. white men	17

*Issei and Nisei are first- and second-generation Japanese migrants, respectively.
From Haenszel W, Kurihara M: Studies of Japanese migrants: I. Mortality from cancer and other disease among Japanese in the United States. J Natl Cancer Inst 40:43–68, 1968.

However, if the disease is environmental in origin, we would expect that over time the risk for such a migrant group would shift toward the lower risk of the adoptive country.

Table 16-13 shows standardized mortality ratios (SMRs) for stomach cancer in Japanese men living in Japan, Japanese men who migrated to the United States (Issei), and the children of the Japanese migrants (Nisei) born in the United States, compared with SMRs of U.S. white males. We see that the SMRs progressively shift toward the lower SMR of U.S. white males. These data strongly suggest that a significant environmental component is involved.

We should bear in mind that when people migrate to their country of adoption, they and their families do not immediately shed the environment of their country of origin. Many aspects of their original culture are retained, including certain dietary preferences. Thus, the microenvironment of the migrant, particularly environmental characteristics related to lifestyle, are generally a combination of those of the country of origin and those of the country of adoption. Another important consideration is the age at which the person migrated; in interpreting the findings from migrant studies, it is important to know how much of the person's life was spent in the country of origin and how much in the country of adoption.

Let us turn to another example. The risk of multiple sclerosis has been shown to be related to latitude: the greater the distance from the equator, the greater the risk. This observation is very intriguing and has stimulated much research. However, ques-

tions remain about the extent to which the relationship to latitude is a result of environmental factors as well as about how we can determine which environmental factors might be involved.

Studies of people who have migrated from high-risk to low-risk areas are ideally suited to answering some of these questions. One country that lent itself nicely to such a study is Israel, which, by latitude, is a low-risk country for multiple sclerosis. Israel had successive waves of immigration during the 20th century. Some of the migrants came from high-risk areas, such as the relatively northerly latitudes of the United States, Canada, and Northern Europe, whereas others came from low-risk latitudes closer to the equator, including areas of North Africa and the Arabian Peninsula.

Table 16-14 shows data for incidence of multiple sclerosis in European, African, and Asian migrants to Israel. The disease is not common; therefore, the sample sizes were small.

First let us look at the rates for African and Asian migrants who moved from one low-risk area to another. Their risk remained low. Now examine the data for European migrants who migrated from a high-risk area (Europe) to a low-risk area (Israel). Europeans who migrated before age 15 years (top row) had a low rate, similar to that of African and Asian migrants. However, Europeans who migrated after age 15 years tended to retain the high rate of their country of origin. These findings suggested that the risk of multiple sclerosis is determined in childhood and that the critical factor is whether childhood years are spent in a high-risk or a low-risk area.

TABLE 16-14. **Incidence of Multiple Sclerosis (MS) per 100,000 among European, African, and Asian Immigrants to Israel by Age at Immigration**

Age at Immigration	INCIDENCE OF MS IN MIGRANTS	
	European	African and Asian
<15 yr	0.76	0.65
15–29 yr	3.54	0.40
30–34 yr	1.35	0.26

Adapted from Alter M, Leibowitz V, Speer J: Risk of multiple sclerosis related to age at immigration to Israel. Arch Neurol 15:234–237, 1966.

A person who spent childhood years in a low-risk area retains a low risk; one who spent childhood years in a high-risk area retains a high risk, even after later migration to a low-risk area. This has suggested that some event in childhood, possibly infectious in origin, may be of importance in the causation of multiple sclerosis; this has led to research on slow virus infections as a possible etiologic agent in this disease.

What are the problems with migrant studies? First, migrants are not representative of the populations of their countries of origin. Therefore, we must ask what factors led certain people to migrate (selection factors)? For example, people who are seriously ill or disabled generally do not migrate. Other factors, including socioeconomic and cultural characteristics, are also related to which persons are likely to migrate and which persons are not. Consequently, given this problem of selection, we must ask whether we can legitimately compare the rates of stomach cancer in Issei and Nisei with the rates in native Japanese. Second, we need to ask what was the age at migration. How many years did the migrants spend in their country of origin and how many in their country of adoption? Third, we should remember that migrants do not completely shed the environment of their country of origin after they migrate.

All these factors must be considered in interpreting the results of migrant studies. There is an obvious parallel with adoption studies, and as seen in Table 16-15, many of the issues that arise in interpreting the findings are similar for the two types of studies.

INTERACTION OF GENETIC AND ENVIRONMENTAL FACTORS

When both genetic and environmental factors are found to have roles in the development of disease, the nature of the relationship of the two types of factors must be elucidated. Certain diseases are largely environmental, whereas others are largely genetic. The distinguished geneticist and pediatrician Dr. Barton Childs has pointed out that in diseases in which most of the cases are environmentally determined, heritability of the disease is seen as low. As environmental causes are successfully addressed and removed, however, we are left with a core of cases in which genetic factors play the major role.[27] He cites lung cancer as an example. Most cases of lung cancer are in smokers and are thus environmentally determined so that the overall heritability of lung cancer today is low. The incidence of lung cancer is decreasing as effective measures are put in place to reduce smoking. As time goes on, the remaining cases will largely be familial cases and the heritability of lung cancer as seen in new cases will appear to be increasing over time.

However, the question of genetic susceptibility to environmental factors and the possibility of interaction between them must also be addressed. In Chapter 14, we discussed the study by Grant and Dawson that described an association of earlier age at onset of alcohol consumption to prevalence of lifetime alcohol abuse (Fig. 16-16). As seen in Figure 16-17, when the subjects were divided into those with a positive family history of alcoholism and those with a negative history, the relationship still held, although the prevalence increased when family history was positive and decreased when family history was negative.[28] This observation suggests that, although the observed relationship of risk of lifetime alcohol abuse to age at onset of alcohol consumption may reflect environmental influences, the effect of family history may suggest either an interaction with genetic factors or the influence of child rearing related to family history of alcohol abuse.

Advances in molecular biology have facilitated the integration of epidemiology and laboratory genetics. For example, oral contraceptive use has long been known to increase a woman's risk of venous thrombosis. Vandenbroucke and colleagues studied the question of whether the factor V Leiden mutation,

---

TABLE 16-15. **Issues in Interpreting the Results of Adoption and Migrant Studies**

Adoption Studies	**Migrant Studies**
• Adoptees are highly selected.	• Migrants are highly selected.
• Age at adoption varies.	• Age at migration varies.
• Adoptees may retain various degrees of contact with their biologic parent(s).	• Migrants may retain many elements of their original environment, particularly those related to culture and lifestyle.

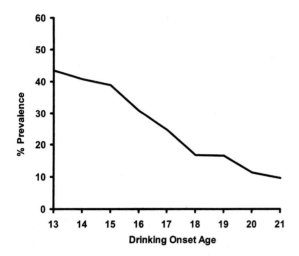

Figure 16-16. Prevalence of lifetime alcohol dependence by age at drinking onset. (Adapted from Grant BF, Dawson DA: Age at onset of alcohol and its association with DSM-IV alcohol abuse and dependence: Results from the national Longitudinal Alcohol Epidemiologic Survey. J Substance Abuse 9:103–110, 1997. With permission from Elsevier, Inc.)

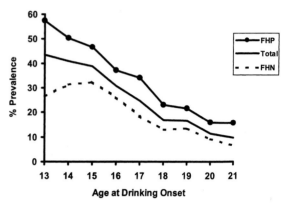

Figure 16-17. Prevalence of lifetime alcohol dependence by age at drinking onset and family history of alcoholism. FHP, family history positive; FHN, family history negative. (Adapted from Grant BF: The impact of a family history of alcoholism on the relationship between age at onset of alcohol use and DSM-IV alcohol dependence: Results from the National Longitudinal Alcohol Epidemiologic Survey. Alcohol Health Res World 22:144–147, 1998.)

which is known to enhance susceptibility to thrombosis, might play a role in the increased risk of thrombosis in women who use oral contraceptives.[29] They conducted a case-control study of 155 premenopausal women who had developed deep venous thrombosis and 169 population-based controls.

As seen in Table 16-16, the risk of thrombosis among carriers of the mutation was increased about sevenfold to ninefold compared with the risk in those without the mutation. Compared with women who were noncarriers of the factor V Leiden mutation and did not use oral contraceptives, women who were both carriers of the mutation and users of oral contraceptives had nearly a 30-fold increase in risk. Because

the findings slightly exceed what would be expected in a multiplicative model, they suggest interaction.

In 1995, Brennan and colleagues reported a study of cigarette smoking and squamous cell cancer of the head and neck.[30] They found that in patients with invasive cancer of the head and neck, smoking was associated with a marked increase in mutations in the p^{53} gene, normally a tumor suppressor. Such mutations are likely to contribute to both the inception and growth of cancers. The investigators studied tumor samples from 127 patients with head and neck cancer and found p^{53} mutations in 42% (54 of 127) of the patients. Patients who smoked at least 1 pack per day for at least 20 years were more than twice as likely to have mutations in p^{53} as patients who were nonsmokers. Patients who smoked and drank more

TABLE 16-16. **Estimated Population Incidence per 10,000 Person-Years of First Venous Thrombosis in Women Aged 15 to 49 Years According to Presence of Factor V Leiden Mutation and Use of Oral Contraceptives**

| | FACTOR V LEIDEN MUTATION | |
	Absent	Present
Did not use oral contraceptives	0.8	5.7
Used oral contraceptives	3.0	28.5

Adapted from Vandenbroucke JP, Koster T, Briët E, et al: Increased risk of venous thrombosis in oral contraceptive users who are carriers of factor V Leiden mutation. Lancet 344:1453–1457, 1994.

Figure 16-18. Association of p^{53} gene mutations with cigarette smoking and alcohol consumption in 129 patients with squamous cell carcinoma of the head and neck. (From Brennan JA, Boyle JO, Koch WM, et al: Association between cigarette smoking and mutation of the p^{53} gene in squamous cell carcinoma of the head and neck. N Engl J Med 332:712–717, 1995.)

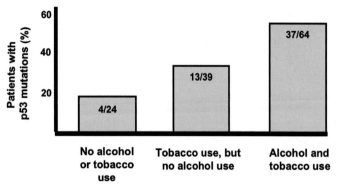

than 1 oz of hard alcohol per day were 3.5 times as likely to have mutations in p^{53} than patients who neither smoked nor drank. As seen in Figure 16-18, p^{53} mutations were found in 58% of patients who both smoked and drank, in 33% of patients who smoked but did not drink, and in 17% of patients who neither smoked nor drank. Furthermore, the type of mutation found in patients who neither smoked nor drank seemed likely to be endogenous rather than exogenous, i.e., caused by environmental mutagens. The findings suggest that cigarette smoking may tend to inactivate the p^{53} tumor suppressor gene and thus provide a molecular basis for the well-recognized relationship of cigarette smoking and head and neck cancer.

A further step in this approach is to identify a specific gene defect that is associated with a certain environmental exposure. An example is seen in findings linking a specific defect in the p^{53} gene to aflatoxin exposure in patients with hepatocellular carcinoma (HCC). In Chapter 15, the positive synergism of hepatitis B virus (HBV) and aflatoxin B_1 exposure in increasing the risk of HCC is discussed. To determine whether the frequency of a specific mutation in the p^{53} tumor suppressor gene (a "hot spot" mutation at codon 249) was related to the risk of aflatoxin exposure, Bressac and coworkers screened HCC samples from 14 countries.[31] The mutation was found in 17% (12/72) of tumor samples from four countries in southern Africa and the southeast coast of Asia but in none of 95 samples from other geographic locations including North America, Europe, the Middle East, and Japan. The four countries in which the mutation was found, China, Vietnam, South Africa, and Mozambique, have most of the cases of HCC in the world and share a similar warm and humid climate, which favors the growth of aflatoxin-producing molds. The rate of HBV carriage was high but did not vary significantly among the countries studied. However, the risk of aflatoxin exposure did vary among these countries and presence of the mutation was found to correlate with the risk of exposure to aflatoxins.

Further support for these findings was provided by Aguilar and colleagues who studied samples of normal liver from three geographic areas that varied in their risk of aflatoxin exposure: negligible levels (United States), low levels (Thailand), and high levels (Qidong, China).[32] The frequency of the mutation paralleled the level of aflatoxin B_1 exposure, suggesting that aflatoxin has a causative and probably early role in the development of liver tumors.

Thus, studies combining epidemiologic and molecular methods may prove invaluable in confirming an etiologic role for certain environmental agents by demonstrating their specific gene effects. Moreover, such studies may also suggest biologic pathways and mechanisms that may be involved in the development of certain cancers and other diseases. However, combined epidemiologic and molecular studies may also help determine that a disease is not primarily caused by environmental factors. For example, Harris pointed out that the exact nature of the p^{53} mutation can be valuable in indicating that a certain cancer did not result from an environmental carcinogen but instead was caused by endogenous mutagenesis, such as was seen in the study just described of patients with head and neck cancers who were nondrinkers and nonsmokers.[33] Germ line mutations in p^{53} can also indicate that a person has an increased susceptibility to cancer as originally proposed by Knudson in 1971 (and discussed earlier in this chapter).[10]

PROSPECTS FOR THE FUTURE

Despite the excitement that accompanies the results of studies such as those described above, in most situations in which both genetic and environmental factors have been implicated, the information currently available is not yet sufficient to delineate the specific nature of their relationship in disease causation, particularly for multifactorial chronic diseases. Enhanced understanding of the molecular changes in cancer resulting from studies of genetic changes in cancer cells should improve our understanding of individual susceptibilities to developing cancers and facilitate the development of specific therapies for the pathways involved in different tumors. These therapies have been called "targeted therapies." By targeting the specific molecular pathways involved in different tumors, as well as the points at which tumor cells may be particularly vulnerable to certain interventions, such therapies should be more effective. They might also have fewer and less severe side effects than many therapies that are currently available which are not sufficiently specific in their cytotoxic effects and therefore affect both abnormal and normal cells.

Childs articulated a concept that encompasses not only the different characteristics of histologically different tumors or other diseases, but also the unique genetic and environmental characteristics of different human beings that may lead to vulnerability to such tumors or diseases.[34] As a result, what might appear at first glance to be the same disease occurring in different individuals should perhaps be considered different diseases with the same phenotype because disease in a person is a "package" of physical, laboratory, and other abnormalities, combined with a unique set of genetically and environmentally determined host susceptibilities. These susceptibilities may often include social and psychological factors in addition to the environmental factors which are often routinely studied. These factors may be operating at the level of the individual, the family, the community, or some other social grouping. Although this combination will differ from one individual to another, by current definitions and classifications of disease, many individuals may appear to have the same illness. Integration of knowledge of all these divergent areas may well provide the foundation for early detection of high-risk individuals and may lead to more effective measures of early prevention in the coming years.

In 2000, Childs and Valle wrote:

The signs and symptoms of a patient today may well have been forged in the developmental and maturational matrix of the past. And in making that characterization, we discern the individuality and

heterogeneity of that which we give the name of a disease. . . .

In medicine we have trouble accepting this kind of individuality. When we see a patient, we think first of the name of a disease and then of the variation expressed in the patient. This way of thinking is typological, and is to be distinguished from "population" thinking in which a population, say, of patients with the "same" disease, consists of variable individuals.[35]

Dalton and Friend published a schematic presentation of the cyclical nature of the process of incorporating new knowledge into therapies that are individualized for each patient (Fig. 16-19) and the process is described in the caption to this figure. Although this approach has great potential, in general, its benefits have not yet been extensively realized in treatment of patients. However, in the coming years, new technologies at the molecular and genetic level are likely to have profound effects on health care and on the development of personalized care, which will include new approaches to disease prevention made possible by technical advances and by the integration

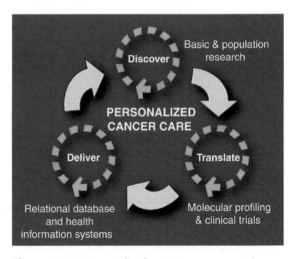

Figure 16-19. Personalized cancer care as a continuous cycle. The cycle starts with the discovery of specific molecular alterations in tumors that are then linked to specific patient outcomes in clinical trials. The ability to capture molecular profiles and clinical information at the level of individual patients allows translation of the information into more personalized cancer care. Available relational databases and health information systems ensure more informed delivery of cancer therapies to future patients and can also guide the discovery of new therapies. (From Dalton WS, Friend SH: Cancer biomarkers—An invitation to the table. Science 312:1165–1168, 2006.)

of new information derived from different biologic and sociologic disciplines.

CONCLUSION

This chapter has described some of the epidemiologic approaches used to assess the relative contributions of genetic and environmental factors to the cause of human disease. The link of epidemiology and genetics has become increasingly recognized, and a field called *genetic epidemiology* has emerged.[15] The Human Genome Project, whose goal was to generate a high-quality reference sequence for the human genome's 3 billion base pairs and to identify all human genes, completed the first working draft of the entire human genome in April 2003, on the 50th anniversary of Watson and Crick's publication of DNA structure. Excellent discussions have been published regarding the impact of the genomic era on epidemiologic research.[36,37]

Most epidemiologic studies are directed at identifying environmental factors in disease, but when designing and conducting studies and interpreting their results, it is important to bear in mind that individuals who are subjects in epidemiologic studies differ not only in environmental exposures but also in their genetic susceptibilities. When appropriate, epidemiologic studies of risk factors, including case-control and other types of studies, should be expanded to include gathering family histories and obtaining biologic samples, if possible. Advances made in the Human Genome Project and genetic markers of susceptibility developed in the laboratory are proving increasingly valuable in epidemiologic studies. They are likely to be increasingly important factors in improving disease prevention in the future.

REFERENCES

1. Eisenberg L: Would cloned humans really be like sheep? N Engl J Med 340:471–475, 1999.
2. Hogben L: Nature and Nurture. New York, WW Norton, 1939.
3. Miki Y, Swensen J, Shattuck-Eidens D, et al: A strong candidate for the breast and ovarian cancer susceptibility gene BRCA1. Science 266:66–71, 1994.
4. Struewing JP, Hartge P, Wacholder S, et al: The risk of cancer associated with specific mutations of BRCA1 and BRCA2 among Ashkenazi Jews. N Engl J Med 336:1401–1408, 1997.
5. Savitsky K, Bar-Shira A, Gilad S, et al: A single ataxia telangiectasia gene with a product similar to PI-3 kinase. Science 268:1749–1753, 1995.
6. Nowak R: Discovery of AT gene sparks biomedical research bonanza. Science 268:1700–1701, 1995.
7. ESTs: Gene discovery made easier. In Just the Facts: A Basic Introduction to the Science Underlying NCBI Resources. National Center for Biotechnology Information, February 10, 2003. http://www.ncbi.nlm.nih.gov/About/primer/est.html.
8. Microarrays: Chipping away at the mysteries of science and medicine. In Just the Facts: A Basic Introduction to the Science Underlying NCBI Resources. National Center for Biotechnology Information, February 10, 2003. http://www.ncbi.nlm.nih.gov/About/primer/microarrays.html.
9. van de Vijver MJ, He YD, van't Veer Lj, et al: A gene-expression signature as a predictor of survival in breast cancer. N Engl J Med 347:1999–2009, 2002.
10. Knudson AG Jr: Mutation and cancer: Statistical study of retinoblastoma. Proc Natl Acad Sci USA 68:820–823, 1971.
11. Cavenee WK, Dryja TP, Phillips RA, et al: Expression of recessive alleles by chromosomal mechanisms in retinoblastoma. Nature 305:779–784, 1983.
12. Benedict WF, Fung WT, Murphree L: The gene responsible for the development of retinoblastoma and osteosarcoma. Cancer 62:1691–1694, 1988.
13. Corder EH, Saunders AM, Strittmatter WJ, et al: Gene dose of apolipoprotein E type 4 allele and the risk of Alzheimer's disease in late onset families. Science 261:921–923, 1993.
14. Childs B, Scriver CR: Age at onset and causes of disease. Perspect Biol Med 29:437–460, 1986.
15. Khoury MJ, Beaty TH, Cohen BH: Fundamentals of Genetic Epidemiology. New York, Oxford University Press, 1993.
16. Kaij L: Studies on the Etiology and Sequels of Abuse of Alcohol. Lund, Hakan Ohlssons Boktryckeri, 1960.
17. Hrubec Z, Omenn GS: Evidence of genetic predisposition to alcoholic cirrhosis and psychosis: Twin concordance for alcoholism and its biological end points by zygosity among male veterans. Alcohol Clin Exp Res 5:207–215, 1981.
18. Murray RM, Clifford C, Gurlin HM: Twin and alcoholism studies. In Galanter M (ed): Recent Developments in Alcoholism, vol 1. New York, Plenum, 1983, pp 25–47.
19. Pickens RW, Svikis DS, McGue M, et al: Heterogeneity in the inheritance of alcoholism: A study of male and female twins. Arch Gen Psychiatry 48:19–28, 1991.
20. MacMahon B: Epidemiology of Hodgkin's disease. Cancer Res 26:1189–1201, 1966.
21. Diehl V, Tesch H: Hodgkin's disease: Environmental or genetic? N Engl J Med 332:461–462, 1995.
22. Gutensohn N, Cole P: Childhood social environment and Hodgkin's disease. N Engl J Med 304:135–140, 1981.
23. Mack TM, Cozen W, Shibata DK, et al: Concordance for Hodgkin's disease in identical twins suggesting genetic susceptibility to the young-adult form of the disease. N Engl J Med 332:413–418, 1995.
24. Tanner CM, Ottman R, Goldman SM, et al: Parkinson disease in twins: An etiologic study. JAMA 281:341–346, 1999.
25. Lichtenstein P, Holm NV, Verkasalo PK, et al: Environmental and heritable factors in the causation of cancer: Analyses of cohorts of twins from Sweden, Denmark, and Finland. N Engl J Med 343:78–85, 2000.

26. Kety SS, Ingraham LJ: Genetic transmission and improved diagnosis of schizophrenia from pedigrees of adoptees. J Psychiatr Res 26:247–255, 1992.

27. Childs B: The entry of genetics into medicine. J Urban Health: Bull NY Acad Medicine 76:497–508, 1999.

28. Grant BF: The impact of a family history of alcoholism on the relationship between age at onset of alcohol use and DSM-IV alcohol dependence: Results from the National Longitudinal Alcohol Epidemiologic Survey. Alcohol Health Res World 22:144–147, 1998.

29. Vandenbroucke JP, Koster T, Briët E, et al: Increased risk of venous thrombosis in oral-contraceptive users who are carriers of factor V Leiden mutation. Lancet 344:1453–1457, 1994.

30. Brennan JA, Boyle JO, Koch WM, et al: Association between cigarette smoking and mutation of the p[53] gene in squamous-cell carcinoma of the head and neck. N Engl J Med 332:712–717, 1995.

31. Bressac B, Puisieux MS, Kew M, et al: p[53] mutation in hepatocellular carcinoma after aflatoxin exposure. Lancet 338:1356–1359, 1991.

32. Aguilar F, Harris CC, Sun T, et al: Geographic variation of p[53] mutational profile in nonmalignant human liver. Science 264:1317–1319, 1994.

33. Harris C: p[53]: At the crossroads of molecular carcinogenesis and risk assessment. Science 262:1980–1981, 1993.

34. Childs B: Genetic Medicine —A logic of disease. Baltimore, Johns Hopkins University Press, 1999.

35. Childs B, Valle D: Genetics, biology and disease. Annu Rev Genom Human Genet 1:1–19, 2000.

36. Millikan R: The changing face of epidemiology in the genomics era. Epidemiology 13:472–480, 2002.

37. Willett WC: Balancing life-style and genomics research for disease prevention. Science 296: 695–698, 2002.

REVIEW QUESTIONS FOR CHAPTER 16

1. If a greater proportion of monozygotic twin pairs are found to be concordant for a certain disease than are dizygotic twin pairs, the observation suggests that the disease is most likely caused by:
   a. Exclusively environmental factors
   b. Exclusively hereditary factors
   c. Hereditary factors almost exclusively, with some nonhereditary factors possibly playing a role
   d. Environmental and genetic factors almost equally
   e. Gender differences in monozygotic twins

Question 2 is based on the information given below:

In a familial study of schizophrenia, the following concordance rates were observed within various pairs of relatives:

Pair	Concordance Rate (%)
Husband–wife	5
Parent–child	40
Monozygotic twins	65
Dizygotic twins	42
Ordinary siblings	40

2. A reasonable conclusion to be drawn from these data is:
   a. Genetic factors are unimportant in the etiology of schizophrenia
   b. The data suggest a potentially important genetic component

   c. The incidence of schizophrenia within relative pairs is highest in monozygotic twins
   d. The prevalence of schizophrenia within relative pairs is highest in monozygotic twins
   e. Twins are less likely to have schizophrenia than are ordinary siblings

Question 3 is based on the information given below:

In a study of Japanese migrants to the United States, the following standardized mortality ratios (SMRs) were found for disease X:

Group	Standardized Mortality Ratio
Native Japanese living in Japan	100
Japanese migrants	105
Children of Japanese ancestry	108
United States whites	591

3. These findings suggest that:
   a. Environmental factors are the major determinants of these SMRs
   b. Genetic factors are the major determinants of these SMRs
   c. Environmental factors associated with the migrant culture are probably involved
   d. Migrants are highly selected and are nonrepresentative of the population in their native country
   e. International differences in coding death certificates for disease X are an important determinant of these SMRs

4. When the incidence of a disease in adopted children is studied and compared with its incidence in biologic relatives and in adoptive relatives, all of the following are relevant concerns *except:*
   a. Age at onset
   b. Amount of contact maintained by the adoptee with his or her biologic parents
   c. Marital status of the biologic parents
   d. Selection factors relating to who is adopted and who is not
   e. *c* and *d*

5. If an association is found between the incidence of a disease and a certain genetically determined characteristic:
   a. The disease is clearly genetic in origin
   b. Genetic factors are at least implicated in all cases of the disease
   c. Genetic factors are implicated in at least some cases of the disease
   d. A role for environmental factors is excluded
   e. Expression of the disease is likely to be unavoidable

Section III

APPLYING EPIDEMIOLOGY TO EVALUATION AND POLICY

In Section II, we reviewed the major types of study designs used in epidemiology and examined how the results of epidemiologic studies are used for demonstrating associations and deriving causal inferences. Although the methodologic issues discussed are interesting and intriguing, much of the excitement in epidemiology stems from the fact that its results have direct application to problems involving human health. The challenges that are therefore involved include deriving valid inferences from the data generated by epidemiologic studies, ensuring appropriate communication of the findings and their interpretations to policy makers and the general public, and dealing with the ethical problems that arise because of the close link of epidemiology to human health and to clinical and public health policy.

This section discusses the uses of epidemiology in evaluating both health services (Chapter 17) and screening programs (Chapter 18). We then turn to some of the specific issues involved in the application of epidemiology to issues of policy (Chapter 19), and finally address some of the major ethical and professional considerations that arise in the context both of conducting epidemiologic investigations and of utilizing the results of epidemiologic studies for improving the health of the community by enhancing the effectiveness of clinical care and public health interventions (Chapter 20).

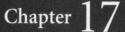

Chapter 17

Using Epidemiology to Evaluate Health Services

Perhaps the earliest example of an evaluation is the description of creation given in the book of Genesis 1:1–4, which is shown in the original Hebrew in Figure 17-1. Translated, with the addition of a few subheadings, it reads as follows:

BASELINE DATA
In the beginning God created the heaven and the earth. And the earth was unformed and void and darkness was on the face of the deep.

IMPLEMENTATION OF THE PROGRAM
And God said, "Let there be light." And there was light.

EVALUATION OF THE PROGRAM
And God saw the light, that it was good.

FURTHER PROGRAM ACTIVITIES
And God divided the light from the darkness.

This excerpt includes all of the basic components of the process of evaluation: baseline data, implementation of the program, evaluation of the program, and implementation of new program activities on the basis of the results of the evaluation. However, two problems arise in this description. First, we are not given the precise criteria that were used to determine whether the program was "good"; we are told only

that God saw that it was good. Second, this evaluation exemplifies a frequently observed problem: the program director is assessing his own program. Both conscious and subconscious biases can arise in evaluation. Furthermore, even if the program director administers the program superbly, he may not necessarily have the specific skills that are needed to conduct a methodologically rigorous evaluation of the program.

Dr. Wade Hampton Frost, a leader in epidemiology in the early part of the 20th century, addressed the use of epidemiology in the evaluation of public health programs in a presentation to the American Public Health Association in 1925.[1] He wrote, in part, as follows:

The health officer occupies the position of an agent to whom the public entrusts certain of its resources in public money and cooperation, to be so invested that they may yield the best returns in health; and in discharging the responsibilities of this position he is expected to follow the same general principles of procedure as would be a fiscal agent under like circumstances. . . .

Since his capital comes entirely from the public, it is reasonable to expect that he will be prepared to explain to the public his reasons for making each investment, and to give them some estimate of the returns which he expects. Nor can he consider it

Figure 17-1. The earliest known evaluation. (Genesis 1:1–4.)

בְּרֵאשִׁית בָּרָא אֱלֹהִים אֵת הַשָּׁמַיִם וְאֵת הָאָרֶץ
וְהָאָרֶץ הָיְתָה תֹהוּ וָבֹהוּ וְחֹשֶׁךְ עַל פְּנֵי תְהוֹם וְרוּחַ
אֱלֹהִים מְרַחֶפֶת עַל פְּנֵי הַמָּיִם וַיֹּאמֶר אֱלֹהִים יְהִי
אוֹר וַיְהִי אוֹר וַיַּרְא אֱלֹהִים אֶת הָאוֹר כִּי טוֹב
וַיַּבְדֵּל אֱלֹהִים בֵּין הָאוֹר וּבֵין הַחֹשֶׁךְ וַיִּקְרָא
אֱלֹהִים לָאוֹר יוֹם וְלַחֹשֶׁךְ קָרָא לַיְלָה וַיְהִי עֶרֶב
וַיְהִי בֹקֶר יוֹם אֶחָד

293

unreasonable if the public should wish to have an accounting from time to time, to know what returns are actually being received and how they check with the advance estimates which he has given them. Certainly any fiscal agent would expect to have his judgment thus checked and to gain or lose his clients' confidence in proportion as his estimates were verified or not. . . .

However, as to such accounting, the health officer finds himself in a difficult and possibly embarrassing position, for while he may give a fairly exact statement of how much money and effort he has put into each of his several activities, he can rarely if ever give an equally exact or simple accounting of the returns from these investments considered separately and individually. This, to be sure, is not altogether his fault. It is due primarily to the character of the dividends from public health endeavor, and the manner in which they are distributed. They are not received in separate installments of a uniform currency, each docketed as to its source and recorded as received; but come irregularly from day to day, distributed to unidentified individuals throughout the community, who are not individually conscious of having received them. They are positive benefits in added life and improved health, but the only record ordinarily kept in morbidity and mortality statistics is the partial and negative record of death and of illness from certain clearly defined types of disease, chiefly the more acute communicable diseases, which constitute only a fraction of the total morbidity.[1]

Dr. Charles V. Chapin commented on Frost's presentation:

Dr. Frost's earnest demand that the procedures of preventive medicine be placed on a firm scientific basis is well timed. Indeed, it would have been opportune at any time during the past 40 years and, it is to be feared, will be equally needed for 40 years to come.

Chapin clearly underestimated the number of years; the need remains as critical today, more than 80 years later, as it was in 1925.

STUDIES OF PROCESS AND OUTCOME

Studies of Process
At the outset, we should distinguish between process and outcome studies. *Process* means that we decide

what constitutes the components of good care. Such a decision is often made by an expert panel. We can then assess a clinic or health care provider, by reviewing relevant records or by direct observation and determine to what extent the care provided meets established and accepted criteria. For example, we can determine what percentage of patients have had their blood pressure measured. The problem with such process measures is that they do not indicate whether the patient is better off; for example, monitoring blood pressure does not ensure that the patient's blood pressure is under control. Second, because process assessments are based on expert opinion, the criteria used in process evaluations may change over time as expert opinion changes. For example, in the 1940s, the accepted standard of care for premature infants required that such infants be placed in 100% oxygen. Incubators were monitored to be sure that such levels were maintained. However, when research demonstrated that high oxygen concentration played a major role in producing a form of blindness in children who had been prematurely born, a condition called retrolental fibroplasia, high concentrations of oxygen were subsequently deemed unacceptable.

Studies of Outcomes
Given the limitations of process studies, the remainder of this chapter focuses on outcome measures. *Outcome* denotes whether or not a patient benefits from the medical care provided. Health outcomes are the domain of epidemiology. Although such measures have traditionally been mortality and morbidity, interest in outcomes research in recent years has expanded the measures of interest to include patient satisfaction, quality of life, degree of dependence and disability, and similar measures.

EFFICACY, EFFECTIVENESS, AND EFFICIENCY

Three terms that are often encountered in the literature dealing with evaluation of health services are *efficacy*, *effectiveness*, and *efficiency*.

Efficacy
Does the agent or intervention "work" under ideal, "laboratory" conditions? We test a new drug in a group of patients who have agreed to be hospitalized and who are observed as they take their therapy. Or a vaccine is tested in a group of consenting subjects. Thus, efficacy is a measure in a situation in which all

conditions are controlled to maximize the effect of the agent.

Effectiveness

If we administer the agent in a "real-life" situation, is it effective? For example, when the vaccine just referred to is tested in a community, many individuals may not come in to be vaccinated. Or, an oral medication may have such an undesirable taste that no one will take it (so that it will prove ineffective), despite the fact that under controlled conditions, when compliance was ensured, the drug was shown to be efficacious.

Efficiency

If an agent is shown to be effective, what is the cost-benefit ratio? Is it possible to achieve our goals in a cheaper and better way? Cost includes not only money, but also discomfort, pain, absenteeism, disability, and social stigma.

If a health care measure has not been demonstrated to be effective, there is little point looking at efficiency, for if it is not effective, the cheapest alternative is not to use it at all. At times, of course, political and societal pressures may drive a program even if it is not effective. However, this chapter will focus only on the science of evaluation and specifically on the issue of effectiveness in evaluating health services.

MEASURES OF OUTCOME

If efficacy of a measure has been demonstrated—that is, if the methods of prevention and intervention that are of interest have been shown to work, we can then turn to evaluating effectiveness. What guidelines should we use in selecting an appropriate outcome measure to serve as an index of effectiveness? First, the measure must be clearly quantifiable; that is, we must be able to express its effect in quantitative terms. Second, the measure of outcome should be relatively easy to define and diagnose. If the measure is to be used in a population study, we would certainly not want to depend on an invasive procedure for assessing any benefits. Third, the measure selected should lend itself to standardization for study purposes. Fourth, the population served (and the comparison population) must be at risk for the same condition for which an intervention is being evaluated. For example, it would obviously make no sense to test the effectiveness of a sickle cell screening program in a white population.

TABLE 17-1. Some Possible Endpoints for Measuring Success of a Vaccine Program

1. Number (or proportion) of people immunized
2. Number (or proportion) of people at (high) risk who are immunized
3. Number (or proportion) of people immunized who show serologic response
4. Number (or proportion) of people immunized and later exposed in whom clinical disease does not develop
5. Number (or proportion) of people immunized and later exposed in whom clinical or subclinical disease does not develop

---

The type of outcome endpoint that we select should depend on the question that we are asking. Although this may seem self-evident, it is not always immediately apparent. Table 17-1 shows possible endpoints in evaluating the effectiveness of a vaccine program. Whatever outcome we select should be explicitly stated so that others reading the report of our findings will be able to make their own judgments regarding the appropriateness of the measure selected and the quality of the data. Whether the measure we have selected is indeed an appropriate one depends on clinical and public health aspects of the disease in question.

Table 17-2 shows possible choices of measures for assessing the effectiveness of a throat culture

---

TABLE 17-2. Some Possible Endpoints for Measuring Success of a Throat Culture Program

1. Number of cultures taken (symptomatic or asymptomatic)
2. Number (or proportion) of cultures positive for streptococcal infection
3. Number (or proportion) of persons with positive cultures for whom medical care is obtained
4. Number (or proportion) of persons with positive cultures for whom proper treatment is prescribed and taken
5. Number (or proportion) of positive cultures followed by a relapse
6. Number (or proportion) of positive cultures followed by rheumatic fever

program in children. Measures of volume of services provided, numbers of cultures taken, and number of clinic visits have been traditional favorites because they are relatively easy to count and are helpful in justifying requests for budgetary increases for the program in the following year. However, such measures are process measures and tell us nothing about the effectiveness of an intervention. We therefore move to other possibilities listed in this table. Again, the most appropriate measures should depend on the question being asked. The question must be specific. It is not enough just to ask how good is the program.

COMPARING EPIDEMIOLOGIC STUDIES OF DISEASE ETIOLOGY AND EPIDEMIOLOGIC RESEARCH EVALUATING EFFECTIVENESS OF HEALTH SERVICES

In classic epidemiologic studies of disease etiology, we examine the possible relationship between a putative cause (the independent variable) and an adverse health effect or effects (the dependent variable). In doing so, we take into account other factors, including health care, that may modify the relationship or confound it (Fig. 17-2A). In health services research, we focus on the health service as the independent variable, with a reduction in adverse health effects as the anticipated outcome (dependent variable) if the modality of care is effective. In this situation, environmental and other factors that may influence the relationship are also taken into account (see Fig. 17-2B). Thus, both etiologic epidemiologic research and health services research address the possible relationship between an independent variable and a dependent variable and the influence of other factors on the relationship. Therefore, it is not surprising that many of the study designs discussed are

common to both epidemiologic and health services research, as are the methodologic problems and potential biases that may characterize these types of studies.

EVALUATION USING GROUP DATA

Regularly available data, such as mortality data and hospitalization data, are often used in evaluation studies. Such data can be obtained from different sources, and such sources may differ in important ways. For example, Figure 17-3 shows discharge rates for short-term hospital stays in the United States from two sources: the National Hospital Discharge Survey (NHDS) and the National Health Interview Survey (NHIS).

Although the trends are similar, the magnitude of the rates differs. The NHDS uses hospital records of inpatients discharged from short-stay non-federal hospitals. The NHIS uses personal interviews, and people tend to forget many of their past hospitalizations. The NHIS also includes discharges from federal hospitals, most of which are Veterans Administration hospitals. The NHDS includes patients who die in the hospital as well as those admitted from nursing homes, two groups not included by the NHIS. The NHDS—but not the NHIS—counts as discharges persons who are hospitalized for less than one day. The point is that in evaluating any modality of health care, we must identify and understand the characteristics of each of the sources of data that will be used, such as who or what is included or excluded, on what variables are data obtained and how the data are categorized. We then assess the impact of these characteristics and the validity of the data obtained, and also examine possible biases that may be introduced. If we are only interested in changes over time—*trends*—the issues may not be critical, but if

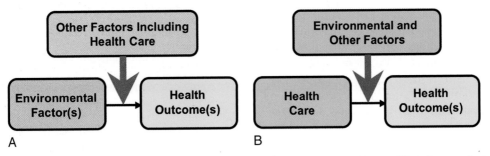

Figure 17-2. A, Classic epidemiologic research into etiology, taking into account the possible influence of other factors, including health care. **B,** Classic health services research into effectiveness, taking into account the possible influence of environmental and other factors.

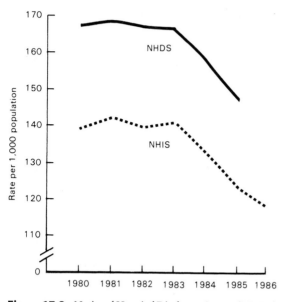

Figure 17-3. National Hospital Discharge Survey (NHDS) and National Health Interview Survey (NHIS) short-stay hospital discharge rates, United States, 1980–1986. (From Moss AJ, Moien MA: Recent declines in hospitalization, United States, 1982–1986. Data from the National Health Interview Survey and the National Hospital Discharge Survey. NCHS Advance Data, Vital and Health Statistics of the National Center for Health Statistics, no. 140, p. 2, 1987.)

we are interested in absolute values, the issues may be important.

Outcomes Research

The term *outcomes research* has been used increasingly in recent years to denote studies comparing the effects of two or more health care interventions or modalities—such as treatments, forms of health care organization, or type and extent of insurance coverage and provider reimbursement—on health or economic outcomes. The health endpoints may include morbidity and mortality as well as measures of quality of life, functional status, and patient perceptions of their health status, including symptom recognition and patient satisfaction. Economic measures may reflect direct or indirect costs, and can include hospitalization rates, outpatient and emergency room visits, lost days of work, child care, and days of restricted activity. Consequently, epidemiology is one of several disciplines needed in outcomes research.

Outcomes research often uses data from large data sets that were derived from large populations. Although in recent years some of the large data sets have been developed from cohorts that were originally set up for different research purposes, many of the data sets used were often originally initiated for administrative or fiscal purposes, rather than for any research goals. Often several large data sets, each having information on different variables, may be linked in order to explore a question of interest.

The advantages of using large data sets are that the data refer to real-world populations, and the issue of "representativeness" or "generalizability" is minimized. In addition, since the data sets exist at the time the research is initiated, analysis can generally be completed and results generated relatively rapidly. Moreover, given the large data sets used, sample size is not usually a problem except when smaller subgroups are examined. Given these considerations, the costs of using existing data sets are generally lower than the costs of primary data collection.

The disadvantages are that, since the data were often initially gathered for fiscal and administrative purposes, they may not be well suited for research purposes and for answering the specific research question addressed in the study. Even when the data were originally gathered for research, our knowledge of the area may now be more complete and new research questions may have arisen that could not even have been conceived of when the original data collection was initiated. In general, data may be incomplete. Data on the independent and dependent variables may be very limited. Data may be missing on clinical details including disease severity and on the details of the interventions, and diagnostic coding may be inconsistent. Data relating to possible confounders may be inadequate or absent since the research now being conducted was often not even possible when the data were originally generated. Because certain variables that today are considered relevant and important were not included in the original data set, investigators may at times create surrogate variables for the missing variables, using certain variables that are included in the data set but that may not directly reflect the variable of interest. However, such surrogate variables vary in the extent to which they are an adequate measure of the missing variable of interest. For all these reasons the validity of the conclusions reached may therefore be in doubt.

Another important problem that may arise with large data sets is that because the necessary variables may be absent in the available data set, the investigator may consciously or subconsciously change the original question he wanted to address to a question

for which the variables that are required for study are present in the data set. Thus, rather than the investigator deciding what research question should be addressed, the data set may be allowed to determine what questions are asked in the study.

Finally, using large data sets, investigators become progressively more removed from the individuals being studied. Over the years, direct interviews and reviews of patient records have tended to be replaced by large computerized databases. Using these sources of data, many personal characteristics of the subjects are never explored and their relevance to the questions being asked is virtually never assessed.

One area in which existing sources of data are often used in evaluation studies is prenatal care. The problems discussed earlier are exemplified in the use of birth certificates. These documents are often used because they are easily accessible and provide certain medical care data, such as the trimester in which prenatal care was begun. However, birth certificates for women with high-risk pregnancies have missing data more often than those for women with low-risk pregnancies. The quality of the data provided on birth certificates also may differ regionally and internationally, and may complicate any comparisons that are made.

An example of outcomes research using large data sets is a study by Gornick et al. of Medicare beneficiaries in the United States.[2] Since Medicare health coverage is provided to virtually all elderly individuals in the United States, it is assumed that if a study population is limited to those who have Medicare coverage, financial obstacles to care and other variables are held constant among different groups such as ethnic subpopulations. However, wide disparities still remain between blacks and whites in utilizing many Medicare services. The authors studied the effects of race and income on mortality and use of services among Medicare beneficiaries. To do this, they linked 1990 census data on median income according to zip code with 1993 Medicare administrative data for 26.3 million beneficiaries 65 years or older. They calculated age-adjusted mortality rates and age- and sex-adjusted rates of various diagnoses and procedures according to race and income and computed black:white ratios.

As seen in Figure 17-4, age-adjusted mortality was higher for black men than for white men (black:white mortality ratio = 1.19), and for black women than for white women (black:white mortality ratio = 1.16). In each of these subgroups, except black women, the highest income group had the lowest

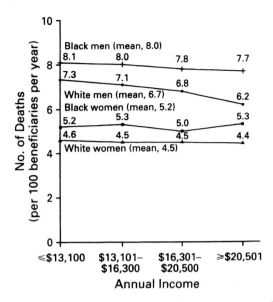

Figure 17-4. Mortality rates according to race, sex, and income among Medicare beneficiaries 65 years or older, 1993. Rates are adjusted for age to the total Medicare population. (From Gornick ME, Eggers PW, Reilly TW, et al: Effects of race and income on mortality and use of services among Medicare beneficiaries. N Engl J Med 335:791–799, 1996. Copyright © 1996 Massachusetts Medical Society. All rights reserved.)

mortality rates and the lowest income group had the highest mortality rates. Many procedures and diagnoses were examined. Use of mammography, for example, varied substantially by race and income (Fig. 17-5). Whites had higher rates of mammography, but in both whites and blacks, less-affluent people had fewer mammograms than did the more affluent. Rates of amputation of part or all of a lower extremity were significantly higher in blacks than in whites (black:white ratio = 3.64) (Fig. 17-6). Among both blacks and whites, amputation rates were highest among the least affluent. These data suggest that these groups of beneficiaries are at higher risk for procedures associated with less than optimal care for chronic conditions such as diabetes.

The authors pointed out that the data set used did not provide information about the health status of individuals and the underlying medical conditions of the beneficiaries, and suggested that lack of such data may limit some of the inferences that can be drawn. Nevertheless, they concluded that race and income substantially affect mortality and use of services among Medicare beneficiaries and that Medicare coverage alone is not sufficient to promote effective patterns of use by all beneficiaries. (Also see "Race

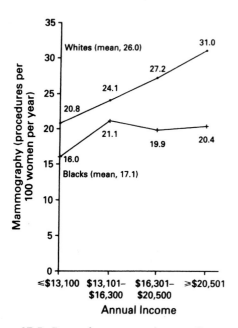

Figure 17-5. Rates of mammography according to race and income among female Medicare beneficiaries 65 years or older, 1993. Rates are adjusted for age to the total female Medicare population. (From Gornick ME, Eggers PW, Reilly TW, et al: Effects of race and income on mortality and use of services among Medicare beneficiaries. N Engl J Med 335:791–799, 1996. Copyright © 1996 Massachusetts Medical Society. All rights reserved.)

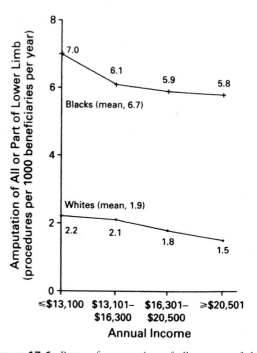

Figure 17-6. Rates of amputation of all or part of the lower limb, according to race and income, among Medicare beneficiaries 65 years or older, 1993. Amputation rates are adjusted for age and sex to the total Medicare population. (From Gornick ME, Eggers PW, Reilly TW, et al: Effects of race and income on mortality and use of services among Medicare beneficiaries. N Engl J Med 335:791–799, 1996. Copyright © 1996 Massachusetts Medical Society. All rights reserved.)

and Ethnicity in Epidemiologic Studies" section in Chapter 20.)

Potential Biases in Evaluating Health Services Using Group Data

Studies evaluating health services using group data are susceptible to many of the biases which characterize etiologic studies as discussed in Chapter 15. In addition, certain biases are particularly relevant for specific research areas and topics. For example, studies of the relationship of prenatal care to birth outcomes are prone to several important potential biases. In such studies the question often addressed is whether prenatal care, as measured by the number of prenatal visits, reduces the risk of prematurity and low birth weight. Several potential biases may be introduced into this type of analysis. For example, other things being equal, a woman who delivers prematurely will have fewer prenatal visits (i.e., the pregnancy was shorter so that there was less time in which it was possible for her to "be at risk" for prenatal visits). The result would be an artifactual relationship between fewer prenatal visits and prematurity, only because the period of gestation was shorter. However,

bias can also operate in the other direction. A woman who begins prenatal care in the last trimester of pregnancy will not have an early premature delivery, as she has already carried the pregnancy to the last trimester. This would lead to an observed association of fewer prenatal visits with a smaller likelihood of early premature delivery. In addition, women who have had medical complications in the past may be so anxious that they come for more prenatal visits, but they may also be at greater risk for a bad outcome. Thus, the potential biases can run in either direction. If such women are at high risk that is not amenable to prevention, an apparent association of more prenatal visits with adverse outcome may be observed.

Finally, such studies are often biased by self-selection—that is, the women who choose to begin prenatal care early in pregnancy are often better educated and from a higher socioeconomic status and have more positive attitudes toward health care. Thus, a population of women, who to begin with are at lower

risk for an adverse birth outcome, select themselves for earlier prenatal care. The result is a potential for an apparent association of early prenatal care with lower risk of adverse pregnancy outcome, even if the care itself is without any true health benefit.

Two Indices Used in Ecologic Studies of Health Services

One index used in evaluating health services using ecologic studies is avoidable mortality. *Avoidable mortality* analyses assume that the rate of "avoidable deaths" should vary inversely with the availability, accessibility, and quality of medical care in different geographic regions. Thus, ideally, avoidable mortality would serve as a measure of the adequacy and effectiveness of care in an area. Changes over time could be plotted and comparisons made with other areas. Unfortunately, the necessary data are lacking for many of the conditions suggested for avoidable mortality analyses. Moreover, data on confounders may not be available and the resulting inferences may therefore be open to question.

A second approach is to use *health indicators*. With this approach, certain sentinel conditions are assumed to reflect the general level of health care, and changes in the incidence of these conditions are plotted over time and compared with data for other populations. The changes and differences that are found are then related to changes in the health service sector and used to derive inferences about causation. However, it is difficult to know what criteria need to be met in order for a given condition to be acceptable as a valid health indicator.

EVALUATION USING INDIVIDUAL DATA

Because of the limitations inherent in studies using group data, that is, studies in which we do not have data on both health care (exposure) and health outcome for each individual, studies using individual data are generally preferable. If we wish to compare two populations, one receiving the care being evaluated and one not receiving it, we must ask the following two questions to be able to derive inferences about the effectiveness of care:

1. Are the characteristics of the two groups comparable—demographically, medically, and in terms of factors relating to prognosis?
2. Are the measurement methods comparable (e.g., diagnostic methods and the way disease is classified) in both groups?

Both issues have been discussed in earlier chapters because they also apply to questions of etiology, prevention, and therapy, and they must therefore be considered in any type of study design.

An important issue in using epidemiology to study outcomes for the evaluation of health services is the need to address prognostic stratification. If a change in health outcome is observed after a certain type of care has been delivered, can we necessarily conclude that the change is due to the health care provided, or could it be a result of differences in prognosis based on comorbidity—preexisting disease which may or may not be specifically related to the disease being studied, in severity, or in other associated conditions that bear on prognosis? To address these issues, such outcome studies must carry out a prognostic stratification by studying case mix and carefully characterizing the individuals studied on the basis of disease severity.

Let us now turn to some *cohort designs* used in evaluation of health services.

Randomized Designs

Randomization eliminates the problem of selection bias that results from either self-selection by the patient or selection of the patient by the health care provider. Usually, study participants are assigned to receive one type of care versus another rather than to receive care versus no care (Fig. 17-7). For many reasons, both ethical and practical, randomizing patients to receive no care usually is not considered.

Let us consider one study that used a randomized design to evaluate different approaches to health care. Early, organized, hospital-based management has been strongly recommended for the care of patients with stroke. However, few data are available from well-conducted controlled studies to compare

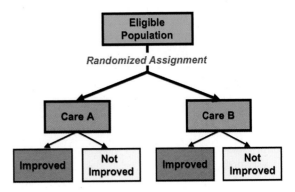

Figure 17-7. Design of a randomized study comparing care A and care B.

4. When the incidence of a disease in adopted children is studied and compared with its incidence in biologic relatives and in adoptive relatives, all of the following are relevant concerns *except:*
   a. Age at onset
   b. Amount of contact maintained by the adoptee with his or her biologic parents
   c. Marital status of the biologic parents
   d. Selection factors relating to who is adopted and who is not
   e. *c* and *d*

5. If an association is found between the incidence of a disease and a certain genetically determined characteristic:
   a. The disease is clearly genetic in origin
   b. Genetic factors are at least implicated in all cases of the disease
   c. Genetic factors are implicated in at least some cases of the disease
   d. A role for environmental factors is excluded
   e. Expression of the disease is likely to be unavoidable

hospital care with specialized care at home (domiciliary care). Furthermore, an alternative to stroke units in the hospital is a specialized stroke team that can provide care anywhere in the hospital where stroke patients may be treated. This consideration is of practical importance because it may not be possible for every hospital to offer all patients who have a stroke care in a specialized unit because of space limitations and other administrative and financial issues.

In order to identify the best organizational structure for the care of patients with stroke, Kalra and colleagues[3] conducted a randomized, controlled trial to compare the efficacy of three forms of care (Fig. 17-8). Patients were randomly assigned to one of the following groups: (1) care provided in a hospital stroke unit by a stroke physician and a multidisciplinary team, (2) care provided by a multidisciplinary stroke team with expertise in stroke management, or (3) care at home (domiciliary care) provided by a specialist team. The outcome was mortality or institutionalization, and was assessed at 3, 6, and 12 months after the onset of a stroke. Data were ana-

lyzed by intention-to-treat. At each of the three time points, patients treated in the stroke unit were less likely to die or to be institutionalized than patients in the group treated by the stroke team or the group receiving domiciliary care. Cumulative survival in the three groups is shown in Figure 17-9. The study supports the use of specialized stroke units for the care of patients with stroke.

As seen in Figure 17-9, an interesting and somewhat surprising finding in this study is that survival was better in patients who were randomized to receive domiciliary care (care at home) than in those randomized to receive care in the hospital by a stroke team.

A possible explanation for this observation is that patients in the domiciliary care group whose condition deteriorated or who had developed new problems were withdrawn from domiciliary care and admitted to a stroke unit. These patients were still analyzed with the domiciliary care group because an intention-to-treat analysis was used that analyzes outcome according to the original randomization. These patients may have benefited from care in the stroke unit, and if so, their outcome would tend to improve the outcome results for the domiciliary care group because of the intention-to-treat analysis.

Drummond and colleagues[4] conducted a 10-year follow-up of a randomized controlled trial of care in

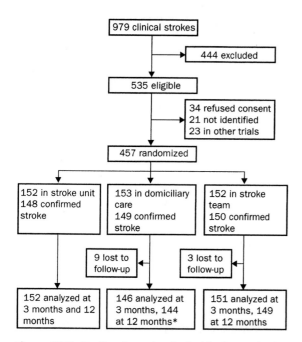

Figure 17-8. Profile of a randomized trial of strategies for stroke care. *Fifty-one patients in this group were admitted to the hospital within 2 weeks of randomization, but are included in the intention-to-treat analysis. (Adapted from Kalra L, Evans A, Perez I, et al: Alternative strategies for stroke care: A prospective randomized controlled trial. Lancet 356:894–899, 2000.)

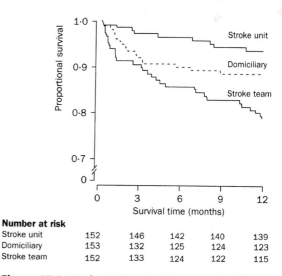

Number at risk					
Stroke unit	152	146	142	140	139
Domiciliary	153	132	125	124	123
Stroke team	152	133	124	122	115

Figure 17-9. Kaplan-Meier survival curves for different strategies of care after acute stroke. (From Kalra L, Evans A, Perez I, et al: Alternative strategies for stroke care: A prospective randomized controlled trial. Lancet 356: 894–899, 2000.)

a stroke rehabilitation unit. They found that management in a stroke rehabilitation unit conferred survival benefits even 10 years after the stroke. The exact reasons are not clear, but the authors suggest that one explanation may be that long-term survival is related to early reduction in disability.

Nonrandomized Designs

All health care interventions cannot be subjected to randomized trials for several reasons. First, such trials are often logistically complex and extremely expensive. Because so many different health care measures are in use at any time, it is not feasible to subject all of them to randomized evaluations. Second, ethical problems are often perceived to occur in randomizing in health services evaluation studies so that randomizing may be viewed as an unacceptable process both by many patients and by health care providers. Third, randomized trials often take a long time to complete, and because programs and health problems change over time, when the results of the study are finally obtained and analyzed, they may no longer be entirely relevant. For these reasons, many health care researchers are looking for alternative approaches that may at least yield some information. One such approach discussed above—*outcomes research*—generally refers to the use of data from nonrandomized studies that often use large existing data sets.

Before-After Design (Historical Controls)

If randomization is not possible or will not be used for any reason, one possible study design to evaluate a program is to compare people who received care before a program was established (or before the health care measure became available) with those who received care from the program after it was established or after the measure became available. What are the problems with this before-after design? First, the data obtained in each of the two periods are frequently not comparable in terms of either quality or completeness. Often, when a new form of health service delivery is developed, a decision is made to evaluate the program by studying people who were treated in the past, before the program began, as a comparison group. As a result, the data available for people after the program was started may be collected using a well-designed research instrument, whereas data for past patients may be available only from health care records that had been designed and used only for clinical or administrative purposes at that time. Hence, if we observe a difference in outcome, we may not know if the observed difference is a result of the effect of the program or of differences in the quality of data from the two time periods.

Second, if we see a difference—for example, mortality is lower after a program was initiated than before the program was initiated—we do not know whether the difference is due to the program itself or to other factors that may have changed over time, such as housing, nutrition, other aspects of lifestyle, or other health services.

Third, a problem of selection exists. Often, it is difficult to know whether the population studied after a program was established is actually similar to that seen before the program was established in terms of other factors that might affect outcome.

Does this mean that before-after studies have no value? No, it does not. But it does mean that such studies only provide a suggestion—and are rarely conclusive—in demonstrating the effectiveness of a health service.

A before-after design was used in a study to assess the impact of the Medicare prospective payment system (PPS) in the United States on quality of care.[5] The study was stimulated by concern that the PPS, with its closely regulated length of hospital stays and incentives for cost-cutting, might have adversely affected the quality of care. The before-after design was selected because the PPS was instituted nationwide, so a prospective cohort design could not be used. Data for almost 17,000 Medicare patients who were hospitalized in 1981–1982 before the PPS was instituted were compared with data for patients hospitalized in 1985–1986 after the PPS was in place. Quality of care was evaluated for five diseases: (1) congestive heart failure, (2) myocardial infarction, (3) pneumonia, (4) cerebrovascular accident, and (5) hip fractures. Outcome findings were adjusted for level of patient sickness on admission to the hospital. Although PPS was not found to be associated with an increase in either 30-day mortality or 6-month mortality, an increase was observed in instability at discharge (defined as the presence of conditions at discharge that clinicians agree should be corrected before discharge or monitored after discharge, and that may result in poor outcomes if not corrected).[6] The authors point out that other factors also may have changed during the time before and after institution of the PPS. Although the before-after design was probably the only design possible for the issue addressed in this study, the study is nevertheless susceptible to some of the problems of this type of design that were discussed earlier.

hospital care with specialized care at home (domiciliary care). Furthermore, an alternative to stroke units in the hospital is a specialized stroke team that can provide care anywhere in the hospital where stroke patients may be treated. This consideration is of practical importance because it may not be possible for every hospital to offer all patients who have a stroke care in a specialized unit because of space limitations and other administrative and financial issues.

In order to identify the best organizational structure for the care of patients with stroke, Kalra and colleagues[3] conducted a randomized, controlled trial to compare the efficacy of three forms of care (Fig. 17-8). Patients were randomly assigned to one of the following groups: (1) care provided in a hospital stroke unit by a stroke physician and a multidisciplinary team, (2) care provided by a multidisciplinary stroke team with expertise in stroke management, or (3) care at home (domiciliary care) provided by a specialist team. The outcome was mortality or institutionalization, and was assessed at 3, 6, and 12 months after the onset of a stroke. Data were analyzed by intention-to-treat. At each of the three time points, patients treated in the stroke unit were less likely to die or to be institutionalized than patients in the group treated by the stroke team or the group receiving domiciliary care. Cumulative survival in the three groups is shown in Figure 17-9. The study supports the use of specialized stroke units for the care of patients with stroke.

As seen in Figure 17-9, an interesting and somewhat surprising finding in this study is that survival was better in patients who were randomized to receive domiciliary care (care at home) than in those randomized to receive care in the hospital by a stroke team.

A possible explanation for this observation is that patients in the domiciliary care group whose condition deteriorated or who had developed new problems were withdrawn from domiciliary care and admitted to a stroke unit. These patients were still analyzed with the domiciliary care group because an intention-to-treat analysis was used that analyzes outcome according to the original randomization. These patients may have benefited from care in the stroke unit, and if so, their outcome would tend to improve the outcome results for the domiciliary care group because of the intention-to-treat analysis.

Drummond and colleagues[4] conducted a 10-year follow-up of a randomized controlled trial of care in

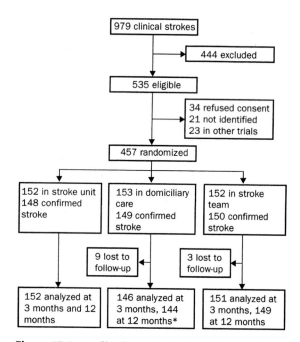

Figure 17-8. Profile of a randomized trial of strategies for stroke care. *Fifty-one patients in this group were admitted to the hospital within 2 weeks of randomization, but are included in the intention-to-treat analysis. (Adapted from Kalra L, Evans A, Perez I, et al: Alternative strategies for stroke care: A prospective randomized controlled trial. Lancet 356:894–899, 2000.)

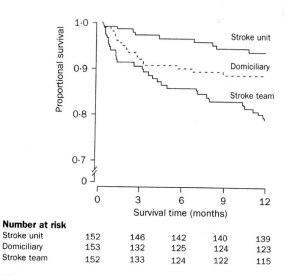

Figure 17-9. Kaplan-Meier survival curves for different strategies of care after acute stroke. (From Kalra L, Evans A, Perez I, et al: Alternative strategies for stroke care: A prospective randomized controlled trial. Lancet 356: 894–899, 2000.)

Simultaneous Nonrandomized Design (Program–No Program)

One option for avoiding the problem of changes that occur over calendar time is to conduct a simultaneous comparison of two populations that are not randomized, in which one population is served by the program and the other is not. This type of design is, in effect, a cohort study in which the type of health care being studied represents the "exposure." As in any cohort study, the problem arises as to how to select exposed and nonexposed groups for study.

In recent years considerable interest has focused on whether higher hospital volume and higher surgeon volume relate to better patient outcomes and many studies have been carried out on these issues. An example of a simultaneous, nonrandomized study of hospital volume is one reported by Jollis and coworkers.[7] This study explored whether differences in patient outcomes in different hospitals related to the volume of hospital procedures performed. The authors studied hospitalizations of patients who underwent percutaneous transluminal coronary angioplasty. They examined the relationship of in-hospital mortality and need for unplanned bypass surgery during the index hospitalization to the volume of angioplasties carried out by the hospital.[7] As seen in Table 17-3, a dose-response relationship was found: the highest in-hospital mortality and the highest rate of unplanned bypass surgery occurred in hospitals that had the smallest volume of angioplasties per year. The finding that hospitals that perform more angioplasties have lower short-term mortality has important potential policy implications and argues for regionalization of angioplasty services.

It is possible that the findings relating higher hospital volumes to better patient outcomes might be due to higher volumes of procedures performed by the surgeons at these hospitals rather than to the overall volumes of procedures performed at these hospitals. Birkmeyer and colleagues addressed this issue.[8] Using Medicare claims data for 1998 and 1999, they examined mortality among all 474,108 patients who underwent one of four cardiovascular procedures or four cancer resection procedures (Fig. 17-10). They found that for most procedures the mortality rate was higher in patients operated on by low-volume surgeons than in patients operated on by high-volume surgeons. This relationship held regardless of the surgical volume of the hospital in which the surgery was performed.

Comparison of Utilizers and Nonutilizers

One approach for a simultaneous, nonrandomized study is to compare a group of people who use a health service with a group of people who do not (Fig. 17-11).

The problems of self-selection inherent in this type of design have long been recognized. Many years ago, Stine and colleagues reported the results of a study of prenatal care provided to women younger than 17 years of age who delivered infants in Baltimore from 1960 to 1961 (Table 17-4).[9]

In this study, 1,397 young women received prenatal care and 315 did not. The neonatal death rate was 30.1 per 1,000 in those who received care and 88.9 per 1,000 in those who did not. The patients were not randomized, but decided themselves whether or not to seek care. As the authors pointed out, in the absence of randomization, we cannot conclude that the care reduced neonatal mortality. For we have the problem of selection: those who came in for care were probably more motivated regarding a broad

---

TABLE 17-3. **In-Hospital Mortality and Rates for Bypass Surgery during Index Hospitalization According to Hospital Volume of Angioplasty Procedures Each Year**

	PROCEDURES		
	<50/yr	**50–100/yr**	**>100/yr**
In-hospital mortality (%)	3.7	3.2	2.7
Bypass surgery during index hospitalization (%)	5.3	4.6	3.5

Adapted from Jollis JG, Peterson ED, DeLong ER, et al: The relation between the volume of coronary angioplasty procedures at hospitals treating Medicare beneficiaries and short-term mortality. N Engl J Med 331:1625–1629, 1994.

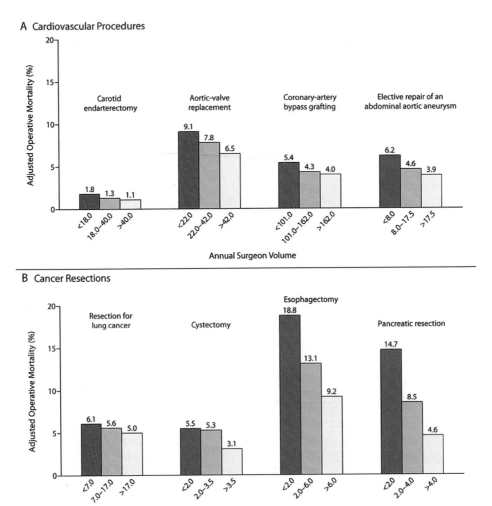

Figure 17-10. Adjusted operative mortality among Medicare patients in 1998 and 1999 according to level of surgeon volume for 4 cardiovascular procedures (panel A) and 4 cancer resection procedures (panel B). Operative mortality was defined as the rate of death before hospital discharge or within 30 days after the index procedure. Surgeon volume was based on the total number of procedures performed. (From Birkmeyer JD, Stukel, TA, Siewers AE, et al: Surgeon volume and operative mortality in the United States. N Engl J Med 349:2117–2127, 2003.)

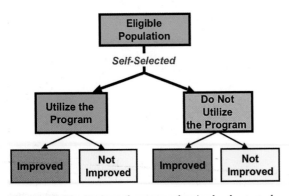

Figure 17-11. Design of a nonrandomized cohort study comparing utilizers with nonutilizers of a program.

array of health and prevention issues compared with those who did not. Consequently, the neonatal mortality difference observed may be due as much to the characteristics of the two groups as to the care provided.

Although we can try to address the selection problem by characterizing the prognostic profile of those who use care and those who do not, so long as the groups are not randomized, we are left with a gnawing uncertainty as to whether some factors were not identified in the study that might have differentiated utilizers and nonutilizers and, therefore, affected the health outcome.

TABLE 17-4. **Relationship of Neonatal Mortality to History of Prenatal Care, Baltimore Residents, Younger Than 17 Years, 1960–1961**

	Received Prenatal Care	Did Not Receive Prenatal Care
Number of births	1,397	315
Number of neonatal deaths	42	28
Neonatal deaths per 1,000 live births	30.1	88.9

Adapted from Stine OC, Rider RV, Sweeney E: School leaving due to pregnancy in an urban adolescent population. J Public Health 54: 1–6, 1964.

Comparison of Eligible and Noneligible Populations

Because of the problem of possible selection biases in comparing groups of utilizers with nonutilizers, another approach compares persons who are eligible for the care being evaluated with a group of persons who are not eligible (Fig. 17-12).

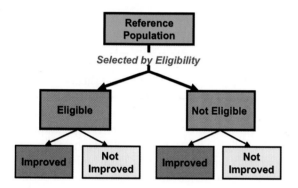

Figure 17-12. Design of a nonrandomized cohort study comparing people eligible with people not eligible for a program.

The assumption being made here is that eligibility or noneligibility is not related to either prognosis or outcome; therefore, no selection bias is being introduced that might affect the inferences from the study. For example, eligibility criteria may include type of employer or census tract of residence. Even with this design, however, one must be on the alert for factors that may introduce selection bias. For example, clearly, census tract of residence may relate to socioeconomic status. The issue of finding an appropriate noneligible population for comparison may be critical.

Combination Designs

As seen in Figure 17-13 (left of figure), in all the nonrandomized study designs that compare the morbidity level in persons who receive care with the morbidity level in those who do not, the assumption is that the original levels of morbidity in the two groups (A_1 and B_1) at time T_1 were comparable before the care was provided to group B. If so, we could interpret the finding of a lower level of morbidity in those receiving the care (B_2) than in those not receiv-

Figure 17-13. Two possible interpretations of an observed difference in morbidity between people receiving a health service and those not receiving the service. (See text.)

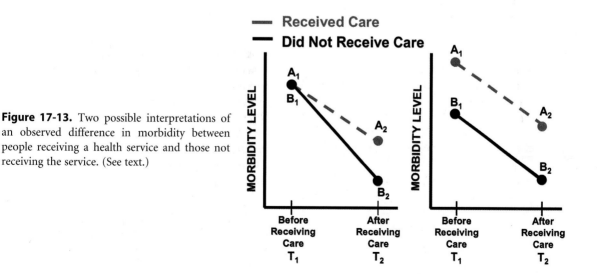

ing the care (A$_2$) at time T$_2$ as likely to have resulted from the care provided.

However, as seen in Figure 17-13 *(right of figure)*, it is possible that the groups might have been different originally and their prognoses may have differed at that time even before the care was provided. If such were the case, any differences in morbidity observed at time T$_2$ (B$_2$ lower than A$_2$) might only reflect the original differences at time T$_1$ and would not necessarily shed any light on the effectiveness of the care provided. Without having data on morbidity levels in the two groups at time T$_1$, the latter explanation of the observations could not be ruled out.

In view of this problem, another approach to program evaluation is to use a *combination design*, which involves both before–after and program–no program designs. This approach is demonstrated in the following example, in which outpatient care for sore throats in children was evaluated.

The study was designed to assess the effectiveness of outpatient care for sore throats in children by determining whether children who were eligible for such care had lower rates of rheumatic fever than did children who were not eligible.[10] The rationale was as follows: "Strep" throats are common in children. Untreated "strep" throats can lead to rheumatic fever. If "strep" throats are properly treated, rheumatic fever can be prevented. Therefore, if these programs are effective in treating "strep" throats, fewer cases of rheumatic fever should occur in the children who received the treatment.

In the mid-1960s, comprehensive care programs for children and youth were established in many inner cities, including Baltimore. Eligibility for care in this program was determined by the census tract of the child's residence. Rheumatic fever had already been shown to cluster in Baltimore's inner city.

It was possible to identify and compare several subgroups of Baltimore children and adolescents and to compare their rates of hospitalization for episodes of acute rheumatic fever with those for all of the city of Baltimore. The groups included residents of census tracts that met eligibility criteria for comprehensive care and residents of census tracts that did not meet these eligibility criteria for comprehensive care. Both were compared with the city of Baltimore as a whole.

Figure 17-14 shows a program–no program comparison of rheumatic fever rates in black children. In children eligible for comprehensive care, the rheumatic fever rate was 10.6 per 100,000, compared with 14.9 per 100,000 in those who were not eligible. Although the rate was lower in the eligible group in

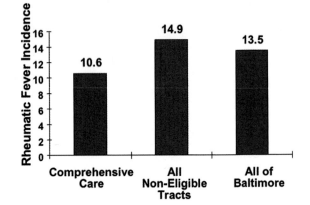

Figure 17-14. Comprehensive care and rheumatic fever incidence per 100,000, 1968–1970; Baltimore, black population, aged 5 to 14 years. (Adapted from Gordis L: Effectiveness of comprehensive-care programs in preventing rheumatic fever. N Engl J Med 289:331–335, 1973.)

this simultaneous comparison, the difference was not dramatic.

The next analysis in this combination design examined changes in rheumatic fever rates over time in both eligible and noneligible populations.

As seen in Figure 17-15, the rheumatic fever rate declined 60% in the eligible census tracts from 1960–1964 (before the programs were established) to 1968–1970 (after the programs were operating). In the noneligible tracts, rheumatic fever incidence was essentially unchanged (+2%). Thus, both parts of the combination design are consistent with a decline related to the care available.

However, because many changes had occurred in the inner city during this time, it was not certain whether the care provided by the programs was indeed responsible for the decline in rheumatic fever. Another analysis was therefore carried out. In a child, a streptococcal throat infection can be either symptomatic or asymptomatic. Clearly, only a child with a symptomatic sore throat would have been brought to a clinic. If we hypothesize that the care in the clinic was responsible for the reduction in rheumatic fever incidence, we would expect the decline in incidence to be limited to children with symptomatic clinical sore throats who would have sought care, and not to have occurred in asymptomatic children who had no clinically apparent infections.

As seen in Figure 17-16, the entire decline was limited to children with prior clinically overt infection; no change in rheumatic fever incidence occurred in those whose sore throats were asymptomatic. These findings are therefore highly consistent with

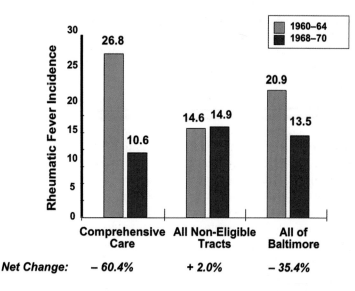

Figure 17-15. Comprehensive care and changes in rheumatic fever incidence per 100,000, 1960–1964 and 1968–1970; Baltimore, black population, aged 5 to 14 years. (Adapted from Gordis L: Effectiveness of comprehensive-care programs in preventing rheumatic fever. N Engl J Med 289:331–335, 1973.)

the suggestion that it was the medical care, or some factor closely associated with it, which was responsible for the decline in rheumatic fever incidence.

Case-Control Studies

The use of the case-control design for evaluating health services, including vaccines and other forms of prevention and screening programs, has elicited increasing interest. Although the case-control design has been applied primarily to etiologic studies, when appropriate data are obtainable, this design can serve as a useful, but limited, surrogate for randomized trials. However, because this design requires definition and specification of cases, it is most applicable

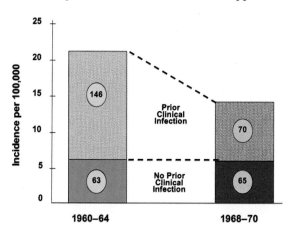

Figure 17-16. Changes in the annual incidence of first attacks of rheumatic fever in relation to preceding clinical respiratory infection. Numbers in circles are numbers of cases of rheumatic fever. (Adapted from Gordis L: Effectiveness of comprehensive-care programs in preventing rheumatic fever. N Engl J Med 289:331–335, 1973.)

to studies of prevention of specific diseases. The "exposure" is then the specific preventive or other health measure that is being assessed. As in most health services research, stratification by disease severity and by other possible prognostic factors is essential for appropriate interpretation of the findings. The methodologic problems associated with such studies (which are discussed extensively in Chapter 10) also arise when the case-control design is used for evaluating effectiveness. In particular, these studies need to address the selection of controls and issues associated with confounders.

CONCLUSION

This chapter has reviewed the application of basic epidemiologic study designs to the evaluation of health services. Many of the issues that arise are similar to those that arise in etiologic studies, although at times they present a different twist. In etiologic studies, we are primarily interested in the possible association of a potential causal factor and a specific disease, and factors such as health services often represent possible confounders that must be taken into account. In health care evaluation studies, we are primarily interested in possible associations of a health care or preventive measure and disease outcome, and factors such as pre-existing disease and other prognostic and risk factors become potential confounders that must be taken into consideration. Consequently, although many of the design issues remain, the focus in evaluation research is often on different issues of measurement and assessment. The randomized trial remains the optimal method for demonstrating the effectiveness of a health intervention. In initiating any evaluation study of health care, we should ask at the outset whether it is biologically and clinically plausible, given our current knowledge, to expect a specific benefit from the care being evaluated.

For practical reasons, nonrandomized observations are also necessary and must be capitalized on in the attempt to expand efforts at evaluation. Critics of randomized trials have pointed out that such studies have included—and can only include—a small fraction of all patients receiving care in the health care system so that generalizability of the results is a potential problem. Although this is true, generalizability is a problem with any study, no matter how large the study population. Nevertheless, even as we further refine the methodology of clinical trials, we also need improved methods to enhance the information that can be obtained even from nonrandomized evaluations of health services.

The study of specific components of care, rather than a care program per se, is essential. In this way, if an effective element can be identified in a mix of many modalities, the others can be eliminated and the quality of care can be enhanced in a cost-effective fashion.

In the next chapter, the discussion of evaluation is extended to a specific type of health services program: screening for disease in human populations.

REFERENCES

1. Frost WH: Rendering account in public health. Am J Public Health 15:394–398, 1925.
2. Gornick ME, Eggers PW, Reilly TW, et al: Effects of race and income and use of services among Medicare beneficiaries. N Engl J Med 335:791–799, 1996.
3. Kalra L, Evans A, Perez I, et al: Alternative strategies for stroke care: A prospective randomized controlled trial. Lancet 356:894–899, 2000.
4. Drummond AE, Pearson B, Lincoln NB, Berman P: Ten year follow-up of a randomized controlled trial of care in a stroke rehabilitation unit. BMJ 331(7515):491–492, 2005.
5. Kahn KL, Rubenstein LV, Draper D, et al: The effects of DRG-based prospective payment system on quality of care of hospitalized Medicare patients: An introduction to the series. JAMA 264:1953–1955, 1990.
6. Kosecroff J, Kahn KL, Rogerts WH, et al: Prospective payment system and impairment at discharge: The "quicker and sicker" story revisited. JAMA 265:1980–1983, 1990.
7. Jollis JG, Peterson ED, DeLong ER, et al: The relation between the volume of coronary angioplasty procedures at hospitals treating Medicare beneficiaries and short-term mortality. N Engl J Med 331:1625–1629, 1994.
8. Birkmeyer JD, Stukel, TA, Siewers AE, et al: Surgeon volume and operative mortality in the United States. N Engl J Med 349:2117–2127, 2003.
9. Stine OC, Rider RV, Sweeney I: School leaving due to pregnancy in an urban adolescent population. J Public Health 54:1–6, 1964.
10. Gordis L: Effectiveness of comprehensive-care programs in preventing rheumatic fever. N Engl J Med 289:331–335, 1973.

REVIEW QUESTIONS FOR CHAPTER 17

1. All of the following are measures of process of health care in a clinic *except*:
   a. Proportion of patients in whom blood pressure is measured
   b. Proportion of patients who have complications of a disease
   c. Proportion of patients advised to stop smoking
   d. Proportion of patients whose height and weight are measured
   e. Proportion of patients whose bill is reduced because of financial need

Question 2 is based on the information given below:

In-Hospital Case-Fatality Rates (CFRs) for 100 Men Not Treated in a Coronary Care Unit (CCU) and for 100 Men Treated in a CCU, According to Three Clinical Grades of Severity of Myocardial Infarction

Clinical Grade	NON-CCU (NO. OF PATIENTS)			CCU (NO. OF PATIENTS)		
	Total	Died	CFR (%)	Total	Died	CFR (%)
Mild	60	12	20	10	3	30
Severe	36	18	50	60	18	30
Shock	4	4	100	30	13	43

The results shown were based on a comparison of the last 100 patients treated before the CCU was installed and the first 100 patients treated within the CCU. All 200 patients were admitted during the same month.

You may assume that this is the *only hospital* in the town and that the natural history of MI was *unchanged* during this period.

2. The authors concluded that the CCU was very beneficial for men with severe MI and for those in shock, because the in-hospital CFRs for these categories were much lower in the CCU. This conclusion:
   a. Is correct
   b. May be incorrect because CFRs were used rather than mortality rates
   c. May be incorrect because of a referral bias of patients to this hospital from hospitals in distant towns
   d. May be incorrect because of differences in the assignment of the clinical severity grade before and after the opening of the CCU
   e. May be incorrect because of failure to recognize a possible decrease in the annual incidence rate of MI in recent years

3. The extent to which a specific health care treatment, service, procedure, program, or other intervention does what it is intended to do when used in a community-dwelling population is termed its:

a. Efficacy
b. Effectiveness
c. Effect modification
d. Efficiency
e. None of the above

4. The extent to which a specific health care treatment, service, procedure, program, or other intervention produces a beneficial result under ideal controlled conditions is its:
   a. Efficacy
   b. Effectiveness
   c. Effect modification
   d. Efficiency
   e. None of the above

5. A major problem in using a historical control design for evaluating a health service using case-fatality rate (CFR) as an outcome is that if the CFR is lower after provision of the health service was started, then:
   a. The lower CFR could be caused by changing prevalence of the disease
   b. The lower CFR may be a result of decreasing incidence
   c. The lower CFR may be an indirect effect of the new health service
   d. The CFR may have been affected by changes in factors that are not related to the new health service
   e. None of the above

Chapter 18

The Epidemiologic Approach to Evaluating Screening Programs

In Chapter 1, we distinguished among primary, secondary, and tertiary prevention. In Section II, we discussed the design and interpretation of studies that aim to identify risk factors or etiologic factors for disease so that disease occurrence can be prevented—*primary prevention*. In this chapter, we address how epidemiology is used to evaluate the effectiveness of screening programs for the early detection of disease—*secondary prevention*. This subject is important in both clinical practice and public health, for there is increasing acceptance of a physician's obligation to include prevention along with diagnosis and treatment as major responsibilities in the care of patients.

The validity and reliability of screening tests were discussed in Chapter 5. In this chapter, we will discuss some of the methodologic issues that must be considered in deriving any inferences about the benefits that may accrue to persons who undergo screening with such tests.

The question of whether patients benefit from early detection of disease includes the following components:

1. Can the disease be detected early?
2. What are the sensitivity and the specificity of the test?
3. What is the predictive value of the test?
4. How serious is the problem of false-positive test results?
5. What is the cost of early detection in terms of funds, resources, and emotional impact?
6. Are the subjects harmed by screening tests?
7. Do the individuals in whom disease is detected early benefit from the early detection, and is there an overall benefit to those who are screened?

In this chapter, we primarily address the last question. Several of the other issues in the preceding list are considered only in the context of this question.

The term *early detection of disease* means detecting a disease at an earlier stage than would usually occur in standard clinical practice. This denotes detecting disease at a presymptomatic stage, at which point the patient has no clinical complaint (no symptoms or signs) and, therefore, no reason to seek medical care for the condition. The assumption in screening is that an appropriate intervention is available for the disease that is detected, and that the intervention can be more effectively applied if the disease is detected at an earlier stage.

At first glance, the question of whether people benefit from early detection of disease may seem somewhat surprising. Intuitively, it would seem obvious that early detection is beneficial and that intervention at an earlier stage of the disease process is more effective and/or easier to implement than a later intervention. In effect, these assumptions represent a "surgical" view; for example, every malignant lesion is localized at some early stage, and at this stage it can be successfully excised before regional spread occurs, or certainly before widespread metastases develop. However, the intuitive attractiveness of such a concept should not blind us to the fact that throughout the history of medicine, deeply felt convictions have often turned out to be erroneous when they were not supported by data obtained from appropriately designed and rigorously conducted studies. Consequently, regardless of the attractiveness of the idea of the beneficial aspects of early disease detection, both to clinicians involved in prevention and therapy and to those involved in community-based prevention programs, the evidence to support the validity of this concept must be rigorously examined.

As in evaluating any type of health service, screening can be evaluated using process or outcome measures. Table 18-1 provides a list of operational measures that includes process measures as well as measurements of yield and information produced by the screening program.

We are particularly interested in the question of what benefit is gained by people who undergo screen-

TABLE 18-1. Assessing the Effectiveness of Screening Programs Using Operational Measures

1. Number of people screened
2. Proportion of target populations screened and number of times screened
3. Detected prevalence of preclinical disease
4. Total costs of the program
5. Costs per case found
6. Costs per previously unknown case found
7. Proportion of positive screenees brought to final diagnosis and treatment
8. Predictive value of a positive test in population screened

Adapted from Hulka BS: Degrees of proof and practical application. Cancer 62:1776–1780, 1988. Copyright © 1988 American Cancer Society. Reprinted by permission of Wiley-Liss, Inc., a subsidiary of John Wiley & Sons, Inc.

TABLE 18-2. Assessing the Effectiveness of Screening Programs Using Outcome Measures

1. Reduction of mortality in the population screened
2. Reduction of case-fatality rate in screened individuals
3. Increase in percent of cases detected at earlier stages
4. Reduction in complications
5. Prevention of or reduction in recurrences or metastases
6. Improvement of quality of life in screened individuals

ing in a screening program. However, just as is the case with evaluation of health services (discussed in Chapter 17), there is little advantage to improving the *process* of screening if persons who are screened derive no benefit. We will therefore examine some of the problems associated with determining whether early detection of disease confers benefits to the individual who undergoes screening (i.e., whether outcome is improved by screening).

What do we mean by *outcome?* To answer the question of whether patients benefit, we must precisely define what we mean by benefit, and what outcome or outcomes are considered to be evidence of patient benefit. Some of the possible outcome measures that might be used are shown in Table 18-2.

THE NATURAL HISTORY OF DISEASE

To discuss the methodologic issues involved in evaluating the benefit of screening, let us examine in further detail the natural history of disease (first discussed in Chapter 6).

We will begin by placing screening in its appropriate place on the timeline of the natural history of disease and will do so in relation to the different approaches to prevention discussed in Chapter 1.

Figure 18-1A is a schematic representation of the natural history of a disease in an individual. At some point, biologic onset of disease occurs. This may be a subcellular change, such as an alteration in DNA, and this point is generally undetectable. At some later

point the disease becomes symptomatic, or clinical signs develop—that is, the disease moves into a clinical phase. The clinical signs prompt the patient to seek care, after which a diagnosis is made and appropriate therapy is instituted, the ultimate outcome of which may be cure, control of the disease, disability, or death.

As seen in Figure 18-1B, the onset of symptoms marks an important point in the natural history of a disease. The period when disease is present can be divided into two phases: The period from the time when signs and symptoms develop to an ultimate outcome such as possible cure, control of the disease, or death is the *clinical phase* of the disease. The period from biologic onset of the disease to the development of signs and symptoms is called the *preclinical phase* of the disease.

As seen in Figures 18-1C and 18-1D, *primary prevention*, that is, preventing the development of disease by reducing exposure to disease-causing agents or by immunization, denotes intervention before a disease has developed. *Secondary prevention*, that is, detecting disease at an earlier stage than usual, such as by screening, takes place during the *preclinical phase* of an illness, that is, after the disease has developed but before clinical signs and symptoms have appeared. *Tertiary prevention* refers to treating clinically ill individuals to prevent complications of the illness including death of the patient.

If we want to detect disease earlier than usual through programs of health education, we could encourage symptomatic persons to seek medical care sooner. But a major challenge lies in identifying persons with disease who are asymptomatic. Our focus in this chapter is on identifying disease in

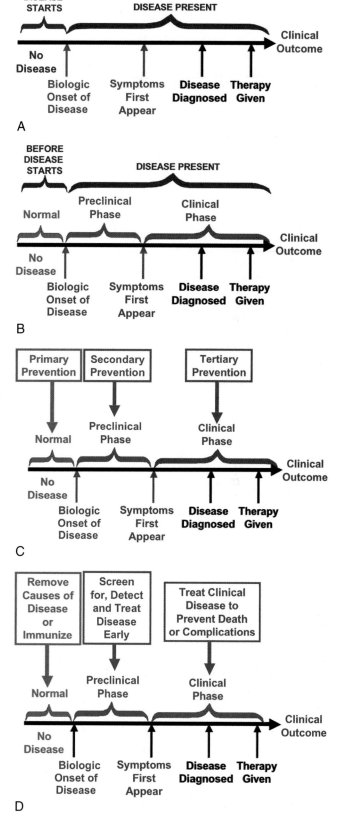

Figure 18-1. A, Natural history of a disease. **B,** Natural history of a disease with preclinical and clinical phases. **C,** Natural history of a disease with points for primary, secondary, and tertiary prevention. **D,** Natural history of a disease with specific primary, secondary, and tertiary prevention measures.

persons who have not yet developed symptoms and who are in the preclinical phase of illness.

Let us now take a closer look at the *preclinical phase* of the disease (Fig. 18-2). At some point during the preclinical phase, it becomes possible to detect the disease by using currently available tests (Fig. 18-2A). The interval from this point to the development of signs and symptoms is the *detectable preclinical phase* of the disease (Fig. 18-2B). When disease is detected by screening, the time of diagnosis is advanced to an earlier point in the natural history of the disease. The *lead time* is defined as the interval by which the time of diagnosis is advanced by screening and early detection of disease compared to the usual time of diagnosis (Fig. 18-2C). The concept of lead time is inherent in the idea of screening and detecting a disease earlier than it would usually be found.

Another important concept in screening is the *critical point* in the natural history of a disease[1] (Fig. 18-3A). This is a point in the natural history before which treatment is more effective and/or less difficult to administer. If a disease is potentially curable, cure may be possible before this point, but not after. For example, in a woman with breast cancer, one critical point would be that at which the disease spreads from the breast to the axillary lymph nodes. If the disease is detected and treated before that point, prognosis is much better than after spread to the nodes has taken place.

As shown in Figure 18-3B, there may be multiple critical points in the natural history of a disease. For example, in the patient with breast cancer, a second critical point may be that at which disease spreads from the axillary nodes to other parts of the body. Prognosis is still better when the disease is confined to the axillary lymph nodes than when systemic spread has occurred.

The critical point is a theoretical concept, and in a given disease we usually cannot identify when the critical point is reached. However, it is a very important idea in screening. For if we cannot envision one or more critical points in the natural history of a disease, there is clearly no rationale for screening and early detection. Early detection presumes that a biologic point exists in the natural history of a disease before which treatment will benefit a person more than if he or she is treated after that point.

THE PATTERN OF DISEASE PROGRESSION

We might expect to see a potential benefit from screening and early detection if the following two assumptions hold:

1. All or most clinical cases of a disease first go through a detectable preclinical phase.
2. In the absence of intervention, all or most cases in a preclinical phase progress to a clinical phase.

Both assumptions are reasonably self-evident. For example, if none of the preclinical cases progress to clinical cases, there is no reason to perform screening tests. Alternatively, if none of the clinical cases passes through a preclinical phase, there is no reason to perform screening tests. Thus, both assumptions are important in assessing any potential benefit from screening.

However, both assumptions are open to question. In certain situations, the preclinical phase may be so short that the disease is unlikely to be detected by any periodic screening program. Also, there is increasing evidence that spontaneous regression may occur in some diseases; therefore, not every preclinical case inexorably progresses to clinical disease.

For example, Figure 18-4A shows the progression from a normal cervix to cervical cancer. We might expect that detection of more cases at the in situ stage would be reflected in a commensurate reduction in the number of cases that progress to invasive disease.

However, evaluating the benefits of cervical cancer screening is complicated by the problem that some cases progress through the in situ stage so rapidly, and the preclinical stage is so brief, that for all practical purposes there is no preclinical stage during which disease can be detected by screening. In addition, nuclear DNA quantitation studies suggest that cervical intraepithelial abnormalities may exist either as a reversible state or as an irreversible precursor of invasive cancer. Data also suggest that some cases of cervical intraepithelial neoplasia detected by a Papanicolaou (Pap) smear regress spontaneously, particularly in the earlier stages, but also in the later stage (carcinoma in situ). In one study, 36% of women with abnormal Pap smears who refused any intervention were later found to have normal Pap smears. In addition, recent data suggest that most, if not all, in situ cervical neoplasias are associated with different types of papillomaviruses. Only neoplasia associated with certain types of papillomavirus progress to invasive cancer, so we may be dealing with heterogeneity of both the causal agent and disease.

Thus, whereas the simple model of progression from normal cervix to invasive cervical cancer seen in Figure 18-4A would suggest that early detection followed by effective intervention would be reflected by a commensurate reduction in the number of invasive lesions that subsequently develop, a more accurate

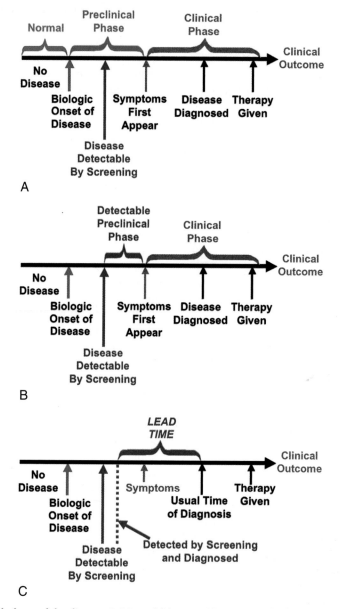

Figure 18-2. Preclinical phase of the disease. **A,** Natural history with point at which disease is detectable by screening. **B,** Natural history with detectable preclinical phase. **C,** Natural history with lead time.

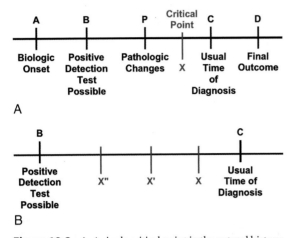

Figure 18-3. **A,** A single critical point in the natural history of a disease. **B,** Multiple critical points in the natural history of a disease. (Adapted from Hutchison GB: Evaluation of preventive services. J Chronic Dis 11:497–508, 1960.)

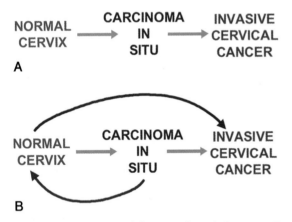

Figure 18-4. **A,** Natural history of cervical cancer: I. Progression from normal cervix to invasive cancer. **B,** Natural history of cervical cancer: II. Extremely rapid progression and spontaneous regression.

presentation of the natural history may be that seen in Figure 18-4B. The extent of both phenomena, spontaneous regression and extremely rapid progression, clearly influences the size of the decrease in invasive disease that might be expected to result from early detection and intervention and must therefore be taken into account in assessing the benefits of screening. Although these issues have been demonstrated for cervical cancer, they are clearly relevant to evaluating the benefits of screening for many diseases.

METHODOLOGIC ISSUES

To interpret the findings in a study designed to evaluate the benefits of screening, certain methodologic

problems must be taken into account. Most studies of screening programs that have been carried out have not been randomized trials, because of the difficulties of randomizing a population for screening. The question is, therefore, why can't we just examine a group of people who have been screened and compare their mortality to that of a group of people who have not been screened—that is, use a cohort design to evaluate the effectiveness of screening?

Let us assume that we compare a population of people who have been screened for a disease with a population of people who have not been screened for the disease. Let us assume further that a treatment is available and will be used for those in whom disease is detected. If we find a lower mortality from the disease in those in whom disease was identified through screening than in those in whom disease was not detected in this manner, can we not conclude that screening and early detection of disease has been beneficial? Let us turn to some of the methodologic issues involved.

Selection Biases
Referral Bias (Volunteer Bias)
In deriving a conclusion about benefits of screening, the first question we might ask is whether there was a selection bias in terms of who was screened and who was not. We would like to be able to assume that those who were screened had the same characteristics as those who were not screened. However, there are many differences in the characteristics of those who participate in screening or other health programs and those who do not. Many studies have shown volunteers to be healthier than the general population and to be more likely to comply with medical recommendations. If, for example, persons whose disease had a better prognosis from the outset were either referred for screening or were self-selected, we might observe lower mortality in the screened group even if early detection played no role in improving prognosis. Of course, it is also possible that volunteers may include many people who are at high risk and who volunteer for screening because they have anxieties based on a positive family history or lifestyle characteristics. The problem is that we do not know in which direction the selection bias might operate and how it might affect the study results.

The problem of selection bias that most significantly affects our interpretation of the findings is best addressed by carrying out the comparison with a randomized experimental study in which care is

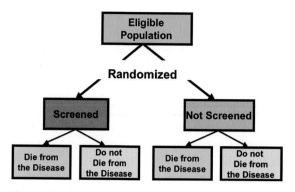

Figure 18-5. Design of a randomized trial of the benefits of screening.

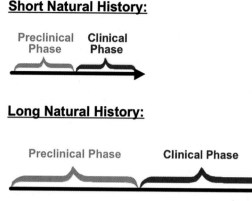

Figure 18-6. Short and long natural histories of disease: relationship of length of clinical phase to length of preclinical phase.

taken that the two groups have comparable initial prognostic profiles (Fig. 18-5).

Length-Biased Sampling (Prognostic Selection)

The second type of selection problem that arises in interpreting the results of a comparison of a screened and an unscreened group is a possible selection bias; this does not relate to who comes for screening but rather to the type of disease that is detected by the screening. The question is: Does screening selectively identify cases of the disease which have a better prognosis? In other words, do the cases found through screening have a better natural history regardless of how early therapy is initiated? If the outcome of those in whom disease is detected by screening is found to be better than the outcome of those who were not screened, and in whom disease was identified during the usual course of clinical care, could the better outcome among those who are screened result from selective identification by screening of persons with a better prognosis? Could the better outcome be unrelated to the time of diagnostic and treatment interventions?

How could this come about? Recall the natural history of disease, with clinical and preclinical phases, shown in Figure 18-1B. We know that the clinical phase of illness differs in length in different people. For example, some patients with colon cancer die soon after diagnosis, whereas others survive for many years. What appears to be the same disease may have a clinical phase of different length in different individuals.

What about the preclinical phase in these individuals? Actually, each patient's disease has a single continuous natural history, which we divide into preclinical and clinical phases (Fig. 18-6) on the basis of

the point in time at which signs and symptoms develop. In some, the natural history is brief and in others the natural history is protracted. This suggests that if a person has a slowly progressive natural history with a long clinical phase, the preclinical phase will also be long. In contrast, if a person has a rapidly progressive disease process and a short natural history, the clinical phase is likely to be short, and it seems reasonable to conclude that the preclinical phase will also be short. There are in fact data to support the notion that a long clinical phase is associated with a long preclinical phase and a short clinical phase with a short preclinical phase.

Remember that our purpose in screening is to detect the disease during the preclinical phase, because during the clinical phase the patient is aware of the problem and even without screening, will seek medical care for symptoms. If we mount a one-time screening program in a community, which group of patients are we likely to identify: those with a short preclinical phase or those with a long preclinical phase?

To answer this question, let us consider a small population that is screened for a certain disease (Fig. 18-7). As shown here, each case has a preclinical and a clinical phase. The figure is drawn so that each preclinical phase is the same length as its associated clinical phase. Patients in the clinical phase will be identified in the usual course of medical care, so the purpose of the screening is to identify cases in the preclinical, presymptomatic state. Note that the lengths of the preclinical phases of cases represented here vary. The longer the preclinical phase, the more likely the screening program is to detect the case

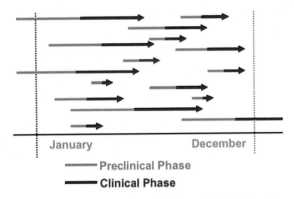

Figure 18-7. Hypothetical population of individuals with long and short natural histories.

while it is still preclinical. For example, if we screen once a year for a disease for which the preclinical phase is only 24 hours long, we will clearly miss most of the cases during the preclinical phase. If, however, the preclinical phase is 1 year long, cases will be identified during that time. Screening tends to selectively identify those cases that have longer preclinical phases of illness. Consequently, even if the subsequent therapy had no effect, screening would still selectively identify persons with a long preclinical phase, and consequently a long clinical phase (i.e., those with a better prognosis). These people would have a better prognosis even if there were no screening program or even if there were no true benefits from screening.

This problem can be addressed in several ways. One approach is to use an experimental randomized design in which care is taken to keep the groups comparable in terms of the lengths of the detectable preclinical phase of illness. However, this may not be easy. In addition, survival should be examined for all members of each group—that is, the screened and unscreened. In the screened group, survival should be calculated for those in whom disease is detected by screening and for those in whom disease is detected between screening examinations, the so-called *interval cases*. We shall return to the importance of interval cases later in this chapter.

Lead Time Bias

Another problem that arises in examining survival in people who are screened and comparing it with survival in those who are not screened is a bias associated with the lead time—how much earlier can the diagnosis be made if the disease is detected by screening compared with the usual timing of the diagnosis if screening were not carried out?

Consider four individuals with a certain disease shown by the four timelines in Figure 18-8. The thicker part of each horizontal line denotes the apparent survival observed. The first timeline (A) shows the usual time of diagnosis and the usual time of death. The second timeline (B) shows an earlier time of diagnosis, but the same time of death. Survival *seems* better because the interval from diagnosis to death is longer, but the patient is not any better off because death has not been delayed. The third timeline (C) shows earlier diagnosis and a delay in death from the disease—clearly a benefit to the patient (assuming that quality of life is good). Finally, the fourth timeline (D) shows earlier diagnosis, with subsequent prevention of death from the disease.

The benefits we seek are delay or prevention of death. Although we have chosen to focus on mortality in this chapter, we could also have used morbidity, recurrences, quality of life, or patient satisfaction as valid measures of outcome.

Lead Time and Five-Year Survival

Five-year survival is a frequently used measure of therapeutic success, particularly in cancer therapy. Let us examine the possible effect of lead time on apparent 5-year survival.

Figure 18-9A shows the natural history of disease in a hypothetical patient with colon cancer, which was diagnosed in the usual clinical context without any screening. Biologic onset of the disease was in 2000. The patient became aware of symptoms in 2008, and had a diagnostic workup leading to a diagnosis of colon cancer. Surgery was performed in 2008 and the patient died of colon cancer in 2010. This patient has survived for 2 years (2008 to 2010) and clearly is not a 5-year survivor. If we use 5-year

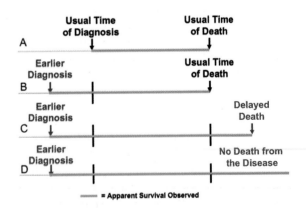

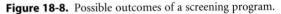

Figure 18-8. Possible outcomes of a screening program.

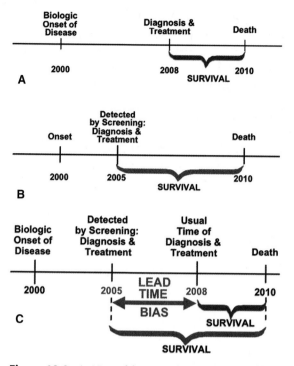

Figure 18-9. **A,** Natural history of a patient with colon cancer without screening. **B,** Disease detected by screening 3 years earlier. **C,** Lead time bias resulting from screening.

survival as an index of treatment success, this patient is a treatment failure.

Consider what might happen to this patient if he resides in a community in which a screening program is initiated (see Fig. 18-9B). For this hypothetical example only, let us assume that there is actually no benefit from early detection—that is, the natural history of colon cancer is unaffected by early intervention. In this case, the patient is asymptomatic but undergoes a routine screening test in 2005, the result of which is positive. In 2005, surgery is performed and the patient dies in 2010. The patient has survived 5 years and is now clearly a 5-year survivor. However, he is a 5-year survivor not because death has been delayed, but because the diagnosis has been made earlier. When we compare this screening scenario with the scenario without screening (see Fig. 18-9A), it is apparent the patient has not derived any benefit from earlier detection in terms of having lived any longer. Indeed the patient may have lost out in terms of quality of life, as the earlier detection of disease by screening gave him an additional 3 years of postoperative and other medical care, and may have deprived him of 3 years of normal life. This problem of an illusion of better survival only because of earlier

detection is called the *lead time bias*, as shown in Figure 18-9C.

Thus, even if there is no true benefit from early detection of a disease, there will *appear* to be a benefit associated with screening, even if death is not delayed, because of an earlier point of diagnosis from which survival is measured. This is not to say that early detection carries no benefit; rather, even without any benefit, the lead time associated with early detection suggests the appearance of a benefit in the form of enhanced survival. Lead time must therefore be taken into account in interpreting the results of nonrandomized evaluations.

Figure 18-10 shows the effect of the bias resulting from lead time on quantitative estimates of survival.

Figure 18-10A shows a situation in which no screening activity is being carried out. Five years after diagnosis, survival is 30%. If we institute a screening program with a 1-year lead time, the entire frame is shifted to the left (see Fig. 18-10B). If we now calculate survival at 5 years from the new time of diagnosis (see Fig. 18-10C), survival appears to be 50%, but only as a result of lead time bias. The problem is that the apparently better survival is not a result of screened people living longer, but it is rather a result of a diagnosis being made at an earlier point in the natural history of their disease.

Consequently, in any comparison of screened and unscreened populations we must make an allowance for an estimated lead time in an attempt to identify any prolongation of survival above and beyond that resulting from the artifact of lead time. If early detection is truly associated with improved survival, survival in the screened group should be greater than survival in the control group *plus the lead time.* We therefore have to generate some estimate of the lead time for the disease being studied.

Another strategy is to compare mortality from the disease in the entire screened group with that in the unscreened group, rather than just the case fatality rate in those in whom disease was detected by screening.

Overdiagnosis Bias

Another potential bias is that of overdiagnosis. At times, people who initiate a screening program have almost limitless enthusiasm for the program. Even cytopathologists reading Pap smears for cervical cancer may become so enthusiastic that they may tend to over-read the smears (i.e., make false-positive readings). If they do over-read, some normal women will be included in the group thought to have positive Pap

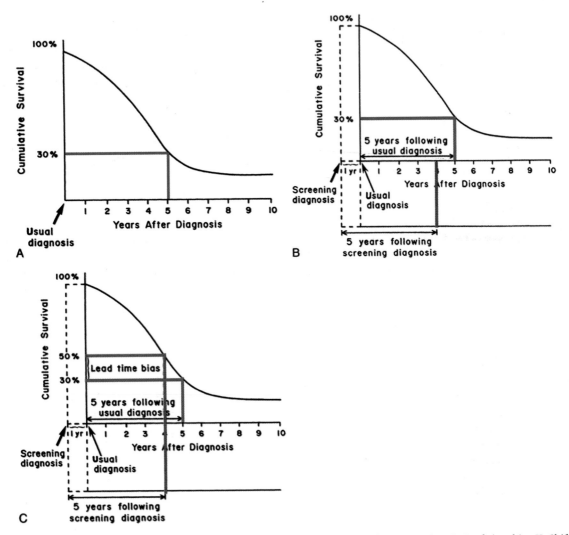

Figure 18-10. A, Lead time bias-I: 5-year survival when diagnosis is made without screening. **B,** Lead time bias-II: Shift of 5-year period by screening and early detection (lead time). **C,** Lead time bias-III: Bias in survival calculation resulting from early detection. (Modified from Frank JW: Occult-blood screening for colorectal carcinoma: The benefits. Am J Prev Med 1:3–9, 1985.)

smears. Consequently, the abnormal group will be diluted with women who are free of cancer. If normal individuals in the screened group are more likely to be erroneously diagnosed as positive than are normal individuals in the unscreened group (that is, labeled as having cancer when in reality they do not), one could get a false impression of increased rates of detection and diagnosis of early-stage cancer as a result of the screening. In addition, because many of the persons with a diagnosis of cancer in the screened group would actually not have cancer, and would therefore have a good survival, the results would represent an inflated estimate of survival after screening in persons thought to have cancer, resulting in a mis-

taken conclusion that screening had been shown to improve survival from cancer in this population.

The possible quantitative impact of overdiagnosis resulting from screening is demonstrated in a hypothetical example shown in Figure 18-11. Figure 18-11A shows Scenario 1, in which there is no screening. In this scenario, 1,000 patients with clinical lung cancer are followed for 10 years. At that point, 900 have died and 100, are alive. The 10-year survival for the 1,000 patients is therefore $\frac{100}{1,000}$ or 10%.

Figures 18-11B and 11C show Scenario 2 in which screening results in overdiagnosis. In this scenario (Fig 11-B), 4,000 people screen positive for lung cancer. Of these, 1,000 are the same patients with clinical lung cancer seen in Fig. 18-11A, and the other 3,000 are people who do not have lung cancer but are overdiagnosed by the screening test as being positive for lung cancer (false positives).

After 10 years (Fig 18-11C), these 3,000 people are still alive, as are the 100 people who had clinical lung cancer and survived as was shown in Figure 18-11A. The result is that of the 4,000 people who screened positive initially, 3,100 have survived for 10 years. As shown in the comparison of Scenario 1 and Scenario 2 in Figure 8-11D, 10-year survival in Scenario 2 is now 78% compared with 10% in Scenario 1 in the original patient population of 1,000 who had clinical lung cancer. However, the apparently "better" survival seen in Scenario 2 is entirely due to the inclusion of 3,000 people who did not have lung cancer but were overdiagnosed by the screening.

In effect, this is a misclassification bias, as discussed in Chapter 15. In this example, 3,000 people without lung cancer have been misclassified by the screening test as having lung cancer. Consequently, it is essential that in such studies of survival, the diagnostic process be rigorously standardized in order to minimize the potential problem of overdiagnosis.

STUDY DESIGNS FOR EVALUATION OF SCREENING

Nonrandomized Studies

In discussing the methodologic issues involved in nonrandomized studies of screening, we have in essence been discussing nonrandomized observational studies of screened and unscreened persons—a cohort design (Fig. 18-12).

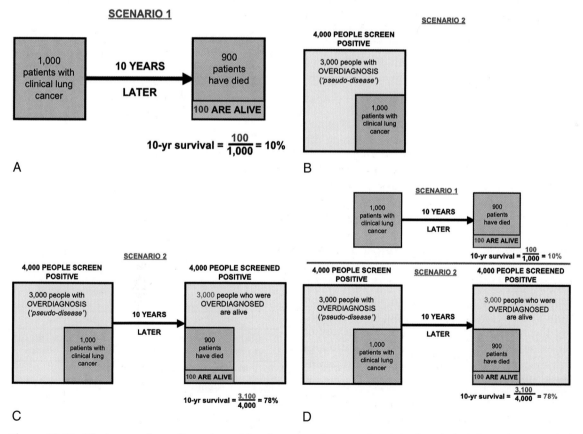

Figure 18-11. The impact of overdiagnosis resulting from screening on estimation of survival. **A,** Scenario 1—survival with no screening. **B,** Scenario 2—when screening results in overdiagnosis—I: Original population screened. **C,** Scenario 2—when screening results in overdiagnosis—II: Survival after 10 years. **D,** Comparison of 10-year survival in Scenario 1 and Scenario 2. (Adapted from Welch HG, Woloshin S, Schwartz LM: Overstating the evidence for lung cancer screening: The International Early Lung Cancer Action Program [I-ELCAP] study. Arch Int Med 167[21]:2289–2295, 2007.)

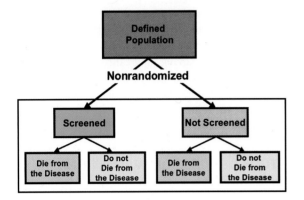

Figure 18-12. Design of a nonrandomized cohort study of the benefits of screening.

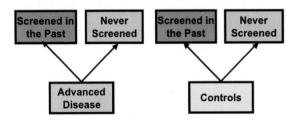

Figure 18-13. Design of a case-control study of the benefits of screening.

In recent years, the case-control design has gained increasing attention as a method of assessing the effectiveness of screening (Fig. 18-13). In this design the "cases" are people with advanced disease—the type of disease we hope to prevent by screening. Several proposals have been made for appropriate controls for such a study. Clearly they should be "noncases"—that is, people without advanced disease. Although the "controls" used in early case-control studies for evaluation of screening were people with disease in an early stage, now many believe that people selected from the population from which the cases were derived are better controls. We then determine the prevalence of a history of screening among both the cases and the controls, so that screening is looked at as an "exposure." If screening is effective, we would expect to find a greater prevalence of screening history among the controls than among those with advanced disease, and an odds ratio can be calculated, which will be less than 1.0 if screening is effective.

Randomized Studies

In this type of study, a population is randomized, half to screening and half to no screening. Such a study is difficult to mount and carry out. Perhaps the best known randomized trial of screening is the trial of screening for breast cancer using mammography that was carried out at the Health Insurance Plan (HIP) of New York.[2] Shapiro and colleagues conducted a randomized trial in women enrolled in the prepaid HIP program. This study has become a classic in the literature in reporting evaluation of screening benefits through a randomized trial design, and it serves as a model for future studies of this type.

The study was begun in 1963. It was designed to determine whether periodic screening using clinical examination and mammography reduced breast cancer mortality in women aged 40 to 64 years. Approximately 62,000 women were randomized into a study group and a control group of about 31,000 each (Fig. 18-14). The study group was offered screening examinations; 65% appeared for the first examination and were offered additional examinations at annual intervals. Most of these women had at least one of the three annual screening examinations that were offered. Screening consisted of physical examination, mammography, and interview. Control women received the usual medical care in the prepaid program. Many reports have been published from this outstanding study, and we will examine only a few of the results here.

Figure 18-15 shows the number of breast cancer deaths and the mortality rates in both the study group (women who were offered mammography) and the control group after 5 years of follow-up.

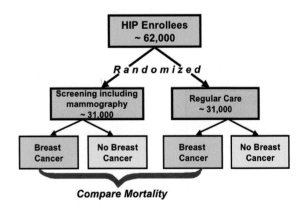

Figure 18-14. Design of the Health Insurance Plan (HIP) randomized controlled trial begun in 1963 to study the efficacy of mammography screening. (Data from Shapiro S, Venet W, Strax P, Venet L (eds): Periodic Screening for Breast Cancer: The Health Insurance Plan Project and Its Sequelae, 1963–1986. Baltimore, Johns Hopkins University Press, 1988.)

Figure 18-15. Numbers of deaths due to breast cancer and mortality rates from breast cancer in control and study groups; 5 years of follow-up after entry into study. Data for study group include deaths among women screened and those who refused screening. (Data from Shapiro S, Venet W, Strax P, et al: Selection, follow-up, and analysis in the Health Insurance Plan Study: A randomized trial with breast cancer screening. Natl Cancer Inst Monogr 67:65–74, 1985.)

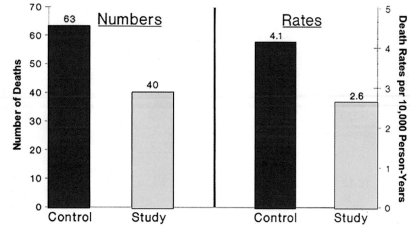

Note that the data for the study group include deaths among women screened and those who refused screening. Recall that in Chapter 7 we discussed the problem of unplanned crossover in randomized trials. In that context, it was pointed out that the standard procedure in data analysis was to analyze according to the original randomization—an approach known as "intention to treat." That is precisely what was done here. Once a woman was randomized to mammography, she was kept in that group for purposes of analysis even if she subsequently refused screening. We see that breast cancer deaths are much higher in the control group than in the study group.

Figure 18-16 shows 5-year case-fatality rates in the women who developed breast cancer in both groups. The case fatality rate in the control group was 40%. In the *total* study group (women who were randomized to receive mammography, regardless of whether or not they were actually screened) the case fatality rate was 29%. Shapiro and coworkers then divided this group into those who were screened and those who refused screening. In those who refused screening, the case fatality rate was 35%. In those who were screened, the case fatality rate was 23%.

Shapiro and colleagues then compared survival in women whose breast cancer was detected at the screening examination with that in women whose breast cancer was identified between screening examinations—that is, no breast cancer was identified at screening, and before the next examination a year later, the women had symptoms that led to the diagnosis of breast cancer. If the cancer had been detected by mammography, the case fatality rate was only 13%. However, if the breast cancer was an *interval case*, that is, diagnosed between examinations, the case-fatality rate was 38%. What could explain this difference in case-fatality rates? The likely explanation is that disease that was found between regular mammographic examinations was rapidly progressive. It was not detectable at the regular mammographic examination, but was identified before the

Figure 18-16. Five-year case-fatality rates among patients with breast cancer. Rates for those in whom detection was due to screening allow for a 1-year lead time. (Data from Shapiro S, Venet W, Strax P, et al: Ten- to 14-year effect of screening on breast cancer mortality. J Natl Cancer Inst 69:349–355, 1982.)

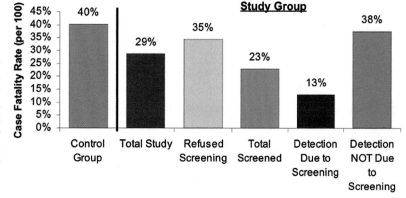

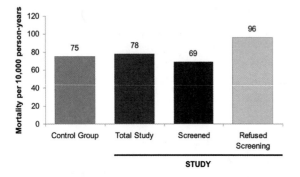

Figure 18-17. Mortality from all causes *excluding breast cancer* per 10,000 person-years, Health Insurance Plan (HIP). (Data from Shapiro S, Venet W, Strax P, et al: Selection, follow-up, and analysis in the Health Insurance Plan Study: A randomized trial with breast cancer screening. Natl Cancer Inst Monogr 67:65–74, 1985.)

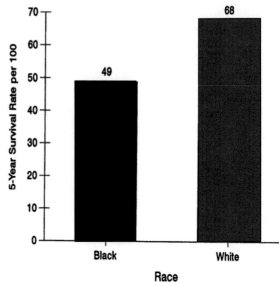

Figure 18-18. Five-year relative survival rates, by race, among women with breast cancer diagnosed 1964–1973 (SEER program). (Data from Shapiro S, Venet W, Strax P, et al: Prospects for eliminating racial differences in breast cancer survival rates. Am J Public Health 72:1142–1145, 1982.)

next regularly scheduled examination a year later because it was so aggressive.

These observations also support the notion discussed earlier in this chapter that a long clinical phase is likely to be associated with a long preclinical phase. Women in whom cancer findings were detected at screening had a long preclinical phase and a case-fatality rate of only 13%, indicating a long clinical phase as well. The women who had normal mammograms and whose disease became clinically apparent before the next examination had a short preclinical phase and, given the group's high case-fatality rate, also had a short clinical phase.

Figure 18-17 shows deaths from causes *other than breast cancer* in both groups over 5 years. Mortality was much higher in those who did not come for screening than in those who did. Because the screening was only directed at breast cancer, why should those who came for screening and those who did not manifest different mortality rates for causes *other* than breast cancer? The answer is, clearly, volunteer bias—the well-documented observation that people who participate in health programs differ in many ways from those who do not: in their health status, attitudes, educational and socioeconomic levels, and other factors. This is another demonstration that for purposes of evaluating a health program, comparison of participants and nonparticipants is not a valid approach.

Before we leave our discussion of the HIP study, we might digress and mention an interesting application of these data carried out by Shapiro and coworkers.[3] Figure 18-18 shows that, in the United States,

5-year relative survival rates from breast cancer are better in whites than in blacks.

The question has been raised whether this is due to a difference in the biology of the disease in blacks and in whites or to a difference between blacks and whites in accessing health care, which may delay the diagnosis and treatment of the disease in black patients. Shapiro and colleagues recognized that the randomized trial of mammography offered an unusual opportunity to address this question. The findings are shown in Figure 18-19. Let us first look only at the survival curves for the control group, blacks and whites (Fig. 18-19A). The data are consistent with those in Figure 18-18: blacks and Hispanics had a worse prognosis than did whites. Now let us also look at the curves for whites and blacks in the study group of women who were screened and for whom there was therefore no difference in access to care or utilization of care, as screening was carried out on a predetermined schedule (Fig. 18-19B). We see considerable overlap of the two curves: essentially no difference. This strongly suggests that the screening had eliminated the racial difference in survivorship, and that the usually observed difference between the races in prognosis of breast cancer is in fact a result of poorer access to care or poorer utilization

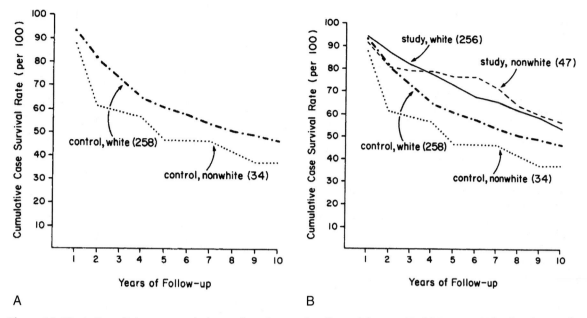

Figure 18-19. **A,** Cumulative case-survival rates, first 10 years after diagnosis by race, Health Insurance Plan (HIP) control groups. **B,** Cumulative case-survival rates, first 10 years after diagnosis by race, Health Insurance Plan (HIP) study and control groups. (From Shapiro S, Venet W, Strax P, et al: Prospects for eliminating racial differences in breast cancer survival rates. Am J Public Health 72:1142–1145, 1982.)

of care among blacks, with a consequent delay in diagnosis and treatment.

Mammography for Women 40 to 49 Years of Age

A major controversy in recent years has centered on the question of whether mammography should be universally recommended for women in their 40s. The data from Shapiro's study as well as from other studies established the benefit of regular mammography examinations for women 50 years and older. However, the data are less clear for women in their 40s. Many issues arise in interpreting the findings of randomized trials carried out in a number of different populations. Although a reduction of mortality has been estimated at 17% for women in their 40s who have annual mammograms, the data available are generally from studies that were not specifically designed to assess possible benefits in this age group. Moreover, many of the trials recruited women in their *late* 40s, suggesting the possibility that even if there are observed benefits, they could have resulted from mammograms performed after age 50.

A related issue is seen in Figure 18-20. When mortality over time is compared in screened and unscreened women *50 years of age or older* (Fig. 18-20A), the mortality curves diverge at about 4 years after enrollment, with the mammography group

showing a lower mortality that persists over time. However, when screened and unscreened *women in their 40s* are compared (Fig. 18-20B), the mortality curves do not suggest any differences in mortality for at least 11 to 12 years after enrollment. Further follow-up will be needed to determine if the divergence observed in the mortality curves will actually persist and represent a true benefit to women who have had mammograms in their 40s. Interpreting these curves is complicated, however, because women who have been followed for 10 or more years in these studies have passed age 50. Consequently, even if mortality in screened women declines after 11 years, any such benefit observed could be due to mammograms that were performed *after* age 50 rather than to mammograms in their 40s. Further follow-up of women enrolled in many of these studies, and newly initiated studies that are enrolling women in their early 40s, may help to clarify these issues.

In 1997, a Consensus Panel was created by the National Institutes of Health to review the scientific evidence for benefits of mammography in women ages 40 to 49. The panel concluded that the data available did not warrant a universal recommendation for mammography for all women in their 40s. The Panel recommended that each woman should decide for herself whether to undergo mammography.[4] Her decision may be based not only on an

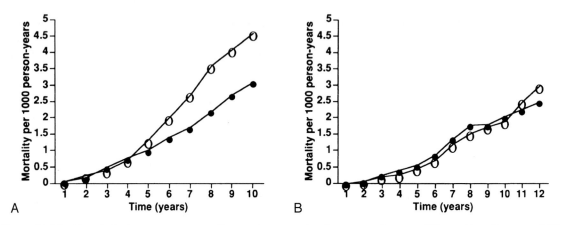

Figure 18-20. Cumulative breast cancer mortality rates in screened and unscreened women (A) ages 50 to 69 years and (B) ages 40 to 49 years. ●, screened; ○, unscreened. (From Kerlikowske K: Efficacy of screening mammography among women aged 40 to 49 years and 50 to 69 years: Comparison of relative and absolute benefit. Natl Cancer Inst Monogr 22:79–86, 1997. **A,** Adapted from Tabar L, Fagerberg G, Duffy SW, et al: Update of the Swedish two-county program of mammographic screening for breast cancer. Radiol Clin North Am 30:187–210, 1992. **B,** Adapted from Nystrom L, Rutqvist LE, Wall S, et al: Breast cancer screening with mammography: Overview of Swedish randomized trials. Lancet 341:973–978, 1993.)

objective analysis of the scientific evidence and consideration of her individual medical history, but also on how she perceives and weighs each potential risk and benefit, the values she places on each, and how she deals with uncertainty. Given both the importance and the complexity of the issues involved in assessing the evidence, a woman should have access to the best possible relevant information regarding both benefits and risks, presented in an understandable and usable form.

The panel added that for women in their 40s who choose to have mammography performed, the costs of the mammograms should be reimbursed by third-party payors or covered by health maintenance organizations so that financial impediments will not influence a woman's decision as to whether or not to have a mammogram. The recommendations of the panel were rejected by the National Cancer Institute which had itself originally requested creation of the panel, and by other agencies. There were clear indications that strong political forces were operating at that time in favor of mammography for women in their 40s.

The controversy over mammography became a broader one with the 2001 publication of a review by Olsen and Gøtzsche of the evidence supporting mammography *at any age.*[5] Among the issues raised by the investigators were concerns about possible inadequacy of the randomization, possible unreliability of assessment of cause of death, their finding that in some trials exclusions of women from the studies were carried out after randomization had

taken place and women with preexisting cancer were excluded only from the screened groups, and their assessment that the two best trials failed to find any benefit.

An accompanying editorial in the issue of the *Lancet* in which the review was published concluded by saying: "At present, there is no reliable evidence from large randomized trials to support screening mammography programmes."[6] However, the U.S. Preventive Services Task Force reviewed the evidence and recommended screening mammography every 1 to 2 years for women 40 years of age and older. Using the methodology described in Chapter 14, they classified the supporting evidence as "fair" on a scale of "good," "fair," or "poor."[7] A 2004 paper countered the arguments raised by Olsen and Gøtzsche and concluded that the prior consensus on mammography was correct.[8] However, the controversy continues unabated. In 2007, the American College of Physicians published new guidelines about mammography for women in their 40s, based on an extensive systematic review that addressed both benefits and potential harms.[9,10] The group concluded that the evidence of net benefit is less clear for women in their 40s than for women in their 50s and that mammography carries significant risks, saying: "We don't think the evidence supports a blanket recommendation."

Thus, the controversy between proponents and critics continues, and is not likely to be settled to everyone's satisfaction by expert pronouncements. The problems in methodology and interpretation are complex and will probably not be resolved by further large trials. Such trials are difficult and expensive to initiate and conduct, and because of the time needed to complete them, these trials are also limited in that the findings often do not reflect the most recent improvements in mammographic technology. However, with so much of the data equivocal and a focus of controversy, progress will most likely come from new technologies for detecting breast cancer. Meanwhile, women are left with a decision-making challenge regarding their own choices concerning mammography, given the major uncertainties in the available evidence.

Screening for Cervical Cancer

Perhaps no screening test for cancer is used more widely than the Pap smear. One would therefore assume that there has been overwhelming evidence of its effectiveness in reducing mortality from invasive cervical cancer. Unfortunately, there has never been a properly designed randomized, controlled trial of cervical cancer screening; and there probably never will be, because cervical cancer screening has been accepted as effective both by health authorities and by the public. This state of affairs is incredible, given the immense resources that have been invested worldwide in screening for cervical cancer.

At this point, one could not ethically do a randomized trial of Pap smears, despite the lack of conclusive evidence as to their effectiveness. In the absence of randomized trials, several alternative approaches have been used. Perhaps the most frequent evaluation design has been to compare incidence and mortality rates in populations with different rates of screening. A second approach has been to examine changes over time in rates of diagnosis of carcinoma in situ. A third approach has been that of case-control studies in which women with invasive cervical cancer are compared with control women, and the frequency of past Pap smears is examined in both groups. All of these studies are generally affected by the methodologic problems raised previously in this chapter.

Despite these reservations, the evidence indicates that many or most carcinomas in situ probably do progress to invasive cancer; consequently, early detection of cervical cancer in the in situ stage would result in a significant saving of life, even if it is lower than many optimistic estimates. Much of the uncertainty we face regarding screening for cervical cancer stems from the fact that no well-designed randomized trial was initially carried out. This observation points out that in the United States, a set of standards

must be met before new pharmacologic agents are licensed for human use, but another, less stringent, set of standards is used for new technology or new health programs. No drug would be licensed in the United States without evaluation through randomized, controlled trials, but no such evaluation is required before screening or other types of programs and procedures are introduced.

Screening for Neuroblastoma

Some of the issues just discussed are encountered in screening for neuroblastoma, which is a tumor that occurs in young children. The rationale for screening for neuroblastoma was outlined by Tuchman and colleagues[11]: (1) Outcome has improved little in the past several decades. (2) Prognosis is known to be better in children who manifest the disease before the age of 1 year. (3) At any age, children in advanced stages of disease have worse prognoses than those in early stages. (4) More than 90% of children presenting with clinical symptoms of neuroblastoma excrete higher than normal amounts of catecholamines in their urine. (5) These metabolites can easily be measured in urine samples obtained from diapers.

These facts constitute a strong rationale for neuroblastoma screening. Figure 18-21 shows data from Japan, where a major effort at neuroblastoma screening had been mounted. The percentages of children younger than 1 year in whom neuroblastoma was detected were compared before and after initiation of screening in Sapporo, a city in Hokkaido, and these data were compared with birth data from the rest of Hokkaido, where no screening program was set up. After initiation of screening, a greater percentage of cases of neuroblastoma in children younger than 1 year was detected in Sapporo than in the rest of Hokkaido.

However, a number of serious problems arise in assessing the benefits of neuroblastoma screening. It is now clear that neuroblastoma is a biologically heterogeneous disease, and there is clearly a better prognosis from the start in some cases than in others. Many tumors have a good prognosis because they regress spontaneously, even without treatment. Furthermore, screening is most likely to detect slow-growing, less malignant tumors and is less likely to detect aggressive, fast-growing tumors.

Thus, it is difficult to show that screening for neuroblastomas is, in fact, beneficial. In fact, two large studies of neuroblastoma screening appeared in 2002. Woods and colleagues[12] studied 476,654 children in Quebec, Canada. Screening was offered to all the children at ages 3 weeks and 6 months. Mortality

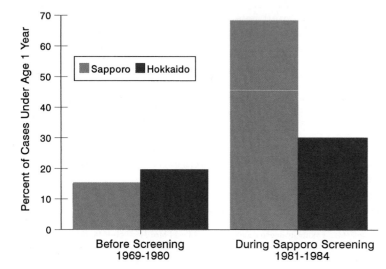

Figure 18-21. Percentage of neuroblastoma cases under 1 year of age in Sapporo and Hokkaido, Japan, before and after screening. (Adapted from Goodman SN: Neuroblastoma screening data: An epidemiologic analysis. Am J Dis Child 145:1415–1422, 1991; based on data from Nishi M, Miyake H, Takeda T, et al: Effects of the mass screening of neuroblastoma in Sapporo City. Cancer 60:433–436, 1987. Copyright © 1987 American Cancer Society. Reprinted by permission of Wiley-Liss, Inc, a subsidiary of John Wiley & Sons, Inc.)

TABLE 18-3. **Rate of Death from Neuroblastoma by 8 Years of Age in the Screened Quebec Cohort, as Compared With the Rates in Four Unscreened Cohorts***

Control Cohort	Number of Deaths Expected in Quebec on the Basis of the Control Cohort	Standardized Mortality Ratio for Quebec (95% CI)
Ontario	19.8	1.11 (0.64–1.92)
Minnesota	24.4	0.90 (0.48–1.70)
Florida	15.7	1.40 (0.81–2.41)
Greater Delaware Valley	22.8	0.96 (0.56–1.66)

*There were 22 deaths due to neuroblastoma in the screened Quebec cohort.
CI, confidence interval.
From Woods WG, Gao R, Shuster JJ, et al: Screening of infants and mortality due to neuroblastoma. N Engl J Med 346:1041–1046, 2002.

from neuroblastoma up to 8 years of age among children screened in Quebec was no lower than among four unscreened cohorts (Table 18-3) and no lower than in the rest of Canada, excluding Quebec, and in two historical cohorts (Table 18-4). Schilling and colleagues[13] studied 2,581,188 children in Germany who were offered screening at 1 year of age. They found that neuroblastoma screening did not reduce the incidence of disseminated disease and did not appear to reduce mortality from the disease, although mortality follow-up was not yet complete. Thus, the data currently available do not support screening for neuroblastoma. The findings in these studies demonstrate the importance of understanding the biology and natural history of a disease and the need to obtain relevant and rigorous evidence regarding the potential benefits or lack of benefits, when screening for any disease is being considered. The ability to detect a disease by screening cannot be equated with a demonstration of benefit to those screened.

PROBLEMS IN ASSESSING THE SENSITIVITY AND SPECIFICITY OF TESTS

New screening programs are often initiated after a screening test first becomes available. When such a test is developed, claims are often made—by manufacturers of test kits, investigators, or others—that the test has high sensitivity and a high specificity. However, as we shall see, from a practical standpoint, this may often be difficult to demonstrate.

Figure 18-22A shows a 2 × 2 table, as we have seen in earlier chapters, tabulating the reality (disease present or absent) against the test results (positive or negative).

To calculate sensitivity and specificity, data are needed in all four cells. However, often only those with positive test results $(a + b)$ (seen in the *upper row* of the figure) are sent for further testing. Data for those who test negative $(c + d)$ are frequently not available, because these patients do not receive further testing.

TABLE 18-4. Rate of Death from Neuroblastoma by 8 Years of Age in the Screened Quebec Cohort, as Compared with the Rates in Unscreened Canadian Cohorts*

Control Cohort	Number of Deaths Expected in Quebec on the Basis of the Control Cohort	Standardized Mortality Ratio for Quebec (95% CI)
Historical cohorts		
Quebec	22.5	0.98 (0.54–1.77)
Canada	21.2	1.04 (0.64–1.69)
Concurrent cohort		
Canada, excluding Quebec	15.8	1.39 (0.85–2.30)

*There were 22 deaths from neuroblastoma in the screened cohort. All data were collected by Statistics Canada.
CI, confidence interval.
From Woods WG, Gao R, Shuster JJ, et al. Screening of infants and mortality due to neuroblastoma. N Engl J Med 346:1041–1046, 2002.

For example, as shown in Figure 18-22B, the Western blot test serves as a gold standard for detecting human immunodeficiency virus (HIV) infection, and those with positive enzyme-linked immunosorbent assay (ELISA) results are sent for Western blot testing.

However, because those with negative ELISA results are generally not tested further, the data needed in the lower cells for calculating sensitivity and specificity of the ELISA are often not available from routine testing. To obtain such data, it is essential that some negative ELISA specimens also be sent for further testing, together with the ELISA-positive specimens.

The situation with the prostate-specific antigen (PSA) test is even more difficult, as shown in Figure 18-22C. This test originally was used to monitor the response to treatment in patients with prostate cancer, but it has been used increasingly to detect prostate cancer. But what are the sensitivity and specificity of the test in detecting prostate cancer?

Men who have elevated PSA levels (positive test results) are often sent for further testing that includes transrectal ultrasound (TRU) and biopsy of the prostate. These procedures are expensive and are associated with pain and discomfort. Again, *only* those who have elevated PSA levels ($a + b$) are sent for further testing, and data are missing for those with negative results ($c + d$). In this case, however, in contrast to the situation for ELISA and Western blot tests, it is hard to conceive of a person with low PSA levels (normal results) being sent for TRU and biopsy solely to complete the data in the lower two cells. Hence, establishing the sensitivity and specificity of the PSA test is difficult at best.

INTERPRETING STUDY RESULTS THAT SHOW NO BENEFIT OF SCREENING

In this chapter thus far we have stressed the interpretation of results that show a difference between screened and unscreened groups. If, however, we are unable to demonstrate a benefit from early detection of disease, any of the following interpretations may be possible:

1. The apparent lack of benefit may be inherent in the natural history of the disease (e.g., the disease has no detectable preclinical phase or an extremely short detectable preclinical phase).
2. The therapeutic intervention currently available may not be any more effective when it is provided earlier than when it is provided at the time of usual diagnosis.
3. The natural history and currently available therapies may have the potential for enhanced benefit, but inadequacies of the care provided to those who screen positive may account for the observed lack of benefit (that is, there is efficacy, but poor effectiveness).

COST-BENEFIT ANALYSIS OF SCREENING

Some people respond to cost-benefit issues by concentrating only on cost, asking, if the test is cheap, why not perform it? However, although the test for blood in the stool, for example, in screening for colon cancer, costs only a few dollars for the filter paper kit and the necessary laboratory processing, to calculate the total cost of such a test we must include the cost of the colonoscopies that are done after the initial

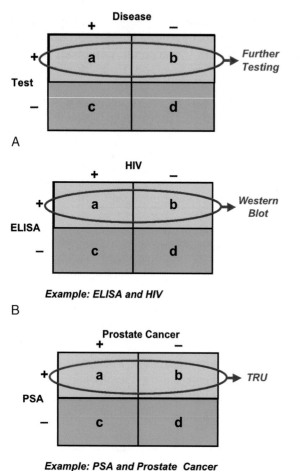

A

B

Example: ELISA and HIV

C

Example: PSA and Prostate Cancer

Figure 18-22. A, Problem of establishing sensitivity and specificity because of limited follow-up of those with negative test results. **B,** Problem of establishing sensitivity and specificity because of limited follow-up of those with negative test results for HIV using the enzyme-linked immunosorbent assay (ELISA) test. **C,** Problem of establishing sensitivity and specificity because of limited follow-up of those with negative test results using the prostate-specific antigen (PSA) test for prostatic cancer. TRU, transrectal ultrasound.

testing as well as the cost of the complications that infrequently result from colonoscopy.

The balance of cost-effectiveness includes not only financial costs, but also nonfinancial costs to the patient, including anxiety, emotional distress, and inconvenience. Is the test itself invasive? Even if it is not, if the test result is positive, is invasive therapy warranted by the test result? What is the false-positive rate in such tests; that is, in what proportion of persons will invasive tests be carried out or anxiety

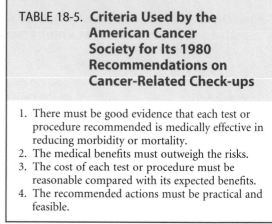

TABLE 18-5. **Criteria Used by the American Cancer Society for Its 1980 Recommendations on Cancer-Related Check-ups**

1. There must be good evidence that each test or procedure recommended is medically effective in reducing morbidity or mortality.
2. The medical benefits must outweigh the risks.
3. The cost of each test or procedure must be reasonable compared with its expected benefits.
4. The recommended actions must be practical and feasible.

be generated despite the reality that the individuals do not have the disease in question? Thus, the "cost" of a test is not only the cost of the test procedure but also the cost of the entire follow-up process that is set in motion by a positive result, even if it turns out to be a false-positive result. These considerations are reflected in the criteria used by the American Cancer Society for its 1980 recommendations on cancer-related check-ups (Table 18-5).

CONCLUSION

This chapter has reviewed some of the major sources of bias that must be taken into account in assessing study findings that compare screened and unscreened populations. The biases of selection for screening and prognostic selection can be addressed, in large part, by using a randomized, controlled trial as the study design. Reasonable estimates of the lead time can be made if appropriate information is available. Few of the methods that are currently used to detect disease early have been subjected to evaluation by randomized, controlled trials, and most are probably not destined to be studied in this way. This is a result of several factors, including the difficulty and expense associated with conducting such studies and the ethical issues inherent in randomizing a population to receive or not receive modalities of care that are widely used and considered effective, even in the absence of strong supporting evidence. Consequently, we are obliged to maximize our use of evidence from nonrandomized approaches, and to do so, the potential biases and problems discussed in this chapter must be considered.

In approaching programs for early disease detection, we need to be able to identify groups who are at high risk. This would include not only those at risk for developing the disease in question, but also those who are "at risk" for benefiting from the intervention. These are the groups for whom cost-benefit calculations will favor benefit. We must keep in mind that, even if the screening test is not in itself invasive (e.g., Pap smear), the intervention mandated by a positive screening test result may be highly invasive (e.g., conization).

The overriding issue is how to make decisions when our data are inconclusive, inconsistent, or incomplete. We face this dilemma regularly, both in clinical practice and in the development of public health policy. These decisions must first consider the existing body of relevant scientific evidence. However, in the final analysis, the decision whether or not to screen a population for a disease is a value judgment that should take into account the incidence and severity of the disease, the feasibility of detecting the disease early, the feasibility of intervening effectively in those with positive screening results, and the overall cost-benefit calculation for an early detection program.

To improve our ability to make appropriate decisions, additional research is needed regarding the natural history of disease and, specifically, regarding the definition of characteristics of individuals who are at risk for a poor outcome. Before new screening programs are introduced, we should argue strongly for well-conducted randomized, controlled trials, so that we will not be operating in an atmosphere of uncertainty at the time in the future when such trials have become virtually impossible to conduct. Nevertheless, given the fact that most medical and public health practice—including early detection of disease—has not been subjected to randomized trials, and that decisions regarding early detection must be made on the basis of incomplete and equivocal data, it is essential that we as health professionals appreciate and understand the methodologic issues involved so that we can make the wisest use of the available knowledge on behalf of our patients. Even the best of intentions and passionate evangelism cannot substitute for rigorous evidence that supports or does not support the benefit of screening.

REFERENCES

1. Hutchison GB: Evaluation of preventive services. J Chronic Dis 11:497–508, 1960.
2. Shapiro S, Venet W, Strax P, Venet L (eds): Periodic Screening for Breast Cancer: The Health Insurance Plan Project and Its Sequelae, 1963–1986. Baltimore, Johns Hopkins University Press, 1988.
3. Shapiro S, Venet W, Strax P, et al: Prospects for eliminating racial differences in breast cancer survival rates. Am J Public Health 72:1142–1145, 1982.
4. Breast Cancer Screening for Women Ages 40–49. NIH Consensus Statement Online. 1997 Jan 21–23, cited 2007, December, 9;15(1):1–35.
5. Olsen O, Gøtzsche C: Cochrane review on screening for breast cancer with mammography. Lancet 358:1340–1342, 2001.
6. Horton R: Screening mammography: An overview revisited. Lancet 358:1284–1285, 2001.
7. U.S. Preventive Services Task Force: Breast cancer screening: A summary of the evidence for the U.S. Preventive Services Task Force. Ann Intern Med 137:347–360, 2002.
8. Freedman DA, Petitti DB, Robins JM: On the efficacy of screening for breast cancer. Int J Epid 33:43–55, 2004.
9. Brewer NT, Salz T, Lillie SE: Systematic review: The long-term effects of false-positive mammograms. Ann Intern Med 146:502–510, 2007.
10. Qaseem A, Snow V, Sherif K, et al: Screening mammography for women 40 to 49 years of age: A clinical practice Guideline from the American College of Physicians. Ann Intern Med 146:511–515, 2007.
11. Tuchman M, Lemieus B, Woods WG: Screening for neuroblastoma in infants: Investigate or implement? Pediatrics 86:791–793, 1990.
12. Woods WG, Gao R, Shuster JJ, et al: Screening of infants and mortality due to neuroblastoma. N Engl J Med 346:1041–1046, 2002.
13. Schilling FH, Spix C, Berthold F, et al: Neuroblastoma screening at one year of age. N Engl J Med 346:1047–1053, 2002.

REVIEW QUESTIONS FOR CHAPTER 18

Questions 1 through 4 are based on the following information:

A new screening program was instituted in a certain country. The program used a screening test that is effective in detecting cancer Z at an early stage. Assume that there is no effective treatment for this type of cancer and, therefore, that the program results in no change in the usual course of the disease. Assume also that the rates noted are calculated from all known cases of cancer Z and that there were no changes in the quality of death certification of this disease.

1. What will happen to the apparent *incidence rate* of cancer Z in the country during the first year of this program?
   a. Incidence rate will increase
   b. Incidence rate will decrease
   c. Incidence rate will remain constant

2. What will happen to the apparent *prevalence rate* of cancer Z in the country during the first year of this program?
   a. Prevalence rate will increase
   b. Prevalence rate will decrease
   c. Prevalence rate will remain constant

3. What will happen to the apparent *case-fatality rate* for cancer Z in the country during the first year of this program?
   a. Case-fatality rate will increase
   b. Case-fatality rate will decrease
   c. Case-fatality rate will remain constant

4. What will happen to the apparent *mortality rate* from cancer Z in the country as a result of the program?
   a. Mortality rate will increase
   b. Mortality rate will decrease
   c. Mortality rate will remain constant

5. The best index (indices) for concluding that an early detection program for breast cancer truly improves the natural history of disease, 15 years after its initiation, would be:
   a. A smaller proportionate mortality for breast cancer 15 years after initiation of the early detection program compared to the proportionate mortality prior to its initiation
   b. Improved long-term survival rates for breast cancer patients (adjusted for lead time)
   c. A decrease in incidence of breast cancer
   d. A decrease in the prevalence of breast cancer
   e. None of the above

6. In general, screening should be undertaken for diseases with the following feature(s):
   a. Diseases with a low prevalence in identifiable subgroups of the population
   b. Diseases for which case-fatality rates are low
   c. Diseases with a natural history that can be altered by medical intervention
   d. Diseases that are readily diagnosed and for which treatment efficacy has been shown to be equivocal in evidence from a number of clinical trials
   e. None of the above

7. Which of the following is *not* a possible outcome measure that could be used as an indicator of the benefit of screening programs aimed at early detection of disease?
   a. Reduction of case-fatality rate in screened individuals
   b. Reduction of mortality in the population screened
   c. Reduction of incidence in the population screened
   d. Reduction of complications
   e. Improvement in the quality of life in screened individuals

Question 8 is based on the information given below:

The diagram at the bottom of the page shows the natural history of disease X:

8. Assume that early detection of disease X through screening improves prognosis. In order for a screening program to be most effective, at which point in the natural history in the diagram must the critical point be?
   a. Between A and B
   b. Between B and C
   c. Between C and D
   d. Anywhere between A and C
   e. Anywhere between A and D

A	B	C	D
Biologic Onset of Disease X	Earliest Possible Detection of Disease X by Any Screening Technique	Usual Time of Diagnosis of Disease X	Usual Time of Death from Disease X

Chapter 19

Epidemiology and Public Policy

All scientific work is incomplete—whether it be observational or experimental.
All scientific work is liable to be upset or modified by advancing knowledge.
That does not confer upon us a freedom to ignore the knowledge we already have, or to
postpone the action that it appears to demand at a given time.[1]
— Sir Austin Bradford Hill, President's Address,
 Royal Society of Medicine, January 14, 1965

Experience is that marvelous thing that enables you to recognize a mistake when you make it
again.[2]
— Franklin P. Jones, legendary American humorist

A major role of epidemiology is to serve as a basis for developing policies that affect human health, including the prevention and control of disease. As seen in previous chapters, the findings from epidemiologic studies may be relevant both to issues in clinical practice and community health, and to population approaches to disease prevention and health promotion. As discussed in Chapter 1, the practical applications of epidemiology are often viewed as being so integral to the discipline that they are incorporated into the very definition of epidemiology. Historically, epidemiologic investigations were initiated to address emerging challenges relating to human disease and the public health. Indeed, one of the major sources of excitement in epidemiology is the direct applicability of its findings to the alleviation of problems of human health. This chapter presents an overview of some issues and problems relating to epidemiology in its application to the formulation and evaluation of public policy.

EPIDEMIOLOGY AND PREVENTION

The importance of epidemiology in prevention has been emphasized in several of the preceding chapters. Identifying populations at increased risk, ascertaining the cause of their increased risk, and analyzing the costs and benefits of eliminating or reducing exposure to the causal factor or factors all require an understanding of basic epidemiologic concepts and of the possible interpretation of the findings of epidemiologic studies. In addition, assessing the strength of the evidence and identifying any limits on the inferences derived or on the generalizability of the findings is of critical importance. Thus, epidemiology can be considered to be the "basic science" of prevention.

How much epidemiologic data do we need to justify a prevention effort? Clearly, there is no easy answer to this question. Some of the issues involved differ depending on whether primary or secondary prevention is being considered. If we are discussing primary prevention, the answer depends on the severity of the condition, on the costs involved (in terms of dollars, human suffering, and loss of quality of life), on the strength of the evidence that implicates a certain causal factor or factors in the etiology of the disease in question, and on the difficulty of reducing or eliminating exposure to that factor.

With secondary prevention, the issues are somewhat different. We must still consider the severity of the disease in question. In addition, however, we must ask whether we can detect the disease earlier than usual by screening, how invasive and expensive such detection would be, whether a benefit accrues to a person who has the disease if treatment is initiated at an earlier-than-usual stage, and whether there are harmful effects associated with screening. Epidemiology is clearly an invaluable approach to resolving many of these issues.

In recent years, considerable attention has been addressed to expanding what has been called the traditional risk factor model of epidemiology in which we explore the relationship of an independent factor such as an exposure to a dependent factor such as a disease outcome (Fig. 19-1). It has been suggested that this approach should be expanded in two ways: First, it should include measurement not only of the adverse outcome—the disease itself—but also of the economic, social, and psychological impacts resulting from the disease outcome on the individual, his or her family, and the community. Second, it is clear that exposure to a putative causal agent is generally not distributed uniformly in a population. The factors that determine whether a person becomes exposed therefore need to be explored if prevention is to be effected by reducing the exposure (Fig. 19-2). The full model is even more complex as seen in Figure 19-3: The relationship is influenced by *determinants of susceptibility* of the individual to the exposure; these include genetic factors together with environmental and social influences. Although such an expanded approach is intuitively attractive and provides an excellent framework in which to analyze public health problems, the need still remains to

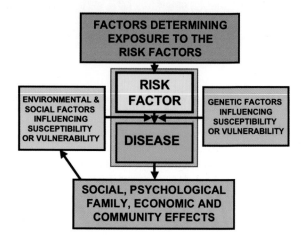

Figure 19-3. Diagram of expanded risk factor epidemiology model to include inter-relationships of factors that determine susceptibility or vulnerability.

demonstrate whether certain exposures or other independent variables are associated with increased risks of specific diseases.

In any case, deciding how much data and what types of data we need for prevention will be societally driven, dependent on a society's values and priorities. Epidemiology, together with other disciplines, can provide much of the necessary scientific data that are relevant to questions of risks and prevention. However, the final decision as to whether to initiate a prevention program will be largely determined by economic and political considerations as well as by societal values. At the same time, it is hoped that such decisions will also be based on a firm foundation of scientific evidence provided by epidemiology and other relevant disciplines.

It is important to distinguish between *macroenvironmental* and *microenvironmental* exposures. Macroenvironmental exposures refer to exposures such as air pollution, which affect populations or entire communities. Microenvironmental exposures refer to environmental factors that affect a specific individual, such as diet, smoking, and alcohol consumption. From the prevention standpoint, macroenvironmental factors are in many ways easier to control and modify, as this can be accomplished by legislation and regulation (e.g., setting environmental standards for pollutants). In contrast, modification of microenvironmental factors depends on modifying individual habits and lifestyle, which is often a much greater challenge.

In dealing with microenvironmental factors, providing scientific evidence and risk estimates is

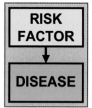

Figure 19-1. Diagram of classic risk factor epidemiology.

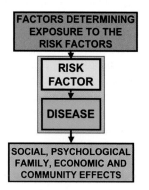

Figure 19-2. Diagram of expanded risk factor epidemiology model to include determinants of exposure as well as social, economic, psychological, and family effects of the disease.

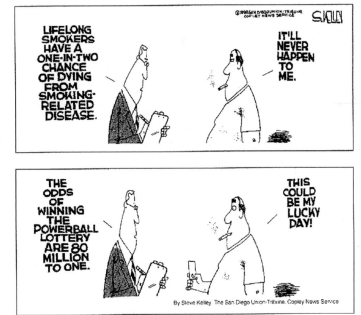

Figure 19-4. Risk of what? How the end-point may affect an individual's perception of risk and willingness to act. (S. Kelley. © 1998 San Diego Union Tribune. Copley News Service.)

frequently not enough to induce individuals to modify their lifestyles to effect prevention. Individuals often differ in the extent to which they are willing to take risks in many aspects of their lives including health. In addition, individual behaviors may differ depending on whether they are confronted with the risk of an adverse outcome or the "risk" of a positive event (Fig. 19-4). In addition, individuals may often place the blame elsewhere for health problems brought on by their own lifestyle. Thus, risk communication, which was mentioned above, must extend beyond communicating risk data to policy makers. It must also deal with communicating with the public in an understandable fashion in the context of people's perceptions of their risk so that individuals will be motivated to accept responsibility and act on behalf of their own health to the greatest extent possible. Epidemiologists should therefore work with health educators in appropriate education of the public in regard to risk issues.

POPULATION VERSUS HIGH-RISK APPROACHES TO PREVENTION

An important question in prevention is whether our approach should target groups that are known to be at high risk or whether it should extend primary prevention efforts to the general population as a whole. This issue was discussed by Rose in 1985[3] and later amplified by Whelton in 1994[4] in a discussion of hypertension prevention and prevention of deaths from coronary heart disease (CHD).

Epidemiologic studies have demonstrated that the risk of death from CHD steadily increases with increases in both systolic and diastolic blood pressure; there is no known threshold. Figure 19-5A shows the distribution of systolic blood pressures in 347,978 men who were screened for the Multiple Risk Factor Intervention Trial (MRFIT).

Figure 19-5B shows the risk of CHD mortality in relation to systolic blood pressure in this group; the risk increases steadily with higher blood pressure levels. Individuals with blood pressures of 180 mm Hg or higher had 5.65 times the risk of CHD death than those whose blood pressure was below 110 mm Hg. Figure 19-5C shows the percentages of excess CHD deaths due to hypertension at each blood pressure level. (Those with blood pressure below 110 mm Hg are defined as having no excess deaths.) Although fewer than one fourth of all individuals had hypertension, they accounted for more than two thirds of the excess CHD deaths. These observations argue for directing our preventive efforts to those at the highest extremes of systolic blood pressure, who have the highest relative risk.

However, almost 80% of the hypertensive persons had blood pressure in the 140 to 159 mm Hg range (stage 1). Stage 1 hypertension accounted for about 43% of the excess risk of dying from CHD in the total population and for almost 64% of the excess CHD

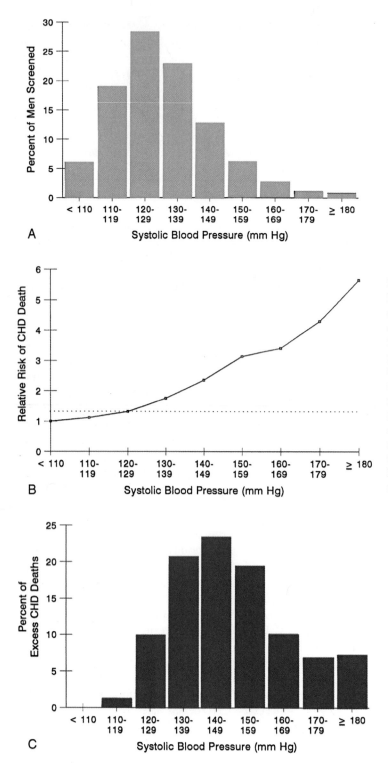

Figure 19-5. **A,** Percent distribution by baseline systolic blood pressure of men screened for MRFIT. **B,** Relative risk of coronary heart disease (CHD) mortality in relation to level of systolic blood pressure in men screened for MRFIT. **C,** Percent distribution of excess CHD deaths by level of systolic blood pressure for men screened for MRFIT. (Adapted from Stamler J, Dyer AR, Shekelle RB, et al: Relationship of baseline major risk factors to coronary and all-cause mortality, and to longevity: Findings from long-term follow-up of Chicago cohorts. Cardiology 82:191–222, 1993.)

death risk among hypertensive subjects. Thus, if we wish to address the overall burden of CHD deaths associated with elevated blood pressure, it is not enough to direct preventive efforts at those with the highest extremes of blood pressure. We also need to focus on those with less marked elevations in blood pressure if we are to prevent most of the excess deaths associated with increased blood pressure.

It therefore seems reasonable to combine a high risk with a population approach: one set of preventive measures addressed to those at particularly high risk and another designed for primary prevention of hypertension and addressed to the population in general.

Such analyses can have significant implications for prevention programs. The types of preventive measures that might be used for high-risk individuals differ from those that are applicable to the general population. Those who are at high risk, and know they are at high risk, are more likely to tolerate more expensive, uncomfortable, and even more invasive procedures. However, in applying a preventive measure to a general population, the measure must have a low cost and be only minimally invasive; it needs to be associated with relatively little pain or discomfort if it is to be acceptable to the general population.

Figure 19-6 shows the goal of a population-based strategy, which is a downward shifting of the entire curve of blood pressure distribution when a blood pressure–lowering intervention is applied to an entire community. Because the blood pressure of most members of the population is above the very lowest levels that are considered optimal, even a small downward shift (shift to the left) in the curve is likely to have major public health benefits. In fact, such a

shift would prevent more strokes in the population than would successful treatment limited to "high-risk" individuals. Furthermore, Rose[3] pointed out that the "high-risk" strategy is an interim expedient that is necessary for the protection of susceptible individuals. Ultimately, however, our hope is to understand the basic causes of the incidence of the disease—in this case, elevated blood pressure—and to develop and implement the necessary means for its (primary) prevention. Rose concluded that

> *Realistically, many diseases will long continue to call for both approaches, and fortunately competition between them is usually unnecessary. Nevertheless, the priority of concern should always be the discovery and control of the causes of incidence.*[3]

EPIDEMIOLOGY AND CLINICAL MEDICINE: HORMONE REPLACEMENT THERAPY IN POSTMENOPAUSAL WOMEN

Epidemiology can be considered the basic science of clinical investigation. Data obtained from epidemiologic studies are essential in clinical decision making in many situations. An understanding of epidemiology is crucial to the process of designing meaningful studies of the natural history of disease, the quality of different diagnostic methods, and the effectiveness of clinical interventions. Epidemiology is highly relevant to addressing many uncertainties and dilemmas in clinical policy, many of which cannot always be easily resolved.

A dramatic example is the use of hormone replacement therapy (HRT) by postmenopausal women. In 1966, a physician, Robert Wilson, published a book entitled *Feminine Forever* that advocated hormone replacement therapy for postmenopausal women.

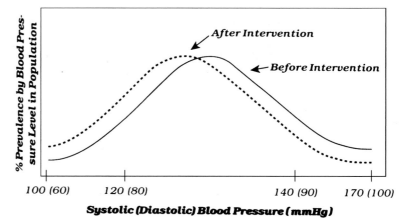

Figure 19-6. Representation of the effects of a population-based intervention strategy on the distribution of blood pressure. (From National Institutes of Health: Working Group Report on Primary Prevention of Hypertension. NIH publication No. 93–2669, p 8. Washington, DC, National Heart, Lung, and Blood Institute, 1993.)

After the publication of this book, millions of post-menopausal women began taking estrogens in the hope of retaining their youth and attractiveness and avoiding the unpleasant symptoms of menopause often encountered, such as hot flashes, night sweats, and vaginal dryness. The medical community largely accepted Wilson's recommendation for estrogen replacement, and even gynecology textbooks supported it. However, in the 1970s, an increased risk of uterine cancer was reported in women taking estrogen replacement. As a result, estrogen was subsequently combined with progestin, which counteracts the effect of estrogen on the uterine endometrial lining. This combination leads to monthly uterine bleeding that resembles a normal menstrual period.

A number of nonrandomized observational studies subsequently appeared and reported other health benefits, such as fewer heart attacks and strokes, less osteoporosis, and fewer hip fractures. Considering the entire body of evidence that had accumulated, support for the conclusion that estrogen protected women against heart disease appeared strong and generally consistent. Women were advised that when they reached 50 years of age, they should discuss with their physicians whether they should begin HRT to protect themselves against heart disease and other conditions associated with aging.

Recognizing that there was little supporting evidence from randomized trials using hard disease endpoints, such as risk of myocardial infarction, two randomized trials were initiated: the Heart and Estrogen/Progestin Replacement Study (HERS) and the Women's Health Initiative (WHI). The HERS study[5] included 2,763 women with known coronary heart disease (CHD). It found that, in contrast to accepted beliefs, combination HRT increased women's risk of myocardial infarctions during the initial years after starting therapy. The study failed to find evidence that HRT offered protection during a follow-up period of almost 7 years (Fig. 19-7).

The WHI[6] was a randomized, placebo-controlled trial of 16,608 women designed in 1991 and 1992 to evaluate HRT as primary prevention for heart disease and other conditions common in the elderly. The planned duration of the trial was 8.5 years. One component (arm) of the study was a randomized, placebo-controlled trial of estrogen plus progestin in postmenopausal women who had an intact uterus. This component of the study was stopped 3 years early because, by that time, results had shown increased risks of heart attack, stroke, breast cancer, and blood clots (Fig. 19-8). Although the study

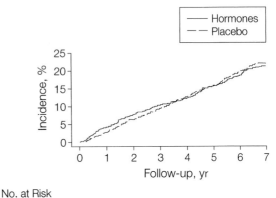

No. at Risk

Hormones	1380	1303	1247	1196	1133	1043	984	354
Placebo	1383	1334	1269	1209	1122	1039	976	336

Figure 19-7. Kaplan-Meier estimates of the cumulative incidence of coronary heart disease events (death and nonfatal myocardial infarctions). (From Grady D et al. for the HERS Research Group: Cardiovascular disease outcomes during 6.8 years of hormone therapy: Heart and estrogen/progestin replacement study follow-up [HERS II]. JAMA 288:49–57, 2002.)

showed reduced incidence of osteoporosis, bone fractures, and colorectal cancer, overall, the dangers from HRT outweighed these benefits.

Only about 2.5% of the enrolled women had adverse events. On the basis of the study results, it has been estimated that, in 1 year, for every 10,000 women taking estrogen plus progestin, we would expect 7 more women to have a heart attack (37 women taking estrogen plus progestin would have a heart attack compared with 30 women taking placebo), 8 more women to have a stroke, 8 more women to have breast cancer, and 18 more women to have blood clots. At the same time, we would expect 6 fewer cases of colorectal cancer and 5 fewer hip fractures.

Many women who had been taking HRT were shocked by the results of the WHI. The findings strongly indicate that, in women taking estrogen plus progestin for protection against heart disease, the risks of cardiovascular endpoints are actually increased. These women were left uncertain as to whether to continue with HRT or whether to seek alternatives. Many also believed that they had been misled by the medical community because, for many years, they had been reassured about the effectiveness and safety of HRT by their physicians, *despite the absence of clear data* from placebo-controlled randomized trials. Complicating the decision-making process for women at the time of menopause is that

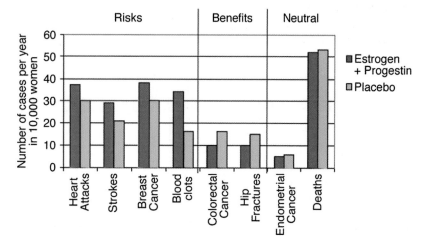

Figure 19-8. Disease rates for women assigned to estrogen plus progestin or to placebo in the Women's Health Initiative (WHI) study. (WHI online: Available at http://www.whi.org/updates_hrt2002.asp)

the WHI did not address the question faced by many women who often take combination HRT for brief periods to prevent and relieve postmenopausal symptoms such as hot flashes.

A major methodologic question is why there was such a discrepancy between the results of the placebo-controlled randomized WHI study regarding risk of heart disease and the results of a large number of nonrandomized, observational studies that previously supported a protective benefit from combination HRT. This issue is of great importance because, in many areas of medicine and public health, we depend on the findings of nonrandomized, observational studies because the costs of randomized trials may be prohibitive, and randomized studies may not be feasible for other reasons.

Several explanations have been offered.[7–9] In the observational studies, the women who were prescribed HRT were often healthier women who had a better cardiovascular risk profile. Women who use HRT are often better educated, leaner, more physically active, less likely to be smokers, more health conscious, and of higher socioeconomic status than women who do not. Often, women who were prescribed HRT were judged to be compliant, and compliers often have other healthy patterns of behavior. Thus, confounding by lifestyle and other factors may have taken place in the observational studies. In addition, in the observational studies, when adverse effects occurred early and led to discontinuation of HRT, these events might not always have been identified in the periodic cross-sectional measurements used. Clearly, in the future it will be essential to address these issues when nonrandomized, observational studies are used as the basis for clinical and public health policy.

RISK ASSESSMENT

A major use of epidemiology in relation to public policy is for risk assessment. Risk assessment has been defined as the characterization of the potential adverse health effects of human exposures to environmental hazards. Risk assessment is viewed as part of an overall process that flows from research to risk assessment and then to risk management, as shown in Figure 19-9. Samet et al[10] reviewed the relationship of epidemiology to risk assessment and described risk management as involving the evaluation of alternative regulatory actions and the selection of the strategy to be applied. Risk management is followed by risk communication, which is the transmission of the findings of risk assessment to those who need to know the findings in order to participate in policy making and to take appropriate risk management actions.

The National Research Council (1983) listed four steps in the process of risk assessment[11]:

1. *Hazard identification:* Determination of whether a particular chemical is causally linked to particular health effects.
2. *Dose-response assessment:* Determination of the relationship between the magnitude of exposure and the probability of occurrence of the health effects in question.
3. *Exposure assessment:* Determination of the extent of human exposure before or after application of regulatory controls.
4. *Risk characterization:* Description of the nature—and often the magnitude—of human risk, including attendant uncertainty.

Clearly, epidemiologic data are essential in each of these steps, although epidemiology is not the only

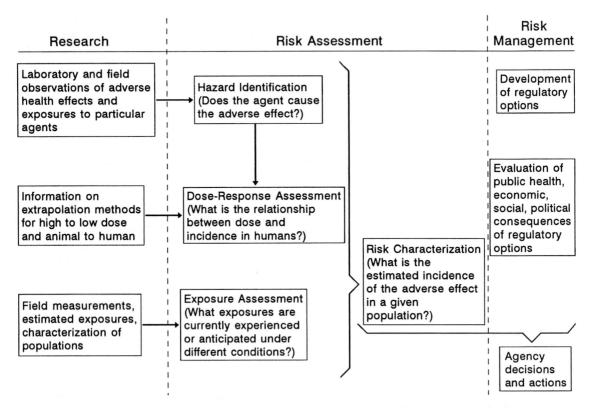

Figure 19-9. Relationships among the four steps of risk assessment and between risk assessment and risk management. (Adapted from Committee on the Institutional Means for Assessment of Risks to Public Health, Commission on Life Sciences, National Research Council: Risk Assessment in the Federal Government: Managing the Process. Washington, DC, National Academy Press, 1983, p 21.)

relevant scientific discipline in the process of risk assessment. In particular, toxicology plays a major role as well, and an important challenge remains to reconcile epidemiologic and toxicologic data when findings from the respective disciplines do not agree.

A number of important methodologic problems affect the use of epidemiology in risk assessment. Because epidemiologic studies generally address the relationship between an environmental exposure and the risk of a disease, rigorous assessment of each variable is critical. Perhaps the most significant problem is assessment of exposure.

Assessment of Exposure

Data regarding exposure generally come from several types of sources (Table 19-1). Each type of source has advantages and disadvantages; the latter include lack of completeness and biases in reporting. Frequently, investigators use several sources of information regarding exposure, but a problem often results when different sources yield conflicting information.

Another problem in exposure assessment is that macroenvironmental factors generally affect many

TABLE 19-1. **Sources of Exposure Data**

1. Interviews
  a. Subject
  b. Surrogate
2. Employment or other records
3. Physician records
4. Hospital records
5. Disease registry records (e.g., cancer registries)
6. Death certificates

individuals simultaneously, so that individual exposures may be difficult to measure. As a result, ecologic approaches are often used in which aggregate rather than individual measurements are used, and the aggregation is often carried out over large areas. The characteristics of the community are therefore ascribed to the individuals residing in that community, but the validity of characterizing an individual exposure by this process is often open to question. Furthermore, personal exposure histories are difficult to obtain either retrospectively or prospectively. In addition, the long latent or induction period between exposure and development of disease makes it necessary to ascertain long-past exposures, which is particularly difficult.

A somewhat parallel set of problems is seen when we try to characterize the occupational exposures of an individual worker and to link an exposure at work to an adverse health outcome. First, because a worker is likely to be exposed to many different agents in an industrial setting, it is often difficult to segregate the risk that can be ascribed to a single specific exposure. Second, because a long latent period often exists between the exposure and the subsequent development of disease, studies of the exposure–disease relationship may be difficult; for example, recall may be poor and records of exposure may have been lost. Third, increased disease risks may occur among those living near an industrial plant, so that it may be difficult to ascertain how much of a worker's risk results from living near the plant and how much is due to an occupational exposure in the work setting itself.

Perhaps the most fundamental problem in measuring exposures in epidemiologic studies is that all of the sources and measures discussed so far are indirect. For example, considerable interest has arisen in recent years over the possible health effects of electromagnetic fields (EMF). This interest followed the article of Wertheimer and Leeper in 1979,[12] which reported increased levels of leukemia in children living near high-voltage transmission lines. Subsequently, many methodologic questions have been raised, and the question of whether such fields are associated with adverse health effects remains unresolved.

In studying EMF, several approaches are used for measuring exposure, including the wiring configuration in the home, spot or 24-hour measurements of the fields, or self-reports of electrical appliance use. However, the results of different studies regarding risk of disease differ depending on the type of exposure measurement that was used. In fact, actual magnetic field measurements, even 24-hour measurements, generate weaker associations with childhood leukemia than do those for wire configuration codes. This observation raises a question about any possible causal link between exposure to magnetic fields and occurrence of disease.

Even the best indirect measure of exposure often leaves critical questions unanswered. First, exposure is generally not dichotomous; data are therefore needed regarding the *dose* of exposure to explore a possible dose–response relationship. Second, it is

important to know whether the exposure was continuous or periodic. For example, in the pathogenesis of cancer, a periodic exposure with alternating exposure and nonexposure periods may allow for DNA repair during the nonexposure periods; in a continuous exposure, no such repair could take place. Finally, information about latency is critical: How long is the latent period and what is its range? This is essential so that we can focus efforts at ascertaining exposure on a time period that seems to be one in which a causal exposure might well have occurred.

Because of these problems in measuring exposure using indirect approaches, much interest has focused on the use of biologic markers of exposures. (Use of such biomarkers has been termed *biochemical epidemiology* or *molecular epidemiology*.) The advantage of using biomarkers is that such use can overcome the problem of limited recall or lack of awareness of an exposure. In addition, biomarkers can overcome errors resulting from variation in individual absorption or metabolism by focusing on a later step in the causal chain.

Biomarkers can be markers of exposure, markers of biologic changes resulting from exposures, or markers of risk or susceptibility. Figure 19-10 exemplifies schematically the different types of exposure we may choose to measure.

We might measure ambient levels of possibly toxic substances in a general environment, the levels to which a specific individual is exposed, the amount of substance absorbed, or the amount of substance or metabolite of the absorbed substance that reaches the target tissue. Biomarkers bring us closer to being able to measure an exposure at a specific stage in the process by which an exposure is linked to human disease. For example, we can measure not only environmental levels of a substance but also DNA adducts that reflect the effect of the substance on biologic processes in the body after absorption.

Nevertheless, despite these advantages, biomarkers generally give us a dichotomous answer—a person was either exposed or not exposed. Biomarkers generally do not shed light on several important questions, such as the following:

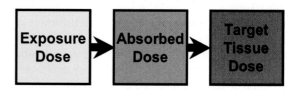

Figure 19-10. What exposures are we trying to measure?

What was the total exposure dose?
What was the duration of exposure?
How long ago did the exposure occur?
Was the exposure continuous or periodic?

The answers to these questions are crucial in properly interpreting the potential biologic importance of a given exposure. For example, in assessing the biologic plausibility of a causal inference being made from observations made of exposure and outcome, we need relevant data that will permit us to determine whether the interval observed between the exposure and the development of the disease is consistent with what we know from other studies about the incubation period of the disease.

It should be pointed out that use of biomarkers is not new in epidemiology. In Ecclesiastes it is written: "There is nothing new under the sun."[13] Even before the revolution in molecular biology took place, laboratory techniques were essential in many epidemiologic studies; these included bacterial isolations and cultures, phage typing of organisms, viral isolation, serologic studies, and assays of cholesterol lipoprotein fractions. With the tremendous advances made in molecular biology, a new variety of biomarkers has become available that is relevant to areas such as carcinogenesis. These biomarkers not only identify exposed individuals, but they also cast new light on the pathogenetic process of the disease in question.

META-ANALYSIS

Several scientific questions arise when epidemiologic data are used for formulating public policy:

1. Can epidemiologic methods detect small increases in risk?
2. How can we reconcile inconsistencies between animal and human data?
3. How can we use incomplete or equivocal epidemiologic data?
4. How can results be interpreted when the findings of epidemiologic studies disagree?

Many of the risks with which we are dealing may be very small, but they may potentially be of great public health importance because of the large numbers of people exposed with a resulting potential for adverse health effects in many people. However, an observed small increase in relative risk above 1.0 may easily result from bias or other methodologic limitations, and such results must therefore be interpreted with great caution unless the results have been replicated and other supporting evidence has been obtained.

Given that the results of different epidemiologic studies may not be consistent, and that at times they may be in dramatic conflict, attempts have been made to systematize the process of reviewing the epidemiologic literature on a given topic. This process is called meta-analysis, and has been defined as "the statistical analysis of a large collection of analysis results from individual studies for the purpose of integrating the findings."[14] Meta-analysis allows for aggregating the results of a set of studies, with appropriate weighting of each study for the number of subjects sampled and for other characteristics. Meta-analysis can increase the statistical power, particularly for certain outcomes and certain subgroups. It can also help to give an overall perspective on an issue when the results of studies disagree.

However, a number of problems and questions are associated with meta-analysis. First, should the analysis include all available studies, or only published studies? Second, how can we address the problem that the reviewed and aggregated studies may vary considerably in quality? Third, when the relative risks or odds ratios from various studies differ, meta-analysis may mask important differences among individual studies. It is therefore essential that a meta-analysis not replace a rigorous examination of each study included in the analysis, including scrutiny of the results and the methodologic limitations of each study. Fourth, the results of meta-analyses themselves are not always reproducible by other analysts. Finally, meta-analysis is subject to the problem of publication bias (discussed later in this chapter). Figure 19-11 shows the type of presentation that is frequently used to show the results of individual studies as well as the results of the meta-analysis.

Meta-analysis is usually applied to randomized trials, but this technique is being used increasingly to aggregate nonrandomized, observational studies, including case-control and cohort studies. In these instances, the studies do not necessarily share a common research design. Hence, the question arises as to how similar must such studies be in order to legitimately include them in a meta-analysis. In addition, appropriate control of biases (such as selection bias and misclassification bias) is essential, but often proves a formidable challenge in meta-analyses. In view of the considerations just discussed, meta-analysis remains a subject of considerable controversy.

A final problem with meta-analysis is that in the face of all the difficulties discussed, putting a quantitative imprint on the estimation of a single relative

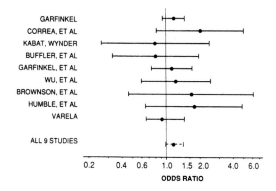

Figure 19-11. Meta-analysis: odds ratios and 95% confidence intervals for nine U.S. epidemiologic studies of the hypothesized association between exposure to environmental tobacco smoke and lung cancer. (From Fleiss JL, Gross AJ: Meta-analysis in epidemiology, with special reference to studies of the association between exposure to environmental tobacco smoke and lung cancer: A critique. J Clin Epidemiol 44:127–139, 1991. Reprinted with permission from Elsevier Science.)

risk or odds ratio from all the studies may lead to a false sense of certainty regarding the magnitude of the risk. People often tend to have an inordinate belief in the validity of findings when a number is attached to them and as a result many of the difficulties that arise in meta-analysis may at times be ignored.

PUBLICATION BIAS

An earlier chapter discussed the use of twin studies as a means of distinguishing the contributions of environmental and genetic factors to the cause of disease. In that discussion it was mentioned that the degree of concordance and discordance in twins is an important observation for drawing conclusions about the role of genetic factors, but that estimates of concordance reported in the literature may be inflated by publication bias, which is the tendency for articles to be published that report concordance for rare diseases in twin pairs.

Publication bias is not limited to studies of twins; it can occur in any area. It is a particularly important phenomenon in publication of articles regarding environmental risks and in publication of the results of clinical trials. Publication bias may occur because investigators do not submit the results of their studies when the findings do not support "positive" associations and increased risks. In addition, journals may select for publication studies that they believe to be of greatest reader interest, and they may not find

studies that report no association to fall in this category. As a result, a literature review that is limited to published articles may preferentially identify studies that report increased risk. Clearly, such a review is highly selective in nature and omits many studies that have obtained what have been called "negative" results (i.e., results showing no effect), which may not have reached publication.

Publication bias therefore has a clear effect on meta-analysis. One approach to this problem is to try to identify unpublished studies and to include them in the analysis. However, the difficulty here is that, in general, unpublished studies are likely not to have passed journal peer review, and as a result, their suitability for inclusion in a meta-analysis may be questionable. Regardless of whether we are discussing a traditional type of literature review or a structured meta-analysis, the problem of potential publication bias must be considered.

EPIDEMIOLOGY IN THE COURTS

As mentioned earlier, litigation has become a major path for policy making in the United States. Epidemiology is assuming an ever-increasing importance in the legal arena. Particularly in the area of toxic torts, it provides one of the major types of scientific evidence that is relevant to the questions involved. Issues such as effects of dioxin, silicone breast implants, and electromagnetic fields are but a few recent examples.

However, the use of data from epidemiologic studies is not without its problems. Epidemiology answers questions about *groups*, whereas the court often requires information about *individuals*. Furthermore, considerable attention has been directed to the court's interpretation of evidence of causality. Whereas the legal criterion is often "more likely than not"—that is, that the substance or exposure in question is "more likely than not" to have caused a person's disease—epidemiology relies to a great extent on the U.S. Surgeon General's guidelines for causal inferences.[15] It has been suggested that an attributable risk greater than 50% might constitute evidence of "more likely than not."[16]

Until recently, evidence from epidemiology was only reluctantly accepted in the courts, but this has changed to a point where epidemiologic data are often cited as the only source of relevant evidence in toxic tort cases. For many years, the guiding principle for using scientific evidence in the courts in the United States was the Frye test, which stated that for a study to be admissible "it must be sufficiently established to have gained general acceptance in the field in which it belongs."[17] Although terms such as "general acceptance" and "field in which it belongs" were left undefined, it did lead to an assessment of whether the scientific opinion expressed by an expert witness was generally accepted by other professionals in the discipline.

In 1993, in *Daubert v. Merrell Dow Pharmaceuticals*,[18] a case in which the plaintiff alleged that a limb deformity at birth was due to ingestion of the drug Bendectin during pregnancy, the U.S. Supreme Court articulated a major change in the rules of evidence. The court ruled that "general acceptance" is not a necessary condition for the admissibility of scientific evidence in court. Rather, the trial judge is now considered a "gatekeeper" and is assigned the task of ensuring that an expert's testimony rests on a reliable foundation and is relevant to the "task at hand." Thus, the judge "must make a preliminary assessment of whether the testimony's underlying reasoning or methodology is scientifically valid and can be properly applied to the facts at issue." Among the considerations cited by the court are whether the theory or technique in question can be and has been tested and whether the methodology has been subjected to peer review and publication.

Given their new responsibilities, judges presiding at trials in which epidemiology is a major source of evidence need to have a basic knowledge of epidemiologic concepts, including, for example, study design, biases and confounding, and causal inferences, if they are to be able to rule in a sound fashion on whether the approach used by the experts follows accepted "scientific method." Recognizing this need, the Federal Judicial Center has published a *Research Manual on Scientific Evidence* for judges that includes a section on epidemiology.[19] Although it is too early to know the ultimate effect of the Daubert ruling, given the tremendous increase in the use of epidemiology in the courts, the ruling will clearly require enhanced knowledge of epidemiology by many parties involved in legal proceedings that use evidence derived from epidemiologic studies.

SOURCES AND IMPACT OF UNCERTAINTY

In 1983, the National Research Council in the United States wrote:

the dominant analytic difficulty [in conducting risk assessments for policy decision making] is

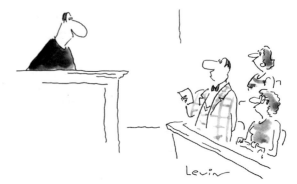

"Your Honor, we, the jury, find this one too close to call."

Figure 19-12. One jury's approach to uncertainty. (©The New Yorker Collection 1996. Arnie Levin from cartoonbank. com. All rights reserved.)

pervasive uncertainty . . . data may be incomplete, and there is often great uncertainty in estimates of the types, probability and magnitude of health effects associated with a chemical agent, of the economic effects of a proposed regulatory action, and of the extent of current and possible future human exposures.[20]

This insight remains as relevant today as when it was originally written. Uncertainty is a reality that we must accept and that must be addressed. Uncertainty is an integral part of science. What we believe to be "truth" today often turns out to be transient. Tomorrow a study may appear that may contradict or invalidate the best scientific information available to us today.

Uncertainty is relevant not only to risk assessments, but also to issues of treatment, to issues of prevention such as screening, and to health economics issues. Clearly it is a relevant concern in the legal setting discussed earlier (Fig. 19-12).

Some of the possible sources of uncertainty are listed in Table 19-2. As seen in this table, the sources of uncertainty may be in the design of the study or in the conduct and implementation of the study, or they may result from the presentation and interpretation of the study findings. Many of these sources have been discussed in earlier chapters.

One issue listed in the table is whether in a study of the effectiveness of a preventive measure, the results are described as a relative risk reduction or an absolute risk reduction. Often a relative risk reduction, such as the *percent* reduction in mortality, is selected because it gives a more optimistic view of the effectiveness of a preventive measure. If, however,

TABLE 19-2. Examples of Possible Sources of Uncertainty in Epidemiology

1. Uncertainty resulting from the design of the study
   a. Study may not have been designed to provide a relevant answer to the question of interest
   b. Biases that were not recognized or not adequately addressed
      i. Selection bias
      ii. Information bias
   c. Measurement errors which may lead to misclassification
   d. Inadequate sample size
   e. Inappropriate choice of analytic methods
   f. Failure to take into account potential confounders
   g. Use of surrogate measures that may not correctly measure the outcomes that are the major dependent variables of interest
   h. Problems of external validity (generalizability to the population of interest): the conclusions regarding potential interventions may not be generalizable to the target population

2. Uncertainty resulting from deficiencies in the conduct and implementation of the study
   a. Observations may be biased if observers were not blinded
   b. Poor quality of laboratory or survey methods
   c. Large proportion of non-participants and/or non-respondents
   d. Failure to identify reasons for non-response and characteristics of non-respondents

3. Uncertainty resulting from the presentation and interpretation of the study findings
   a. How were the results expressed?
   b. If the study assessed risk and possible etiology, were the factors involved described as risk factors or causal factors?
   c. If the study assessed the effectiveness of a proposed preventive measure, was the benefit of the measure expressed as relative risk reduction or absolute risk reduction? Why was it chosen to be expressed as it was, and how was the finding interpreted?

absolute risk reduction is used, such as the *number of individuals per 1,000* whose lives would be saved, the result appears less impressive. If the rate of adverse events, such as mortality from the disease that is observed without screening, is low, a relative risk reduction will always seem more impressive than an absolute risk reduction because the *number* of events that could potentially be prevented is small even if the *percent* reduction is higher.

Another issue that contributes to uncertainty in policy making but is not generally related to specific epidemiologic studies is how we deal with *anecdotal evidence,* such as that provided by a person who states that she was screened for breast cancer 10 years earlier, received early treatment, and is alive and apparently well 10 years after the screening. There is often a tendency to accept such evidence as supporting the effectiveness of the screening in reducing mortality from the disease. However, anecdotal evidence has two major problems: First, it does not take into account slow-growing tumors that might have been detected by screening but might not have affected survival even if the patient had not been screened; and second, it does not take into account

very fast growing tumors that screening would have missed so that the person would not have received early treatment. That is, for those giving anecdotal evidence of survival after screening, there is no comparison group of individuals who were screened but did *not* survive. As an unknown sage has said, "The plural of *anecdote* is not 'data.'" Nevertheless, despite these major limitations, anecdotal evidence given by patients who have survived serious illness may have a strong emotional impact which may significantly influence policy makers.

Ultimately, the impact of scientific uncertainty on the formulation of public policy will depend on how the major stakeholders deal with uncertainty. Among the different groups of stakeholders are scientists (including epidemiologists), policy makers, politicians, and the public (or the target populations). Each of these groups may have different levels of sophistication, different levels and types of self-interest, and may view data differently and be influenced to varying degrees by colleagues, friends, and various constituencies in society. Moreover, individuals have different personalities with different levels of risk tolerance and different ways of dealing with

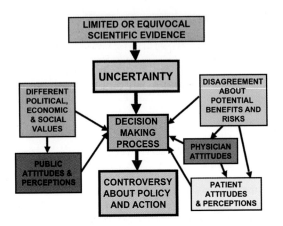

Figure 19-13. Schematic presentation of some of the factors involved in the impact of uncertainty on the decision-making process for health policy.

uncertainty. Furthermore, an important mediator is the set of values that every individual has relating to issues such as the value of a human life and the principles that should guide the allocation of limited resources in a society. The result is a complex interaction of uncertainty resulting from characteristics of a study, interacting with a network of relationships relating to the elements just described. A schematic of some of the inter-relationships influencing the effect of uncertainty on public policy is shown in Figure 19-13. These factors are clearly major concerns in formulating appropriate public health and clinical policy. It is important that they be taken into account if a plan of action is to be successfully developed and implemented to address health issues in the population.

POLICY ISSUES REGARDING RISK: WHAT SHOULD THE OBJECTIVES BE?

Public policy is often recognized to be largely made through the processes of legislation and regulation. As discussed earlier, in the United States, litigation has also become an important instrument for developing and implementing public policy. Ideally, each of these processes should reflect societal values and aspirations.

Certain major societal issues must be considered in making decisions about risk. Among the questions that must be confronted are the following:

1. What percentage of the population should be protected by the policy?
2. What level of risk is society willing to tolerate?

3. What level of control of risk is society willing to pay for?
4. Who should make decisions about risk?

At first glance, it might seem appealing to protect the entire population from any amount of risk, but, realistically, this is difficult—if not impossible—to accomplish. Regardless of what we learn from risk data about populations, there are clearly rare individuals who are extraordinarily sensitive to minute concentrations of certain chemicals. If the permissible amount of a chemical is to be set at a level that protects *every* worker, it is possible that entire manufacturing processes may be halted. Similarly, if we demand zero risk for workers or for others who may be exposed, the economic base of many communities might be destroyed. Policy making therefore requires a balance between what *can* be done and what *should* be done. The degree of priority attached to elimination of all risk and the decision as to what percent of risk should be eliminated clearly are not scientific decisions but rather depend on societal values. It is hoped that such societal decisions will capitalize on available epidemiologic and other scientific knowledge in the context of political, economic, ethical, and social considerations.

CONCLUSION

The objectives of epidemiology are to enhance our understanding of the biology and pathogenesis of disease to improve human health and to prevent and treat disease. A thorough understanding of the methodologic issues that arise is needed in order to interpret epidemiologic results properly as a basis for formulating both clinical and public health policy. The appropriate and judicious use of the results of epidemiologic studies is fundamental to an assessment of risk to human health and to the control of these risks. Such use is therefore important to both primary and secondary prevention. Policy makers are often obliged to develop policy in the presence of incomplete or equivocal scientific data. In clinical medicine, both in the diagnostic and the therapeutic processes, decisions are often made with incomplete or equivocal data; this has perhaps been more of an overt impediment in public health and community medicine. No simple set of rules can eliminate this difficulty. As H. L. Mencken wrote: "There is always an easy solution to every human problem—neat, plausible, and wrong."[21] A major challenge remains to develop the best process for formulating rational policies under such circumstances, both in clinical medicine and public health.

REFERENCES

1. Hill AB: The environment and disease: Association or causation? Proc R Soc Med 58:295–300, 1965.
2. Jones FB, Saturday Evening Post, November 29, 1953.
3. Rose G: Sick individuals and sick populations. Int J Epidemiol 14:22–38, 1985.
4. Whelton PK: Epidemiology of hypertension. Lancet 344:101–106, 1994.
5. Grady D et al. for the HERS Research Group: Cardiovascular disease outcomes during 6.8 years of hormone therapy: Heart and estrogen/progestin replacement study follow-up (HERS II). JAMA 288:49–57, 2002.
6. The Women's Health Initiative: Risks and benefits of estrogen plus progestin in healthy postmenopausal women: Principal results. The Women's Health Initiative randomized controlled trial. JAMA 288:321–333, 2002.
7. Grodstein F, Clarkson TB, Manson JE: Understanding the divergent data on postmenopausal hormone therapy. N Engl J Med 348:645–650, 2003.
8. Michels KB: Hormone replacement therapy in epidemiologic studies and randomized clinical trials—Are we checkmate? Epidemiology 14:3–5, 2003.
9. Whittemore AS, McGuire V: Observational studies and randomized trials of hormone replacement therapy: What can we learn from them? Epidemiology 14:8–10, 2003.
10. Samet JM, Schnatter R, Gibb H: Epidemiology and risk assessment. Am J Epidemiol 148:929–936, 1998.
11. National Research Council Committee on the Institutional Means for Assessment of Risks to Public Health: Risk Assessment in the Federal Government: Managing the Process. Washington, DC, National Academy Press, 1983, p 21.
12. Wertheimer N, Leeper E: Electrical wiring configurations and childhood cancer. Am J Epidemiol 109:273–284, 1979.
13. Ecclesiastes 1:9.
14. Glass GV: Primary, secondary and meta-analysis of research. Educ Res 5:3–8, 1976.
15. United States Department of Health, Education and Welfare: Smoking and Health: Report of the Advisory Committee to the Surgeon General. Washington, DC, Public Health Service, 1964.
16. Black B, Lilienfeld DE: Epidemiology proof in toxic tort litigation. Fordham Law Rev 52:732–785, 1984.
17. *Frye v. United States*, 293F. 1013 (D. C. Cir. 1923).
18. *Daubert v. Merrell Dow Pharmaceuticals, Inc.,* 113 S. Ct. 2786 (1993).
19. Green M, Freedman M, Gordis L: Reference guide on epidemiology. In Reference Manual on Scientific Evidence, 2nd ed. Washington, DC, Federal Judicial Center, 2000.
20. National Research Council Committee on the Institutional Means for Assessment of Risks to Public Health: Risk Assessment in the Federal Government: Managing the Process. Washington, DC, National Academy Press, 1983, p 11.
21. Mencken HL: The divine afflatus. The New York Evening Mail, Nov 16, 1917. (Essay reprinted in Mencken HL: Prejudices, series 2. New York, Alfred A. Knopf, 1920.)

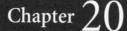

Ethical and Professional Issues in Epidemiology

No man is an Island, entire of itself;
every man is a piece of the Continent, a part of the main . . .
any man's death diminishes me, because I am involved in Mankind;
And therefore never send to know for whom the bell tolls;
It tolls for thee.
— John Donne, English clergyman and poet (1572–1631), Meditation XVII

In these lines John Donne emphasized the interconnection of all people. Epidemiology also teaches us major lessons about connections and relationships. The previous chapters have demonstrated that disease does not arise in a vacuum. Many contagious diseases clearly depend on human contacts for transmission and for propagation of epidemics. Moreover, in recent years, more and more diseases that were long thought not to have an infectious etiology are being identified as being of infectious origin to varying degrees. For example, the micro-ogranism *Helicobacter pylori* has been implicated in the etiology of peptic ulcer and gastric cancer (see Chapter 14). Many cases of cancer of the cervix are linked to human papillomavirus (HPV), especially types 16 and 18, and the foundation thus exists for developing prevention programs through immunization against HPV.

Furthermore, a major focus of epidemiology is on the impact of the environment on the risk of human disease. This reflects a combination of factors: First, we are at risk from effects of nature, including flooding and other natural disasters such as the Indian Ocean earthquake and tsunami that primarily affected Indonesia, Thailand, and Sri Lanka in 2004, and Hurricane Katrina, which affected New Orleans, Louisiana, and the surrounding region in the United States in 2005. Second, we are also vulnerable to environmental and ecologic damage that results from certain human attitudes, lifestyles, and behaviors. The negative impact that human activities have on our planet are often not adequately considered. These activities and effects include air pollution, depletion of the ozone layer, global warming, pollution of

natural water supplies, deforestation, and overdevelopment, among many others. The negative effects of many of these types of problems are only now beginning to be fully understood and the legacy of environmental damage being left to future generations is being increasingly recognized. As these are studied, increased understanding is also needed of individual variations in genetically determined human vulnerability to environmental agents.

Another aspect of interdependence that is relevant to epidemiologists is their need to develop collaborative relationships with other epidemiologists as well as with professionals in other fields. We have learned that many epidemiologic investigations require multidisciplinary approaches so that professionally, epidemiologists cannot be most productive and effective as "islands." Thus, the lesson of "connectedness" expressed in John Donne's lines seems integral both to the dynamics of the diseases and conditions investigated by epidemiologists and to the practice of epidemiology. It also applies to the participation of epidemiologists in formulating and implementing health-related policy, as demonstrated by the story of Semmelweis presented in Chapter 1.

Today, we live in a depersonalized era in which individuals often consider their own advancement to be life's major goal. A sense of community and concern for others is often lost. John Donne's worldview stressing the interdependence of people at times seems alien to some current views of the world, one of which is humorously seen in Figure 20-1. One of the best articulations of the need to simultaneously balance the competing interests and needs of the individual and the community was given by Hillel, a

349

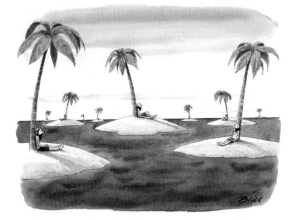

Figure 20-1. "No man is an island"—a different view. (© The New Yorker Collection 2007 Harry Bliss, from cartoonbank.com. All rights reserved.)

Talmudic sage who lived some 2,000 years ago. He said: "If I am not for myself [If I don't take care of myself], who will be for me, but if I am only for myself [i.e., if I take care only of myself], what am I worth? And if not now, when?"

Another factor with impact on epidemiology and epidemiologists is the rapid pace of societal change and technological progress. A story is told of Adam and Eve in the Garden of Eden. After being expelled from Eden, Adam turned to Eve and said, "Eve, my dear, we are living in a time of change."[1] In the 21st century, we too are living in a time of dramatic changes. The rapidly evolving social and scientific context in which epidemiologic research is being conducted has led to new challenges for those working in epidemiology, for those who use the results of epidemiologic studies, and for the general public. In addition, major technological advances, including tremendous increases in computing capacity and dramatic advances in laboratory technology, have made it possible to rapidly analyze large numbers of samples and maintain very large data sets. In so doing, they have made possible many population-based studies that would not have been conceivable even a decade or two ago. At the same time, these technological advances have also introduced new and different issues related to privacy, confidentiality, and the individual.

In the light of the preceding discussion, this chapter briefly reviews some ethical and professional issues that are critical for epidemiologic research and for applying the results of this research to the improvement of human health. The issues to be discussed include several that relate to the actual conduct of epidemiologic studies and others that relate to broader societal issues and go beyond the actual epidemiologic research itself.

ETHICAL ISSUES IN EPIDEMIOLOGY

Clearly, in any scientific pursuit, fraud, deceit, or misrepresentation elicits universal disapproval and condemnation from other members of the discipline, other professionals, and the lay public. Such issues are not discussed in this chapter. Today, some of the most difficult ethical dilemmas in epidemiology are likely to be more subtle, involving judgments, philosophies, attitudes, and opinions, for which consensus may be more difficult to obtain.

Does epidemiology differ from other scientific disciplines with regard to ethical issues? Although epidemiology shares many characteristics with other scientific disciplines, it differs in some important ways. It is a discipline that largely grew out of medicine and public health, and even in its earliest years, its findings had immediate policy implications for clinical care or public health action. John Snow's studies of cholera in London and his removal of the pump handle of the Broad Street pump, which his studies had implicated in the outbreak, whether actually done before or after the crest of the outbreak, reflected the clear policy implications of his work.

The ultimate objective of epidemiology is to improve human health; epidemiology is the basic science of disease prevention. Hence, the relationship of epidemiology to the development of public policy is integral to the discipline. As a result, the ethical and professional issues go beyond those that might apply to a scientific discipline, such as biophysics or physiology, and must be viewed in a broader context. First, epidemiologic findings have direct and often immediate societal relevance. Second, epidemiologic studies are generally funded from public resources and often have major implications for allocation of limited societal resources. Third, epidemiologic research involves human subjects in some way, and subjects who participate in epidemiologic studies generally derive no personal benefit from the results of these studies.

INVESTIGATORS' OBLIGATIONS TO STUDY SUBJECTS

What are the investigators' obligations to the subjects in the nonrandomized observational studies with which most epidemiologists generally deal? First, to the greatest extent possible, a truly informed consent, which is consistent with the principle of individual autonomy, should be obtained from every subject. But can a truly informed consent be obtained from a subject in an epidemiologic study? If we believe that a full disclosure to the subjects of the study's objectives and hypotheses will introduce a response bias or other type of bias, clearly the consent will not be a fully "informed" one. Another issue in consent relates to privacy and confidentiality. For many years, in good conscience, epidemiologists assured subjects that their data would be kept confidential, and that this commitment was unqualified. However, research data have become subject to subpoena in recent years, with only a few exceptions. Therefore, the assurance of confidentiality given in informed consent statements must now include qualifications to allow for breaches in confidentiality that could be legally mandated and that would therefore be beyond the control of the investigator. New privacy regulations went into effect in the United States in 2003, which significantly affect the rights of patients regarding health information. We return to the subject of privacy and confidentiality later in this chapter.

Another issue pertains to balancing the rights of the individual and the welfare of society. In a study of men at high risk for HIV infection, participants were assured of confidentiality. In the interview that was subsequently administered, subjects were asked whether they had donated blood during the previous 2 years. Several subjects who were found to be HIV-positive reported having given blood within the 2 years prior to the HIV testing. The concern that emerged was that the donated blood might have been used in a transfusion. Although the blood may have been discarded by the blood bank, there was no way to check on this without breaching confidentiality and violating the original commitment to the subjects. Perhaps the investigators should have anticipated such a problem at the time the interview was developed, before obtaining the subjects' informed consent. But even with foresight, such problems arise. In this case, how do we balance the original commitment to the subjects with a need to determine whether anyone had received blood from these donors, so that further transmission of HIV might be prevented?

A third obligation to the subjects relates to communicating the study findings to them. Our approach to this issue may differ depending on whether the subject has been found to have developed a health problem linked to an exposure being studied or whether the subject has only been found to be at increased risk for future development of disease as a result of the exposure. In either case, communicating

the results regarding risk to the subjects can be viewed as a possible expression of the ethical principle of beneficence—the obligation of the investigator to help the subjects further their important legitimate interests, such as disease prevention and control, for themselves and their families. However, according to this principle, we not only must provide the benefits such as prevention of disease but also must balance the benefits and costs or harm (principle of utility).

If, for example, a subject has been exposed to a factor that is shown in a study to be a strong risk factor for cancer of the pancreas, should the subject be given this information? On the one hand, given that no effective treatment for pancreatic cancer is available and that there is no strong evidence that early detection of the disease is beneficial, might we be increasing a person's anxieties by transmitting this information without providing any benefit to that person? On the other hand, we could argue that a participant in any study is entitled to receive the findings of the study even if the findings have no direct bearing on the person's health or even if they may lead to heightened anxiety. Indeed, many epidemiologists now offer all participating subjects the option of requesting a report of the study findings when the study has been completed.

PRIVACY AND CONFIDENTIALITY

Concerns about privacy and confidentiality in our society have increased with the increasing erosion of individual privacy through computerized records. Protection of privacy and confidentiality within the framework of medical investigation, including epidemiologic research, has become an important issue. The origins of such concerns are quite old. Hippocrates wrote in the now commonly used Oath of Physicians:

that whatsoever I shall see or hear . . . of the lives of men and women . . . which is not fitting to be spoken . . . I will keep inviolably secret.

As Hippocrates qualified "whatsoever I shall see or hear" with the phrase "which is not fitting to be spoken," he apparently considered certain types of information to be of a nature that *is* "fitting to be spoken." Presumably then, under certain circumstances, Hippocrates would have advocated the carefully monitored sharing of personal information in the interest of societal benefit. For example, if a case of smallpox were reported in an American city, Hippocrates would probably support the reporting of this case to health authorities. Thus, individual autonomy regarding privacy and confidentiality is an important principle, but it is not unlimited.

In regard to privacy and confidentiality in epidemiologic studies, attention has focused on use of medical records. Let us ask, first, why medical records are needed in epidemiologic studies. These records are needed for two main purposes:

1. To generate aggregate data or validate information obtained by other means without contacting patients.
2. To identify individual patients for subsequent follow-up using means such as interviews or blood tests.

Because epidemiology's objectives of improving human health are clearly laudable, one might be tempted at first glance to dismiss any concerns about misuse of medical record data and about intrusions into individual privacy by epidemiologists. However, the words of Supreme Court Justice Louis D. Brandeis ring as true today as when they were first written in 1928:

> Experience should teach us to be most on guard to protect liberty when the Government's purposes are beneficent. Men born to freedom are naturally alert to repel invasion of their liberty by evil-minded rulers. The greatest dangers to liberty lurk in insidious encroachment by men of zeal, well-meaning but without understanding.[2]

The ethical principle of autonomy argues strongly for a meaningful informed consent in many areas related to research, including privacy and confidentiality. Therefore, concerns about protection of confidentiality in the research arena are valid. Over the years, they have led to two major legislative proposals that look reasonable at first but in actuality would seriously damage epidemiologic research and impede progress in both public health and clinical practice. The two proposals are as follows:

1. Patient consent should be required before investigators are allowed access to medical records.
2. Data from medical records should be made available to investigators without any information that would identify an individual.

Both proposals are consistent with the ethical principle of *nonmaleficence*—doing no harm—to the subjects participating in a research study. However, if society has a vested interest in the findings from epidemiologic and other biomedical studies, it is necessary to strike a balance between the interests of the individual and those of the community.

Let us consider these two proposals separately. Why would the first proposal, which requires patient consent before investigators are allowed access to medical records, make many studies impossible?

- As a first step in a study, records must be reviewed to identify which patients meet the study criteria (for example, which patients have the disease in question and are therefore eligible for inclusion in a case-control study).
- Many studies are conceived of only many years after a patient was hospitalized, so informed consent could not have been obtained from the patient at that time. By the time the study is later developed, many patients may have died or are not traceable.
- Certain patients refuse to be interviewed in epidemiologic studies, but the nonparticipants can be characterized using data in their medical records so that any biases resulting from their nonparticipation can be assessed. If records were not available because of patient refusals, a potential selection bias would be introduced, the magnitude and direction of which could not be assessed.

Turning to the second proposal, why is information from medical records that identifies individuals essential for most epidemiologic studies?

- Review of medical records is often the first step in identifying a group of persons with a disease who will receive subsequent follow-up.
- Identifying information is essential for linking the records of specific individuals from different sources (such as hospital records, physicians' records, employment records, and death certificates in studies of occupational cancer).

As seen in Figure 20-2, linkage of records is critical for generating unbiased and complete information about each subject, not only in occupational studies (as shown here) but in many types of epidemiologic investigations.

Thus, we see that the use of medical records is essential for epidemiologic studies. Indeed, many significant advances in protecting human health that resulted from epidemiologic research could not have been made if access to medical records had been restricted.[3] At the same time, however, we must be concerned about protecting individual privacy and confidentiality. For many years, epidemiologic studies have used the following procedures designed to protect the confidentiality of subjects:

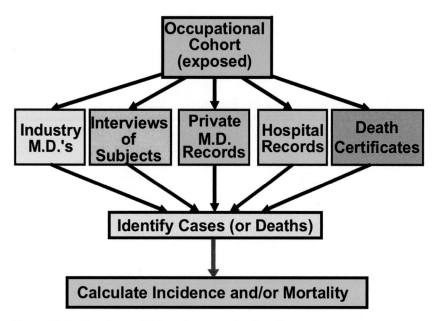

Figure 20-2. Use of record linkage in occupational studies.

- Informed consent is required for all phases of research, except review of medical records.
- All data obtained are stored under lock and key.
- Only study numbers are used on data forms. The key for linking these numbers to individual names is kept separately under lock and key.
- Individual identifying information is destroyed at the end of the study unless there is a specific justification for retaining this information. Such retention must be approved by the institutional review board (IRB) or committee on human research.
- All results are published only in aggregate or group form so that individuals are never identified.
- Unless it is essential for the study, individual identifying information is not entered in computer files, and individual identifiers are not included in routine tabulations generated from computerized data.
- The importance of maintaining privacy and confidentiality is regularly emphasized to the research staff.

When people consent to participate in epidemiologic studies, they have voluntarily agreed to some invasion of their privacy for the common good of society, hoping for advances in health promotion and disease prevention as a result of the studies they are making possible. Therefore, investigators have an ethical obligation to protect the privacy and confidentiality of the subjects in these studies to the greatest extent possible. The policies described earlier that are currently in force have been highly successful in achieving this goal.

Recognizing the importance of the use of medical records in epidemiologic research and the effectiveness of current measures to protect privacy and confidentiality, the Privacy Protection Study Commission recommended that patient consent not be required for the use of medical records in epidemiologic research.[4] However, on April 14, 2003, the picture changed dramatically in the United States, when new federal privacy regulations went into effect pursuant to the Health Insurance Portability and Accountability Act of 1996 (HIPAA).[5] The Act was introduced in response to increasing public concern about lack of individual control over medical information and the general erosion of individual privacy in the United States. Electronic transfer of medical information and fears about potential misuse of genetic information made available by new laboratory methods also led to the development of these new regulations.

The HIPAA regulations provide the first systematic nationwide privacy protection for health information in the United States. The regulations give patients more control over their health information and set boundaries for the use and release of health records. With some exceptions, individual signed authorization is now required for the release of protected health information for many purposes. Protected health information can be disclosed to public health authorities for public health purposes, including—but not limited to—public health surveillance, investigations, and interventions. Protected health information can also be released for health research without individual authorization under certain conditions, including the following: (1) if an Institutional Review Board (IRB) has provided a waiver, (2) for activities preparatory to initiation of research, and (3) for research on a decedent's information.[6] The regulations are extremely complex. It will take time before the full impact of the new regulations on clinical and public health investigations and activities and on epidemiologic research can be assessed. Extensive discussions of the regulations have been published.[7-9]

ACCESS TO DATA

When a study has been completed, who "owns" the data? Who should have access to the data—either "raw" or partially "cooked"—and under what conditions? We live in an era in which we can be confident that virtually any research data generated that deal with a controversial issue will be reanalyzed by real or alleged experts who support different positions. Some of the relevant questions regarding sharing of data include the following:

- At what point has a study truly been completed?
- Should the policy on sharing research data be dependent on who has paid for the study?
- Should the policy depend on who is requesting the data and on that person's possible motivations in making the request?
- Under what conditions should identifiers be included with the data?
- How can the investigator's interests be protected?
- Who will pay for the expenses involved?

The challenge is to strike an appropriate balance between the interests of the investigator on the one hand, and those of society on the other hand, for they do not inevitably coincide.

RACE AND ETHNICITY IN EPIDEMIOLOGIC STUDIES

An important issue that has received increasing attention in recent years is the use of race and ethnicity designations in epidemiologic studies. These variables are used both to describe populations and to test hypotheses in which race may serve as an independent variable.

As a descriptor, race is often used to characterize the individuals who are studied in clinical trials or to describe inclusions and exclusions of populations in different types of epidemiologic studies. Race and ethnicity variables can be very useful for this purpose and may be important for assessing the potential generalizability of the findings beyond the population studied.

When variables that designate race or ethnicity are included in studies designed to test hypotheses, the focus is often on possible associations of race with certain health outcomes. However, as Bhopal and Donaldson[10] have pointed out, biologically, race is ill defined and poorly understood, and may be of questionable validity. DNA research indicates that genetic diversity is a continuum with no clear breaks that can delineate racial groups.[11] Race has been described as "an arbitrary system of visual classification" that does not demarcate distinct subgroups of the human population.[12] Beginning with the 2000 U.S. census, new guidelines permit respondents to identify themselves with more than one racial group. In the future, this policy may complicate the use of census data on race in epidemiologic studies.

An alternate approach is to use ethnicity rather than race. However, classifying people by ethnicity also is not simple. Ethnicity is a complex variable that implies shared origins or social backgrounds; shared culture and traditions that are distinctive, maintained between generations, and lead to a sense of identity and group; or shared language or religious tradition.[13] What have been the results of using racial designations in epidemiologic research? Many believe that, given the ambiguities involved in defining race, research using disease rates according to race has not significantly advanced our fundamental understanding of the causes and pathogenesis of human disease.[14] However, some have argued that even if such designations have not enhanced our understanding of the biologic mechanisms of disease, the use of racial variables in research has helped to identify subgroups—particularly minority and immigrant groups—to whom additional health care resources need to be directed. For example, race-specific mortality data in the United States have shown that[15]:

- A black infant is more than twice as likely as a white infant to die in the first year of life.
- Death rates for most causes of death are much higher for black people than for white people.

In studies relating to health needs and health care priorities of various populations, the race of a population group may be described, an explicit comparison may be made with other racial and ethnic groups, or a comparison may be implied, but not explicitly stated. Death rates by race are frequently used for setting national and state health objectives. The Centers for Disease Control and Prevention stated that, "death rates by race and Hispanic origin are important for monitoring the health status of these population groups and for informing policies and programs directed to reducing disparities."[15]

One problem in using racial variables is that in so doing, even well-meaning investigators may inadvertently stigmatize certain population subgroups. As a result, certain racial designations may, in effect, become surrogates for undesirable lifestyle characteristics such as criminal behavior and drug abuse. As Bhopal has pointed out, "by emphasizing the negative aspects of the health of ethnic minority groups, research may have damaged their social standing and deflected attention from their health priorities."[14]

What conclusions can we draw? No variable, including race, should be included uncritically as a matter of routine in any epidemiologic study. Perhaps the best approach in planning any epidemiologic study in which race will be addressed is to ask a number of questions, including the following:

- "Why is race being studied?"
- "On what basis will study participants be classified by race?"
- "How valid will the designations of race be, and how will they contribute to increasing our biologic knowledge of the disease in question or to enhancing preventive activities in certain disadvantaged groups?"
- "If race is being used as a surrogate for certain lifestyle factors, such as diet, could information on diet or other lifestyle factors be obtained directly, without using race as a surrogate?" At the same time, we should also ask whether any damage may be done by using racial designations in a given study and whether such designations may unintentionally serve as virtual surrogates for undesirable lifestyles or characteristics.

In any study, racial variables that are used should have a definite purpose that can be precisely articulated and should meet the same standards of validity that we would expect of any other variables we study. The potential benefit of using such variables in a study should clearly exceed any potential harm that may result. Race may be an appropriate and potentially valuable variable to address in epidemiologic studies provided the above issues have been adequately considered and addressed.

CONFLICT OF INTEREST

Both actual and perceived biases may result from conflict of interest. Such conflict can arise at each stage of a study, from an initial decision as to whether a specific study should be undertaken in the first place through analysis and interpretation of the data and dissemination of the results. Most epidemiologic work in the United States today is performed by epidemiologists who work in academia, industry, or government. These three environments differ in several ways. Funding for epidemiologic research in government and industry is generally internal, whereas academic epidemiologists must seek outside financial support. As a result, research performed by academic epidemiologists is generally subjected to more rigorous peer review as part of the grant application process. Even more important, however, is that the employer of the academic epidemiologist generally has no vested interest in what the results of the study may be. This contrasts with other settings in which the employer may be significantly affected—politically, economically, or legally—by the nature of the findings. Consequently, overt or subtle pressure by an employer not to initiate a study or to prolong the process leading to reporting of the results can introduce a serious bias into reviews of the literature concerning issues such as occupational hazards. Moreover, these biases may be impossible to assess.

The potential bias resulting from such studies that have not been conducted and that might well have revealed associations of specific exposures with adverse outcomes has not been named. In this context, some may be reminded of a dialogue in Sir Arthur Conan Doyle's Sherlock Holmes story *Silver Blaze* in which Holmes investigates the disappearance of a race horse with that name and the murder of its trainer. As Holmes is about to leave the village during the investigation, the local inspector turns to him and asks:

> "Is there any point to which you wish to draw my attention?"
> "To the curious incident of the dog in the night time." [replies Holmes]
> "The dog did nothing in the night time."
> "That was the curious incident," remarked Sherlock Holmes.[16]

(Holmes later described how he successfully identified the villain. He explained that when the intruder entered the stable "the dog did nothing in the night time" and did not even bark much, indicating that "obviously, the midnight visitor was someone whom the dog knew well.")

With the above conversation in mind, the potential bias introduced by studies that are not done, might be called *Silver Blaze bias.* Holmes understood why the dog failed to act and was able to apply this knowledge to solving the problem at hand. Similarly, there may be much to learn when a manufacturer fails to conduct what seems to be a clearly needed study of possible adverse effects of a product. But when such an association has been suggested, it is often difficult to determine whether certain epidemiologic studies were not initiated because of vested interests and concerns about the potential results of the study. In the absence of evidence documenting an explicit decision not to conduct a certain study, this type of bias is often difficult or impossible to quantify or even detect.

Although academic settings are not immune to their own problems and pressures, problems relating to epidemiologic research that arise in an academic setting are less likely to be linked to the potential impact of the study's specific findings. Nevertheless, the possibility of conflict of interest relating to any epidemiologic study must be considered, regardless of the specific setting in which the research was conducted. Indeed, such conflict may be related more to sources of funding than to the research setting itself. However, the possibility must be recognized that infrequently institutional as well as individual conflicts of interest may influence publication and dissemination of the results. Efforts should be expended to ensure that the results of the study—whatever they may turn out to be—are published in a peer-reviewed journal in a timely fashion. Sponsorship of the study should be clearly acknowledged in the article that reports the results of the study, as should any financial or other interests of the investigators or their families that may be affected by the study results.

INTERPRETING FINDINGS

Many of the most critical issues regarding how epidemiologic studies are conducted arise in connection with the appropriateness of the study design and the interpretation and reporting of findings. Epidemiologists have often been accused of endlessly reporting new risks, many of which are not confirmed in subsequent studies. The result is that the public finds many reported but often unconfirmed risks in the media, which leads them to become skeptical of newly reported risks because they are unable to sort out true and important risks from unconfirmed or trivial ones (Fig. 20-3); they frequently become unwilling to take responsibility for their own health care.[17] The question again arises: How do we assess the importance of a single study that shows an

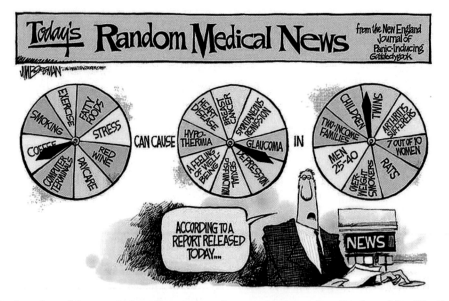

Figure 20-3. One view of the seemingly endless stream of reported risks confronting the public. (Jim Borgman. The Cincinnati Enquirer. 1997. Reprinted with special permission of King Features Syndicate.)

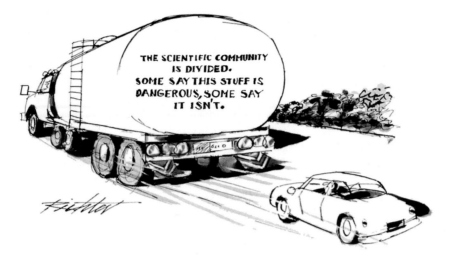

Figure 20-4. Dealing with scientific uncertainty. (© The New Yorker Collection 1988 Mischa Richter, from cartoonbank. com. All rights reserved.)

increased risk? How many confirmatory studies are needed?

An additional problem is that in earlier years, initial solitary epidemiologic findings or scientific controversies were generally addressed and often resolved within the scientific community before findings were disseminated to the public. Today, both initial unconfirmed reports and scientific controversies are often aired in the press or on television, even before the studies have appeared in peer-reviewed journals (Fig. 20-4). The dilemma is that although enhanced public education and increased public awareness of scientific issues are laudable, anxiety levels are often unjustifiably raised by single studies that are widely reported and that may later be refuted. The problem is exacerbated by a reported bias in newspapers against reporting the results of studies that show no effect.[18]

Furthermore, significant uncertainty is associated with the findings regarding certain questions such as whether mammography is beneficial for women in their 40s, whether prostate-specific antigen testing is beneficial to men with localized prostate cancer, and whether postmenopausal use of hormone replacement therapy is beneficial. Dealing with uncertainty is difficult—and often painful—for people who are struggling to make a decision about any of these interventions. Epidemiologists should assist the public with understanding uncertainty and help people cope with the challenge of making decisions in the face of equivocal and incomplete information. Other issues relating to uncertainty are discussed in Chapter 19.

An additional question is: "At what point does a reported trivial increase in risk ratio, even if it is statistically significant, become a biologically significant risk that merits public concern?" This question relates to the overall issue of public perceptions of risk. These perceptions are reflected in Tables 20-1

TABLE 20-1. **Involuntary Risks**	
Involuntary Risk	**Risk of Death per Person per Year**
Struck by automobile (United States)	1 in 20,000
Struck by automobile (United Kingdom)	1 in 16,600
Floods (United States)	1 in 455,000
Earthquake (California)	1 in 588,000
Tornadoes (Midwest)	1 in 455,000
Lightning (United Kingdom)	1 in 10 million
Falling aircraft (United States)	1 in 10 million
Falling aircraft (United Kingdom)	1 in 50 million
Release from an atomic power station	
At site boundary (United States)	1 in 10 million
At 1 km (United kingdom)	1 in 10 million
Flooding of a dike (The Netherlands)	1 in 10 million
Bites of venomous creatures (United Kingdom)	1 in 5 million
Leukemia	1 in 12,500
Influenza	1 in 5,000
Meteorite	1 in 100 billion

From Dinman BD: The reality and acceptance of risk. JAMA 244:1226, 1980. Copyright 1980, American Medical Association.

TABLE 20-2. Voluntary Risks

Voluntary Risk	Risk of Death per Person per Year
Smoking: 20 cigarettes/day	1 in 200
Drinking: 1 bottle of wine/day	1 in 13,300
Soccer, football	1 in 25,500
Automobile racing	1 in 1,000
Automobile driving (United Kingdom)	1 in 5,900
Motorcycling	1 in 50
Rock climbing	1 in 7,150
Taking oral contraceptive pills	1 in 5,000
Power boating	1 in 5,900
Canoeing	1 in 100,000
Horse racing	1 in 740
Amateur boxing	1 in 2 million
Professional boxing	1 in 14,300
Skiing	1 in 430,000
Pregnancy (United Kingdom)	1 in 4,350
Abortion: Legal < 12 wk	1 in 50,000
Abortion: Legal > 14 wk	1 in 5,900

From Dinman BD: The reality and acceptance of risk. JAMA 244:1226, 1980. Copyright 1980, American Medical Association.

and 20-2. For many of the risks listed, the degree of public concern and the change in behavior do not seem commensurate with the magnitude of the risk.

If the absolute risk is low, even if the relative risk in exposed individuals is significantly increased, the actual risk to exposed individuals will still be very low. It is interesting that the public often prefers to address "hot" issues (such as a reported risk from alar in apples) for which the evidence may be tenuous while ignoring well-established risk factors such as smoking, alcohol consumption, and sun exposure, for which lifestyle changes that are dependent on individual initiative have been clearly warranted by the available evidence.

Epidemiologists have a major function in communicating health risks and in interpreting epidemiologic data for nonepidemiologists; if epidemiologists do not participate in this activity, it will be left to others with far less training and expertise. This is an essential part of the policy-making process. Studies of human populations often yield different findings, and epidemiologists often hesitate to draw conclusions on the basis of existing data. In academic settings, epidemiologists can criticize studies and recommend additional research to resolve an issue. However, policy makers working at the front lines do not have this luxury of delay; they must make immediate decisions (e.g., to regulate or not to regulate). Even a decision not to regulate at this time represents a policy decision. Such decisions should ideally capitalize on epidemiologic information. However, policy makers cannot act in a rational fashion by merely waiting for findings from future studies to direct their actions regarding current pressing health issues. Epidemiologists must therefore draw the best conclusions possible on the basis of currently available data, fully realizing that a better study, or even a perfect study, may appear tomorrow and may contradict today's conclusions.

Epidemiologists have several roles in the process of policy making, including generating and interpreting the data, presenting specific policy options, projecting the impact of each option, developing specific policy proposals, and evaluating the effects of policies after they have been implemented. Should an epidemiologist be both a researcher and an advocate for a specific policy? Does advocacy for a position imply a loss of objectivity and of scientific credibility? These are difficult questions, but many clear issues, such as the health hazards resulting from cigarette smoking, urgently need the participation of epidemiologists in the struggle to eliminate the source of the danger to the public's health. The question then is not only whether it is ethical for an epidemiologist to be an advocate, but whether it is ethical for an epidemiologist to *not* be an advocate when the evidence of risk is so convincing. Thus, the epidemiologist must serve as an educator as well as a researcher. The epidemiologist's educational efforts are directed at many target populations, including other scientists, other health professionals, legislators, policy makers, lawyers, judges, and the public. Each group must be dealt with differently, depending on its specific needs and on the objectives toward which the educational effort is directed. Epidemiologists must learn to work with the media, including radio, television, magazines, and newspapers, in order to further their educational efforts. Epidemiologists should also familiarize themselves with what is known about how risks are perceived by patients, health care providers, and the general public so that they can help these groups deal with the findings of epidemiologic studies and with their implications for preventive measures including lifestyle changes.[19]

CONCLUSION

The ethical and professional issues facing epidemiology primarily reflect epidemiologists' obligations to participants in epidemiologic and clinical studies and the challenges resulting from the major position that the discipline occupies at the interface of science and public policy. The issues are complex, often subtle, and without simple answers. Given the pivotal position of epidemiology in the development of both clinical and public health policy, and its implications for environmental regulation, individual lifestyle changes, and modifications in clinical practice, the findings from epidemiologic studies attract widespread attention and high public visibility. As new questions are addressed by epidemiology in the future, the ethical and professional dilemmas facing the discipline will also continue to evolve. Therefore, a critical need exists for a continuing dialogue between epidemiologists and those who use the results of epidemiologic studies, including physicians and policy makers, as well as those who will be affected by new health and prevention policies in the coming years.

REFERENCES

1. Cited in Strong WS: Copyright in a time of change. J Electronic Pub 4(3), 1999. Accessed at http://www.press.umich.edu/jep/04-03/strong.html, May 27, 2007.
2. Brandeis L: Dissenting opinion in *Olmstead v. United States*, 277 U.S. 438 (1928).
3. Gordis L, Gold E: Privacy, confidentiality, and the use of medical records in research. Science 207:153–156, 1980.
4. The Report of the Privacy Protection Study Commission: Personal Privacy in an Information Society. Washington, DC, US Government Printing Office, 1977.
5. Health Insurance Portability and Accountability Act of 1996. Pub. L. No. 104–191, 110 Stat. 1936 (1996).
6. Centers for Disease Control and Prevention: HIPAA Privacy Rule and public health: Guidance from CDC and the U.S. Department of Health and Human Services. MMWR 52 (Suppl):1–20, 2003.
7. Gostin LO: National health information privacy: Regulations under the Health Insurance Portability and Accountability Act. JAMA 285:3015–3021, 2001.
8. Gostin LO, Hodge JG Jr: Personal privacy and common goods: A framework. Minnesota Law Review 86:1439–1480, 2002.
9. Kulynych J, Korn D: The new federal medical privacy rule. N Engl J Med 347:1122–1134, 2002.
10. Bhopal R, Donaldson L: White, European, Western, Caucasian, or what? Inappropriate labeling in research on race, ethnicity and health. Am J Public Health 88:1303–1307, 1998.
11. Marshall E: DNA studies challenge the meaning of race. Science 282:654–655, 1998.
12. Fullilove MT: Abandoning "race" as a variable in public health research—An idea whose time has come. Am J Public Health 88:1297–1298, 1998.
13. Senior PA, Bhopal R: Ethnicity as a variable in epidemiological research. BMJ 309:327–330, 1994.
14. Bhopal R: Is research into ethnicity and health, racist, unsound or important science? BMJ 314:1751–1756, 1997.
15. Rosenberg HM, Maurer KD, Sorlie PD, et al: Quality of death rates by race and Hispanic origin: A summary of current research, 1999. National Center for Health Statistics. Vital Health Stat 2(128):1–13, 1999.
16. Doyle AC: Silver Blaze. In: The Complete Sherlock Holmes. New York, Doubleday, 1930.
17. Taubes G: Epidemiology faces its limits. Science 269:164–169, 1995.
18. Koren G, Klein N: Bias against negative studies in newspaper reports of medical research. JAMA 13:1824–1826, 1991.
19. Klein MP, Stefanek, ME: Cancer risk elicitation and communication: Lessons from the psychology of risk perception. CA Cancer J Clin 57:147–167, 2007.

Answers to Review Questions

*Note to reader: To find complete rationales for all answer options, please go to www.studentconsult.com and activate/access your full online version of the book and ancillary content.

CHAPTER 2
1. b
2. a
3. b
4. d
5. c

CHAPTER 3
1. e
2. 10%
3. c
4. c
5. d
6. b
7. c

CHAPTER 4
1. 5/1,000
2. 30%
3. e
4. b

5. b
6. d
7. d
8. 9.6/1,000
9. e
10. a
11. 2.5 or 250%

CHAPTER 5
1. 72.0%
2. 84.0%
3. 69.2%
4. d
5. d
6. b
7. 3.3%
8. b
9. 70.0%
10. 57.1%
11. 0.40
12. b

CHAPTER 6
The answers to questions 6–8 are based on calculating and completing the table provided as shown below.
1. c
2. 54.7%
3. c
4. b
5. c
6. 0.982 or 98.2%
7. 0.006 or 0.6%
8. c

CHAPTERS 7 AND 8
1. e
2. e
3. c
4. b

5. b
6. a
7. 57
8. c

CHAPTER 9
1. d
2. a
3. c
4. a
5. c

CHAPTER 10
1. c
2. a
3. c
4. b
5. c
6. d
7. e
8. d

For questions 6–8 in Chapter 6:

Survival of Patients with AIDS Following Diagnosis

(1) Interval Since Beginning Treatment (months)	(2) Alive at Beginning of Interval	(3) Died During Interval	(4) Withdrew During Interval	(5) Effective Number Exposed to Risk of Dying During Interval: Col (2) − $\frac{1}{2}$[Col (4)]	(6) Proportion Who Died During Interval: $\frac{\text{Col (3)}}{\text{Col (5)}}$	(7) Proportion Who Did Not Die During Interval: 1 − Col (6)	(8) Cumulative Proportion Who Survived From Enrollment to End of Interval: Cumulative Survival
x	l_x	d_x	w_x	l'_x	q_x	p_x	P_x
1–12	248	96	27	234.5	0.4094	0.5906	0.5906
13–24	125	55	13	118.5	0.4641	0.5359	0.3165
25–36	57	55	2	56.0	0.9821	0.0179	0.0057

CHAPTER 11

1. 15.2
2. e
3. d
4. e
5. 4.5
6. 6.3
7. 1:7 (.0143)
8. e
9. e

CHAPTER 12

1. b
2. 27.5/1,000
3. 84.6%
4. 3.6/1,000
5. 78.3%

CHAPTER 14

1. c
2. a
3. e
4. c
5. b
6. d

CHAPTER 15

1. e
2. c
3. 12
4. 18.7
5. 9
6. 6.2
7. d
8. b

CHAPTER 16

1. c
2. b
3. b
4. c
5. c

CHAPTER 17

1. b
2. d
3. b
4. a
5. d

CHAPTER 18

1. a
2. a
3. b
4. c
5. b
6. c
7. c
8. b

Index

Note: Page numbers followed by the letter f refer to figures; those followed by t refer to tables.

DMF index, 9, 10f
DNA analysis
    of autosomal dominant disorders, 273, 274f
    of autosomal recessive disorders, 273, 274f
DNA microarrray technology, 268
DNA repair, alternating exposure and nonexposure periods
    and, 341
DNA sequencing, 268
DNA transcription, 267
Dose-response relationship, causation and, 236–237, 237f
Down syndrome, diseases associated with, 266, 267t
Drop-ins, in randomized trials, 144
Dropouts, in randomized trials, 144
Drug(s), new, phases in testing of, 156–157
Duodenal ulcers, *Helicobacter pylori* infection and, 239–241,
    240t

E
Ecologic fallacy, 229
Ecologic study(ies), 228, 300
Ectopic pregnancy, 68, 68f. *See also* Pregnancy.
Effectiveness, in health services evaluation, 295
Efficacy
    in health services evaluation, 294–295
    of agent, expression of, 152
Efficiency, in health services evaluation, 295
Electromagnetic fields (EMF), 341
Eligible-noneligible populations, in health services evaluation,
    comparison of, 305, 305f
Emphysema, smoking and, 183
Endemic disease, 22–23, 23f
Environmental factors, interaction of, in genetic disease,
    283–285, 284f, 284t, 285f
Enzyme-linked immunosorbent assay (ELISA), 329
Eosinophilia-myalgia syndrome, 190, 237, 238f
Epidemic curve, definition of, 27
Epidemic disease, 22–23, 23f
Epidemiologic triad, of disease, 19, 19f
Epidemiology, 3–17
    and prevention, 6–7, 6t, 333–335, 334f, 335f. *See also*
        Prevention; Screening test(s).
    community health problems and, 4–5, 4f–6f, 5t
    definition of, 3
    ethical issues in, 350. *See also* Ethical issue(s).
    from observations to preventive actions, 9–17
    in clinical practice, 7–8, 8f
    in evaluation of health services, 293–308. *See also* Health
        services evaluation.
    objectives of, 3
Esophageal cancer, cigarette smoking and, 255, 255f
Ethical issue(s), 349–359
    access to data as, 354
    conflict of interest as, 355–356
    ethnicity as, 354–355
    in epidemiology, 350
    in randomized trials, 157–158
    interpretation of findings as, 356–358, 356f, 357f, 357t, 358t
    obligation to study subjects as, 350–351
    privacy and confidentiality as, 351–354, 353f
    race as, 354–355
Ethnicity, 354–355

Etiology. *See also* Causation.
    approaches to, 228, 228f
    study of, 228–230, 229f, 230t
Exclusion bias, 248–249
Exposure(s)
    assessment of, 340–342, 340t, 341f
    biomarkers of, 341, 341f
    cessation of, 237, 238f
    data regarding, sources of, 339–340, 340t
    disease risk and, 202–203, 202t, 203t. *See also* Attributable
        risk; Relative risk.
    attributable, 215–217, 216f, 217f
        calculation of, 218, 218t, 221t
    in case-control study, 190–191, 191f
    macroenvironmental, 334
    microenvironmental, 334–335
    susceptibility to, 334, 334f
External validity, of randomized trials, 153, 153f

F
Factor A, 251, 255
Factor V Leiden mutation, 283–284, 284t
Factorial design, of randomized trials, 143–144, 143f, 144f
False negative result, 87t, 88
False positive result, 87t, 88
Familial adenomatous polyposis, colon cancer and, 266, 267t
Family study(ies), of genetic disease, 272–281
    adoption data for, 279–281, 279t, 280t
    application of molecular biologic methods in, 272–273,
        273f, 274f
    in first-degree relatives, 272, 272f
    in twins, 273, 275–279, 275f–278f, 275t, 276t, 277t, 278t,
        279t. *See also* Twin study(ies).
Fat(s), dietary, breast cancer and, 229, 229f
Febrile seizures, in children, 127, 127f
α-Fetoprotein, 98, 98f
First-degree relatives, risk of disease in, 272, 272f
Fluoridation, dental caries and, 8–9, 9f
Follow-up loss bias, in cohort studies, 174
Foodborne disease, outbreak of, 201, 202t
Food-specific attack rate, 34t
    calculation of, 28
Framingham Study, 171, 171t, 204, 205t
Frequency matching, in case-control studies, 186

G
Gastric cancer, *Helicobacter pylori* infection and, 239–241, 241f
Gastroenteritis, outbreaks of, on cruise ships, 23–24, 24f
Gene(s). *See also specific gene.*
    disease susceptibility of, 272–273, 273f
    regulation of expression of, 267–268
Genetic disease, 265–287
    age of onset of, 268–271, 270f, 271f
    family studies of, 272–281
        adoption data for, 279–281, 279t, 280t
        application of molecular biologic methods in, 272–273,
            273f, 274f
        in first-degree relatives, 272, 272f
        in twins, 273, 275–279, 275f–278f, 275t, 276t, 277t, 278t,
            279t. *See also* Twin study(ies).
    future prospects for, 285–287, 286f